Prenatal and Postnatal Health: A Woman-Centered Approach

Prenatal and Postnatal Health: A Woman-Centered Approach

Editor: Nicola Morse

AMERICAN MEDICAL PUBLISHERS
www.americanmedicalpublishers.com

AMERICAN
MEDICAL PUBLISHERS
www.americanmedicalpublishers.com

Cataloging-in-Publication Data

Prenatal and postnatal health : a woman-centered approach / edited by Nicola Morse.
p. cm.
Includes bibliographical references and index.
ISBN 978-1-63927-165-8
1. Prenatal care. 2. Postnatal care. 3. Maternal health services. 4. Preconception care.
5. Women's health services. I. Morse, Nicola.
RG801 .P74 2022
618.24--dc23

American Medical Publishers,
41 Flatbush Avenue,
1st Floor, New York,
NY 11217, USA

ISBN 978-1-63927-165-8 (Hardback)

Contents

Preface

Pregnancy presents substantial health risks. Inspite of advances in obstetrics and gynecology, maternal mortality remains a major problem. Obstructed labor, hemorrhage, sepsis, eclampsia, and unskilled abortion are some of the causes of maternal deaths. Good medical care is vital for improving pregnancy outcomes. Prenatal care along with prenatal screening and diagnosis are vital for minimizing the risks of maternal death, miscarriages, neonatal infections, birth defects, etc. The mother should receive necessary immunizations and prenatal nutrition. The psychological health of the mother is also of utmost importance. Several psychological disorders may emerge during the postpartum period, such as post-traumatic stress disorder, postpartum depression and puerperal psychosis. The early diagnosis and management of these are vital both for the mother and child. This book presents a woman-centered approach to prenatal and postnatal health. While understanding the long-term perspectives of the topics, the book makes an effort in highlighting their impacts in reducing maternal mortality across the globe. For all those who are interested in obstetrics, this book can prove to be an essential guide.

This book is the end result of constructive efforts and intensive research done by experts in this field. The aim of this book is to enlighten the readers with recent information in this area of research. The information provided in this profound book would serve as a valuable reference to students and researchers in this field.

At the end, I would like to thank all the authors for devoting their precious time and providing their valuable contribution to this book. I would also like to express my gratitude to my fellow colleagues who encouraged me throughout the process.

Editor

1

Emotional and cognitive experiences during the time of diagnosis and decision-making following a prenatal diagnosis: a qualitative study of males presented with congenital heart defect in the fetus carried by their pregnant partner

Tommy Carlsson[1,3*] and Elisabet Mattsson[1,2]

Abstract

Background: Expectant fathers consider the second-trimester obstetric ultrasound examination as an important step towards parenthood, but are ill prepared for a detection of a fetal anomaly. Inductive research is scarce concerning their experiences and needs for support. Consequently, the aim of this study was to explore the emotional and cognitive experiences, during the time of diagnosis and decision-making, among males presented with congenital heart defect in the fetus carried by their pregnant partner.

Methods: Twelve expectant fathers were consecutively recruited through two tertiary referral centers for fetal cardiology in Sweden, after they had been presented with a prenatal diagnosis of congenital heart defect in the fetus carried by their pregnant partner. The respondents were interviewed via telephone, and the interviews were analyzed using inductive qualitative content analysis.

Results: The respondents experienced an intense emotional shock in connection with detection. However, they set their own needs aside to attend to the supportive needs of their pregnant partner, and stressed the importance of an informed joint decision regarding whether to continue or terminate the pregnancy. When terminating the pregnancy, they experienced a loss of a wanted child, an emotionally intense termination procedure, needs of support neglected by professionals, and worries about the risk of recurrence in future pregnancies. When continuing the pregnancy, they tried to keep a positive attitude about the coming birth, but were simultaneously worried about the postnatal situation.

Conclusions: The findings illustrate the importance of inclusive care and adequate follow-up routines for both expectant parents following a prenatal diagnosis. This includes the initial emotional shock, the decisional process, and depending on decision reached, the termination or continuation of the pregnancy. Expectant fathers presented with a fetal anomaly need adequate follow-up routines to address worries about risk of recurrence in future pregnancies and worries about the postnatal situation.

Keywords: Congenital heart defects, Fathers, Partners, Pregnancy, Prenatal diagnosis

* Correspondence: tommy.carlsson@kbh.uu.se
[1]Department of Women's and Children's Health, Uppsala University, SE-75237 Uppsala, Sweden
[3]BMC, Husargatan 3, D11:1, SE-75237 Uppsala, Sweden
Full list of author information is available at the end of the article

Background

Expecting a child is a life-transforming event [1], and expectant fathers go trough a process of adaptation to a parental role during the course of pregnancy, with increased emotional involvement as the pregnancy progresses [2–4]. This process of adaptation may be experienced as a stressful period, involving a number of psychological difficulties. The lack of tangible evidence of the pregnancy may make it feel unreal, resulting in attachment difficulties for expectant fathers. They experience a change in the relationship with their pregnant partner, with a discrepancy of the expectations and needs within the couple. Moreover, the situation requires a change in their core identity, with an adjustment to a new role as a parent, rather than a partner [4]. Although the needs of both expectant parents are acknowledged as equally important in healthcare, expectant fathers often feel excluded from the prenatal care, calling attention to the need for organizational changes and studies that address their specific experiences [5].

The obstetric ultrasound examination of pregnant persons in the second trimester of pregnancy, which involve the possibility to detect fetal anomalies, have been implemented as a part of maternity care in many countries around the world [6]. Expectant fathers consider the this examination an important step in their journey to become a parent [7], and desire to be involved in these pregnancy-related activities [5, 8, 9]. The examination is viewed by expectant parents as an opportunity to get a visual confirmation of the pregnancy, and considered an obvious choice because of the longing for the child [8]. However, many lack knowledge about the medical purposes of prenatal screening procedures [10, 11] and are thus often ill prepared for adverse findings, such as a prenatal diagnosis of a fetal anomaly [11–16].

Congenital heart defects are the most common of the fetal anomalies [17], and approximately one in five cases are diagnosed during pregnancy [17]. However, there is a great variation in the severity and prognosis depending on the nature of the defect [18, 19], and most of the severe defects are today prenatally diagnosed [17]. Research has shown that pregnant persons faced with a prenatal diagnosis of fetal anomaly experience a major life crisis [16, 20], involving a loss of the joy of being pregnant as well as the expected health of the fetus [16, 21]. Following the detection of a fetal anomaly, expectant parents may be presented with the option of terminating the pregnancy, a decision-making process that involves many informational and ethical considerations [22–27]. When told about the diagnosis, expectant parents move to a phase of trying to gain meaning and knowledge in order to reach an informed decision whether to continue or terminate the pregnancy [13]. However, an informed decision requires interpretation of complex medical information [28], and many persons who terminate the pregnancy experience the decision difficult to reach [22]. Expectant parents consider the decision to terminate the pregnancy to contradict deep parental instincts to protect one's unborn child [29]. The decision entails a combination of chosen loss and lost choices, as the pregnancy is wanted while the fetal malformation is not [16]. Those faced with a prenatal diagnosis of fetal anomaly in the fetus carried by their pregnant partner show high levels of psychological distress and depression at the time of the diagnosis [30, 31]. When the pregnancy is terminated, a considerable proportion show symptoms of post-traumatic stress and depression, up to several months after the abortion [32, 33]. Expectant parents who continue the pregnancy show high levels of anxiety and depression during pregnancy [31], with expressions of intensive and varied positive as well as negative emotions [34, 35].

Research is scarce concerning the needs of support among expectant fathers [4] and their experiences when faced with a prenatal diagnosis of a fetal anomaly [20, 36]. Previous research has primarily focused on their role as supporters, rather than their own feelings and experiences [36]. Consequently, inductive qualitative research is needed to gain deeper insights into the experiences of these individuals. With this study, we wanted to address the scarcity of inductive research on the needs of care among this population, by giving attention to their own experiences in connection to the diagnosis and decision-making regarding whether to continue or terminate the pregnancy. Thus, the aim of this study was to explore the emotional and cognitive experiences, during the time of diagnosis and decision-making, among males presented with congenital heart defect in the fetus carried by their pregnant partner.

Methods

Study design

We conducted an inductive qualitative descriptive study, as we wanted to provide straight descriptions of the phenomenon and stay close to the collected material [37].

Study context

In Sweden, midwives have primary responsibility for providing care to expectant parents with medically uncomplicated pregnancies and childbirths. The maternity care is a cost-free service that most expectant parents use. It consists of regular visits with the overall purpose to assess the status and progression of pregnancy, as well as to prepare expectant parents for childbirth and parenthood. At approximately 18 weeks of gestation, all expectant parents are offered a second-trimester obstetric ultrasound examination, with the medical purpose to estimate the gestational age, localize the placenta, assess the number of carried fetuses, and screen for fetal anomalies. When detected, suspected congenital heart defects are referred to a fetal cardiologist at a tertiary center for a specialist consultation. If a congenital heart defect is detected, the specialist offers information on a broad variety of topics related to the diagnosis, including the option of terminating the pregnancy. Before 18 completed weeks, pregnant persons may freely decide to terminate the pregnancy, and at later gestations approval for termination needs to be applied to the National Board of Health and Welfare. In clinical practice, pregnancy terminations are very seldom performed after 22 completed weeks [38].

Sample

Respondents were consecutively recruited between March and November 2014 at two tertiary referral centers for fetal cardiology in central Sweden. To be eligible, participants needed to speak Swedish well enough to be interviewed and be presented with a prenatal diagnosis of major congenital heart defect in the fetus carried by their partner, diagnosed before 22 completed weeks of gestation. We define major congenital heart defect as in need of surgical repair within the child's first year of life. During the inclusion period, 24 expectant fathers presented with a prenatal diagnosis of major congenital heart defect in the fetus were consulted at the centers. When approached face-to-face by the last author or a specialist nurse who worked at one of the sites, 20 consented to be contacted via telephone by the first author 5-15 weeks after the diagnosis. Four were not reached via telephone and four declined participation when contacted. Consequently, the final sample consisted of 12 respondents. Table 1 presents the characteristics of the sample. Among the terminated pregnancies (n = 7), four fetuses were diagnosed with univentricular defects, two with atrioventricular septal defects with associated trisomy 21, and one with pulmonary atresia/ventricular septal defect and major aortopulmonary collateral arteries. Among the continued pregnancies (n = 5), one fetus was diagnosed with a univentricular defect, three with tetralogy of fallot, and one with coarctation of the aorta. The fetuses were diagnosed between 17 and 20 weeks of gestation.

Table 1 Characteristics of the sample (n = 12)

Characteristic	Category	Terminated pregnancy (n = 7), n	Continued pregnancy (n = 5), n	Total (n = 12), n
Age	20-29	2	1	3
	30-39	3	3	6
	>39	2	1	3
Born children	0	2	2	4
	1	4	3	7
	2	1	0	1
Country of birth	Sweden	5	5	10
	Other	2	0	2
Highest education	Senior high school	3	2	5
	University/ College	4	3	7

Interviews

The respondents were interviewed via the telephone 5-15 weeks after the diagnosis (mean = 12 weeks). Semi-structured interviews were conducted by the first author, and lasted on average 35 min (range = 23-47) among those who continued the pregnancy and 37 min (range = 20-56) among those who terminated the pregnancy. Handwritten notes were kept during the course of the interviews, which were used to summarize it for the respondents. The interviews were digitally audio-recorded and transcribed verbatim. An interview guide was used to stay relevant to the aim (Table 2). Probes, such as "Can you please tell me more?", were used to explore experiences further. At the end of the interview, the first author summarized his initial observations and asked if the participant wanted to correct or add anything. No repeat interviews were conducted.

Analysis

The transcribed material was analyzed with inductive qualitative content analysis, a method to discover patterns in written texts [39] without preconceived theories or models to guide the analysis [40]. Nvivo version 10.2.0 (QSR International, Doncaster, Victoria, Australia) was used to structure the analytic process. The first author was responsible for the analysis. Initially, the transcripts were read several times to get a sense of the overall content. Meaning units were identified in the transcripts, defined as pieces of the text that represented a single item of content that corresponded to the aim of this study. The identified meaning units were condensed and then assigned a code, defined as a label that described the core of the meaning unit. The codes were abstracted to preliminary major themes, defined as overarching threads in the data that represent the underlying interpreted meaning. On account of the intertwined nature of human experiences, themes did not have to be mutually exclusive. Thus, codes could be placed in several themes [39]. Only the first author coded the transcripts. As more themes were identified, the last author was involved through discussions about

Table 2 Interview guide

Main question	Sub-question
What was it like to be informed about the malformation?	What were your thoughts and feelings at that moment?
Could you describe how it was for you to make the decision to continue or terminate the pregnancy?	Was it difficult to make the decision?
	How would you describe your feelings and thoughts at the time?
	How did you feel when you were faced with the decision?
	Was there anything that was particularly difficult/easy?
Could you describe how you feel today?	What are your thoughts today about what happened?

the main findings and thematization. The analysis involved a continuous interpretive process that moved back and forth dialectically. For ethical reasons, no member checks took place. Table 3 presents examples of the analytic process.

Research team and reflexivity

The authors are researchers, specialist nurses and midwives. The first author identifies himself as male and is in his 30's, while the last author identifies herself as female and is in her 50's. The first author had no contact with the respondents before the data collection. Before the interviews were initiated, the first author presented himself and stated the aim of the study. At the time of recruitment, the last author worked as a nurse-midwife at one of the units for fetal cardiology and was in charge of the recruitment from this site. The first author had no clinical experience of prenatal diagnostics before conducting the interviews. Both authors have previous experience of, and formal training in, interviews and qualitative content analysis.

Results

The findings are portrayed through five themes: (1) Trying to support the partner during an emotional shock, (2) the importance of reaching an informed and joint decision, (3) the loss of a wanted child through an emotionally intense pregnancy termination, (4) ambivalent feelings of anticipation and worries about the birth, and (5) worries of recurrence in future pregnancies.

Trying to support the partner during an emotional shock

The initial detection had been a complete emotional shock, described as a heartbreaking tragedy. When told about the suspected anomaly at the initial ultrasound examination, the respondents felt shocked, panicked, and disoriented. The wait between the initial detection and the consultation with the fetal cardiologist was described as very difficult, involving sleepless nights and many worries. When the fetal cardiologist confirmed the defect, respondents experienced the diagnosis surreal and unfair. While all reacted with shock to the initial detection, some distanced themselves from their own emotional reactions to cope with the situation. The expectant fathers mentioned the importance of supporting their pregnant partner, and because of this set their own needs aside to be attentive to the needs of their partners.

> *I felt that I needed to be stable for my fiancée's sake; depending on how she reacted I felt that I needed to be... more supportive than if I, if I broke down myself, if I put it like that...* (R6, pregnancy continued)

The importance of reaching an informed and joint decision

The respondents emphasized the importance of being offered enough information in order to reach an informed decision whether to continue or terminate the pregnancy. Most considered they had reached the

Table 3 Examples of the analytic process

Meaning unit	Condensed meaning unit	Code	Theme
A heart defect is serious, of course, it really is, and I sound very calm about it but that is because there's no reason not to believe it will go fine. That's how we see it. Because if you don't, you just can't take it, I reckon	It is serious, and I sound very calm because there's no reason not to believe it will go fine. That's how we see it. If you don't, you just can't take it.	Expecting anything else than all will go well would not be possible to manage	Ambivalent feelings of anticipation and worries about the birth
That was really the thing that you pondered about the most, how it will, how will it feel to leave the child, what would happen if there's chaos with the trains as there is every summer, things like that. What happens if we're stranded, who has responsibility for us then.	That was the thing you pondered about most, how will it feel to leave the child, what happens if there's chaos with the trains, things like that. What happens if we're stranded, who has responsibility for us.	Pondering about the time after the birth	
It went like this, we had to deliver and that kind of thing, it became rather... emotional, still.	We had to deliver, it became rather emotional.	The pregnancy termination was emotional	The loss of a wanted child through an emotionally intense pregnancy termination
In part bad conscience I think. It feels like you terminate... someone else, so to say, you take away someone's chance to live so to say.	In part bad conscience. Feels like you terminate... someone else, you take away someone's chance to live.	Bad conscience to terminate a life	

decision with certainty and did not regard any other option than the one they decided upon. Those who terminated the pregnancy perceived no other choice in order to protect their expected child from future suffering. On the contrary, respondents who continued the pregnancy regarded the severity of the heart defect as mild enough not to impose on the quality of life for the child and thus did not consider pregnancy termination.

> *We would be happy to take over his pain ten-fold if that would make him pain-free. [...] It wasn't particularly difficult bearing in mind that I don't want to subject someone else to such pain.* (R10, pregnancy terminated)

> *We haven't really begun to think about if we should terminate the pregnancy, it doesn't feel as if we have thought really hard along those lines actually, or so deeply about it, but it has always felt as if this will be OK in the end.* (R1, pregnancy continued)

The importance of reaching a joint decision together with their partner was brought up. It seemed that most couples came to a joint decision, and did not have any regrets over the final decision. However, some described not feeling included in the decision, which they in hindsight felt sad about.

> *I wanted to go on but my girl preferred not to. [...] I wanted to do everything to make her feel good, so I went along with most things. So it was more...her decision you might say in that respect. Unfortunately.* (R3, pregnancy terminated)

The loss of a wanted child through an emotionally intense pregnancy termination

All respondents with experience of pregnancy termination described the situation as painful and emotionally stressful, involving complex ethical and existential issues. To terminate the pregnancy was described as a life-long burden, involving an alternative that no expectant parent should ever have to deliberate about. The expected child was deeply desired by respondents, who at the time of the diagnosis had started to look forward to becoming a parent. Thus, the alternative to terminate the pregnancy was regarded as a decision that partly contradicted their instincts to protect their unborn child. Simultaneously, they came to the conclusion that the decision was reached as a deed to spare the child from future postnatal suffering. Considering the existential aspects in play during the deliberation about the life-or-death options presented in connection to the diagnosis, the decision-making process was regarded as an inhumane situation, involving too great responsibilities for one person or couple to handle.

> *I am playing God now. That is what I thought, playing God and deciding who was going to live and who was not going to live...* (R5, pregnancy terminated)

The pregnancy termination involved considerable emotional stress and the loss of a wanted child, likened by respondents to an execution and a murder. Some expressed negative experiences of abortion care. One referred to the pregnancy termination as a catastrophe, with unprofessional and stressed caregivers. Another drew attention to his vulnerable situation, and felt that the professionals had not been attentive to his needs.

> *For something like this, the termination of a pregnancy, I have a bit of a feeling that they are not quite as good at taking care of the other partner. [...] You feel a little bit like an appendage, to one side, but of course the partner is also in a helluva position.* (R8, pregnancy terminated)

Respondents who decided to view the fetus after the expulsion described it in both negative and positive terms. While an emotionally stressful moment, it also made the fetus feel more real, facilitated emotional recuperation, and brought closure. However, these respondents would have appreciated more time to deliberate about whether or not to view the fetus, as it was considered difficult to reach a decision when not presented with the option before the termination took place. Residual emotional scars and psychological consequences were experienced after the abortion, and thoughts about the loss of their expected child were often experienced among respondents. Moreover, they described feelings of guilt and shame over their decision, and pondered over how their situation would have been if the pregnancy had been continued.

> *I'm still psychologically affected by it, naturally. I think most about the day when we had the abortion done.. It is that day in particular that comes back to my mind.* (R2, pregnancy terminated)

Ambivalent feelings of anticipation and worries about the birth

Respondents with experience of a continued the pregnancy expressed ambivalent feelings about the future, as the birth of their child was anticipated and longed for, but accompanied by worries about the postnatal situation. Overall, the expectant fathers tried to keep a positive attitude towards the birth, as a way to cope with the situation. They were hopeful about the prognosis for the child, and relied on competent health care professionals to take care of their child once it was born.

> *A heart defect is serious, of course, it really is, and I sound very calm about it but that is because there's no reason not to believe it will go fine. That's how we see it. Because if you don't, you just can't take it, I reckon [...] It weighs you down a bit, of course, but... But... you have to see it as ... perfectly normal and not at all dangerous.* (R9, pregnancy continued)

However, many worries about the postnatal situation were also expressed. For example, these worries included the status of the child after birth, risks of planned surgeries, and managing the care of siblings during the critical postnatal periods. To deal with their worries and feel more in control, expectant fathers wished to be involved in the health care planning of the postnatal situation. One described his many thoughts and worries about taking care of the siblings after the child was born.

> *It would just have been much easier if everything is ready here, like, you come down here as a family, stay here, we solve the problem... But it's also like this, if there is room you can have your children and thoughts like that [...] If you consider things you worry about, perhaps it's in that area. How is he [the sibling] going to take it, like, will it be chaos, panic at home if we're gone for a few days, as he's so small.* (R1, pregnancy continued)

Worries of recurrence in future pregnancies

Respondents with experience of a terminated pregnancy and one father whose child died shortly after birth described worries about the risk of recurrence in future pregnancies. These worries were very difficult to cope with, as new pregnancies were simultaneously longed for. As a way to deal with these worries, they expressed a need for expanded prenatal examinations in future pregnancies. To have experienced a prenatal detection of a fetal anomaly changed their views about obstetric ultrasound examinations, raising awareness of its medical purposes and influencing their feelings about the examination in future pregnancies.

> *You're a bit afraid that it, how can I put it, that next time, if there is a next time, that it will be another baby. You'll, you can feel it even now, you'll go and worry all the way up to the first ultrasound [...] You feel that a bit even today, so to speak, a bit afraid that it will happen again.* (R10, pregnancy terminated)

Discussion

The respondents experienced emotional distress in connection to the diagnosis and emphasized the importance of an informed joint decision. When the pregnancy was terminated, the procedure was described as emotionally painful, with health professionals not attentive to their needs for support. When the pregnancy was continued, respondents described worries related to the postnatal situation and wished to be involved in the planning of the postnatal care. Regardless of the decision to continue or terminate the pregnancy, respondents described that they tried to set their own needs aside to support their partner. According to previous studies, male partners faced with a prenatal detection of fetal anomaly hide their anxiety and grief in order to be strong for the pregnant person [12], resulting in concealment of their actual needs for support [41]. The results of this study confirm this, and bring to light that they, similar to pregnant persons, experience emotional distress following a prenatal diagnosis. The fact that expectant fathers put their feelings aside to be attentive to the supportive needs of their pregnant partner calls attention to the risk of overlooking their need for professional psychosocial support.

Previous studies report that women who terminate the pregnancy due to a fetal anomaly need compassionate care, but occasionally experience insensitivity and non-responsiveness from health professionals [15]. The findings of this study indicate that some male partners experience similar issues, and do not feel included in the abortion care. Moreover, the findings raise awareness of their vulnerable situation during pregnancy terminations, which is an incentive for health professionals to systematically assess and attend to the needs of both the pregnant person and their partner during this stressful process in their lives. A limited amount of research has been conducted concerning the psychological consequences of perinatal loss among male partners. The few reports that exist show that they grieve after a perinatal loss, although with less intensity and with other types of coping mechanisms than those of women [42]. Studies report that women suffer from psychological consequences years after a pregnancy termination due to a fetal anomaly [29, 32, 43]. This study provides an understanding about the emotional reactions among males faced with a prenatal diagnosis, namely the loss of a wanted child and worries about the risk of recurrence in future pregnancies. Considering the fact that we interviewed respondents a few weeks after the diagnosis, we cannot conclude the presence of complicated grief, defined as symptoms of grief that last at least 6 months [44]. However, continuity of care and adequate follow-up routines have previously been identified as important aspects of care for women terminating a pregnancy due to a fetal anomaly [45, 46]. The findings reflect that males need to be included in adequate follow-up routines, and illustrate the need for care that expands beyond the initial period following a pregnancy termination due to a fetal anomaly. To promote reproductive health and realistic expectations concerning the risk of recurrence, health professionals should take steps to address the thoughts and worries concerning future pregnancies. An example of an initiative that might promote reproductive health after a pregnancy termination due to a fetal anomaly is interconceptional counseling for couples, in other words care that focuses on the time between the termination and a new pregnancy or an informed decision not to conceive [47]. More research is needed to investigate appropriate timing of such counseling and its potential effects of promoting reproductive health among women and their partners after a pregnancy termination due to a fetal anomaly.

In line with other studies [21, 48, 49] expectant fathers with a continued pregnancy expressed ambivalent feelings about the birth of their child, suggesting the need for continuous care and support during the remainder of the pregnancy. Among expectant parents to prenatally diagnosed infants, gender differences may exist in the early postdiagnosis stage, with regard to psychological distress and quality of life. Nonetheless, both mothers and fathers show high levels in comparison to parents to healthy infants [31]. Moreover, 1 month after the disclosure, no gender differences exist with regard to emotional reactions [35, 50], and intracouple congruence of emotional reactions is frequent [50]. Consequently, health professionals must recognize that the diagnosis may result in an increased risk of developing psychopathological symptoms for both expectant parents when the pregnancy is continued, and include both of them in their assessments of the need for psychosocial support. Following the diagnosis, expectant parents move from grief to preparation as the pregnancy progresses [51] and are concerned or worried about various issues [21, 48]. In summary, the findings illustrate the importance of including both of the expectant parents in the health care planning of the postnatal situation, and the need for team-based efforts that address the worries of the postnatal situation expressed by the respondents.

Strengths and limitations

The strength of this study is that it included males with experience of continuation and termination of pregnancy following a prenatal diagnosis of congenital heart defect in the fetus. Respondents with different ages, educational levels and fetal diagnoses were represented in the sample. Recruitment took place at two different tertiary units, indicating that the sample corresponds to different clinical settings. However, we did not use purposeful sampling to reach a sample of maximum variation [52], and half of the eligible persons declined participation or were not reached. We have no details regarding the characteristics of persons in the group who did not participate in the study. Consequently, it is possible that the interviewed respondents do not represent a varied sample from the complete population. For example, we failed to recruit any immigrants who continued the pregnancy. We acknowledge that the findings may have limited transferability to other settings and populations.

The material was collected using telephone interviews, a method that may promote respondents to feel more relaxed during the interview, increase anonymity, and lead to less influence from social pressure [53–56]. On the other hand, it may be more difficult to create a trusting atmosphere, use social cues [55], and it is impossible to observe nonverbal communication [56] via the telephone. During data collection, it became clear that the respondents appreciated the practical advantages of the chosen method. Further, we argue that it facilitated recruitment and helped participants to feel more relaxed when talking about the subject in question, which may have been a personal and intimate subject for some of the respondents. However, we cannot disregard the possibility that face-to-face-interviews may have generated richer data.

We acknowledge that this qualitative analysis is a product of using a single researcher as the primary instrument for analysis. To strengthen the credibility of the analysis, the first author kept a reflective journal about his preconceptions during the course of the data collection and analysis. Furthermore, the analytic process was discussed with the last author. This allowed for different perspectives and insights during the analytic process. Nevertheless, it is impossible to disregard the probability that our preconceptions had an impact on the analysis, and the findings needs to be interpreted with this in mind.

Recommendations for future research

The findings implicate a need to longitudinally investigate the need for emotional support among expectant fathers faced with a prenatal diagnosis of fetal anomaly. Special attention needs to be directed towards couples that do not reach a joint decision regarding the future of the pregnancy. Research should also address worries of recurrence in future pregnancies and its potential impact on reproductive health. Moreover, research should explore how expectant parents that continue the pregnancy following the diagnosis most appropriately can be supported, so as to deal with their worries about the postnatal situation.

Conclusions

This qualitative study adds insights into the existing literature, with regard to the emotional and cognitive experiences during the diagnosis and decision-making among males presented with congenital heart defect in the fetus carried by their pregnant partner. The findings illustrate the importance of inclusive care and adequate follow-up routines for both expectant parents following a prenatal diagnosis of congenital heart defect in the fetus. Despite experiencing an emotional shock in connection to the diagnosis, expectant fathers may put their own needs aside to support their pregnant partners. Consequently, they are at risk of not being adequately supported, and we suggest that professionals must always offer professional support to both expectant parents faced with a prenatal diagnosis of congenital heart defect in the fetus. This includes the initial emotional shock, the decisional process and, depending on decision reached, the termination or continuation of the pregnancy. Those with experience of pregnancy termination consider their decision as an option without alternatives, and describe the decision as an inhumane choice that contradicts their instincts to protect their unborn child. The experiences of insufficient support in connection to the termination calls attention to a need for abortion care that is inclusive, to adequately meet the emotional needs of males who experience a prenatal loss. Subsequent to the termination, these persons express worries of recurrence in future pregnancies, which needs to be addressed and followed up in order to promote realistic expectations about their reproductive futures. When the pregnancy is continued, partners express worries about the postnatal situation, raising awareness of the importance of continuous support during the remainder of the pregnancy. They need to be actively involved in the health care planning of the postnatal care, to feel prepared for the birth of the expected child.

Acknowledgements

The authors thank the respondents for their willingness to share their experiences.

Funding

Tommy Carlsson was financed by Uppsala County Council, Uppsala, Sweden ("ALF"). The funders had no role in design of the study, data collection, analysis, interpretation of data or writing of the manuscript.

Authors' contributions

TC conceived and designed the study, collected the data, analyzed the data and wrote the manuscript. EM conceived and designed the study, contributed to the thematization and wrote the manuscript. Both authors have read and approved the final version of this manuscript.

Competing interests

The authors declare that they have no competing interests.

Author details

[1]Department of Women's and Children's Health, Uppsala University, SE-75237 Uppsala, Sweden. [2]Department of Health Care Sciences, Ersta Sköndal University College, SE-10061 Stockholm, Sweden. [3]BMC, Husargatan 3, D11:1, SE-75237 Uppsala, Sweden.

References

1. Mercer RT. Becoming a mother versus maternal role attainment. J Nurs Scholarsh. 2004;36:226–32.
2. May KA. Three phases of father involvement in pregnancy. Nurs Res. 1982; 31:337–42.
3. Habib C, Lancaster S. Changes in identity and paternal–foetal attachment across a first pregnancy. J. Reprod. Infant Psychol. 2010;28:128–42.
4. Genesoni L, Tallandini MA. Men's psychological transition to fatherhood: an analysis of the literature, 1989-2008. Birth Berkeley Calif. 2009;36:305–18.
5. Wells MB. Literature review shows that fathers are still not receiving the support they want and need from Swedish child health professionals. Acta Paediatr. 2016;105:1014–23.
6. Campbell S. A short history of sonography in obstetrics and gynaecology. Facts Views Vis ObGyn. 2013;5:213–29.
7. Draper J. "It"s the first scientific evidence': men's experience of pregnancy confirmation. J Adv Nurs. 2002;39:563–70.
8. Ekelin M, Crang-Svalenius E, Dykes A-K. A qualitative study of mothers' and fathers' experiences of routine ultrasound examination in Sweden. Midwifery. 2004;20:335–44.
9. Widarsson M, Engström G, Tydén T, Lundberg P, Hammar LM. "Paddling upstream": fathers' involvement during pregnancy as described by expectant fathers and mothers. J Clin Nurs. 2015;24:1059–68.
10. Åhman A, Runestam K, Sarkadi A. Did I really want to know this? Pregnant women's reaction to detection of a soft marker during ultrasound screening. Patient Educ Couns. 2010;81:87–93.
11. Garcia J, Bricker L, Henderson J, Martin M-A, Mugford M, Nielson J, et al. Women's views of pregnancy ultrasound: a systematic review. Birth. 2002;29:225–50.
12. Åhman A, Lindgren P, Sarkadi A. Facts first, then reaction—expectant fathers' experiences of an ultrasound screening identifying soft markers. Midwifery. 2012;28:e667–75.
13. Lalor J, Begley CM, Galavan E. Recasting hope: a process of adaptation following fetal anomaly diagnosis. Soc Sci Med. 2009;68:462–72.
14. Lalor JG, Devane D, Begley CM. Unexpected diagnosis of fetal abnormality: women's encounters with caregivers. Birth. 2007;34:80–8.
15. McCoyd JLM. What do women want? Experiences and reflections of women after prenatal diagnosis and termination for anomaly. Health Care Women Int. 2009;30:507–35.
16. Sandelowski M, Barroso J. The travesty of choosing after positive prenatal diagnosis. J Obstet Gynecol Neonatal Nurs. 2005;34:307–18.
17. Dolk H, Loane M, Garne E. The prevalence of congenital anomalies in Europe. Adv Exp Med Biol. 2010;686:349–64.
18. Allan LD, Huggon IC. Counselling following a diagnosis of congenital heart disease. Prenat Diagn. 2004;24:1136–42.
19. Warnes CA. The adult with congenital heart disease: born to be bad? J Am Coll Cardiol. 2005;46:1–8.
20. Wool C. Systematic review of the literature: parental outcomes after diagnosis of fetal anomaly. Adv. Neonatal Care. 2011;11:182–92.
21. McKechnie AC, Pridham K. Preparing heart and mind following prenatal diagnosis of complex congenital heart defect. Qual Health Res. 2012;22:1694–706.
22. Asplin N, Wessel H, Marions L, Georgsson Öhman S. Pregnant women's perspectives on decision-making when a fetal malformation is detected by ultrasound examination. Sex. Reprod. Healthc. 2013;4:79–84.
23. Carlsson T, Bergman G, Wadensten B, Mattsson E. Experiences of informational needs and received information following a prenatal diagnosis of congenital heart defect. Prenat Diagn. 2016;36:515–22.
24. Chenni N, Lacroze V, Pouet C, Fraisse A, Kreitmann B, Gamerre M, et al. Fetal

heart disease and interruption of pregnancy: factors influencing the parental decision-making process. Prenat Diagn. 2012;32:168–72.
25. Howe D. Ethics of prenatal ultrasound. Best Pract Res Clin Obstet Gynaecol. 2014;28:443–51.
26. Carlsson T, Bergman G, Karlsson AM, Wadensten B, Mattsson E. Experiences of termination of pregnancy for a fetal anomaly: A qualitative study of virtual community messages. Midwifery. 2016;41:54–60.
27. Tararbit K, Bui TTT, Lelong N, Thieulin A-C, Goffinet F, Khoshnood B. Clinical and socioeconomic predictors of pregnancy termination for fetuses with congenital heart defects: a population-based evaluation. Prenat Diagn. 2013; 33:179–86.
28. Carlsson T, Bergman G, Melander Marttala U, Wadensten B, Mattsson E. Information following a diagnosis of congenital heart defect: experiences among parents to prenatally diagnosed children. PLoS One. 2015;10:e0117995.
29. Heba H. Women's long-term life experience after pregnancy termination for fetal abnormality: interpretive phenomenological study. Ontario: Electronic Thesis and Dissertation Repository; 2015.
30. Fonseca A, Nazaré B, Canavarro MC. Parental psychological distress and quality of life after a prenatal or postnatal diagnosis of congenital anomaly: a controlled comparison study with parents of healthy infants. Disabil Health J. 2012;5:67–74.
31. Kaasen A, Helbig A, Malt UF, Naes T, Skari H, Haugen GN. Paternal psychological response after ultrasonographic detection of structural fetal anomalies with a comparison to maternal response: a cohort study. BMC Pregnancy Childbirth. 2013;13:147.
32. Korenromp MJ, GCML P-C, van den Bout J, EJH M, JAM H, CMA P, et al. A prospective study on parental coping 4 months after termination of pregnancy for fetal anomalies. Prenat Diagn. 2007;27:709–16.
33. Korenromp MJ, Page-Christiaens GCML, van den Bout J, Mulder EJH, Hunfeld JAM, Bilardo CM, et al. Psychological consequences of termination of pregnancy for fetal anomaly: similarities and differences between partners. Prenat Diagn. 2005;25:1226–33.
34. McKechnie AC, Pridham K, Tluczek A. Preparing heart and mind for becoming a parent following a diagnosis of fetal anomaly. Qual Health Res. 2015;25:1182–98.
35. Fonseca A, Nazaré B, Canavarro MC. Patterns of parental emotional reactions after a pre- or postnatal diagnosis of a congenital anomaly. J Reprod Infant Psychol. 2011;29:320–33.
36. Locock L, Alexander J. "Just a bystander"? Men's place in the process of fetal screening and diagnosis. Soc Sci Med. 2006;62:1349–59.
37. Sandelowski M. Whatever happened to qualitative description? Res. Nurs. Health. 2000;23:334–40.
38. The National Board of Health and Welfare. Statistics on induced abortions 2014. 2015 [cited 2016 Feb 8]. Available from: https://www.socialstyrelsen.se/Lists/Artikelkatalog/Attachments/19915/2015-9-4.pdf
39. Graneheim UH, Lundman B. Qualitative content analysis in nursing research: concepts, procedures and measures to achieve trustworthiness. Nurse Educ Today. 2004;24:105–12.
40. Elo S, Kyngäs H. The qualitative content analysis process. J Adv Nurs. 2008; 62:107–15.
41. Dheensa S, Metcalfe A, Williams RA. Men's experiences of antenatal screening: a metasynthesis of the qualitative research. Int J Nurs Stud. 2013;50:121–33.
42. Kersting A, Wagner B. Complicated grief after perinatal loss. Dialogues Clin Neurosci. 2012;14:187–94.
43. Korenromp MJ, Page-Christiaens GCML, van den Bout J, Mulder EJH, Visser GHA. Adjustment to termination of pregnancy for fetal anomaly: a longitudinal study in women at 4, 8, and 16 months. Am J Obstet Gynecol. 2009;201:160.e1–7.
44. Zhang B, El-Jawahri A, Prigerson HG. Update on bereavement research: evidence-based guidelines for the diagnosis and treatment of complicated bereavement. J Palliat Med. 2006;9:1188–203.
45. Asplin N, Wessel H, Marions L, Georgsson Öhman S. Pregnancy termination due to fetal anomaly: women's reactions, satisfaction and experiences of care. Midwifery. 2014;30:620–7.
46. Asplin N, Wessel H, Marions L, Georgsson ÖS. Pregnant women's experiences, needs, and preferences regarding information about malformations detected by ultrasound scan. Sex Reprod Healthc. 2012;3:73–8.
47. Moore T, Parrish H, Black BP. Interconception care for couples after perinatal loss: a comprehensive review of the literature. J Perinat Neonatal Nurs. 2011; 25:44–51.
48. Bratt E-L, Järvholm S, Ekman-Joelsson B-M, Mattson L-Å, Mellander M. Parent's experiences of counselling and their need for support following a prenatal diagnosis of congenital heart disease - a qualitative study in a Swedish context. BMC Pregnancy Childbirth. 2015;15:171.
49. Hedrick J. The lived experience of pregnancy while carrying a child with a known, nonlethal congenital abnormality. J Obstet Gynecol Neonatal Nurs. 2005;34:732–40.
50. Fonseca A, Nazaré B, Canavarro MC. Clinical determinants of parents' emotional reactions to the disclosure of a diagnosis of congenital anomaly. J Obstet Gynecol Neonatal Nurs. 2013;42:178–90.
51. Askelsdóttir B, Conroy S, Rempel G. From diagnosis to birth: parents' experience when expecting a child with congenital anomaly. Adv Neonatal Care. 2008;8:348–54.
52. Patton MQ. Qualitative research & evaluation methods. 3rd ed. London: Sage publications; 2002.
53. Kavanaugh K, Ayres L. "Not as bad as it could have been": assessing and mitigating harm during research interviews on sensitive topics. Res. Nurs. Health. 1998;21:91–7.
54. Novick G. Is there a bias against telephone interviews in qualitative research? Res Nurs Health. 2008;31:391–8.
55. Opdenakker R. Advantages and disadvantages of four interview techniques in qualitative research. Forum Qual Soc Res. 2006;7:11.
56. Sturges JE, Hanrahan KJ. Comparing telephone and face-to-face qualitative interviewing: a research note. Qual Res. 2004;4:107–18.

2

Barriers to identifying eating disorders in pregnancy and in the postnatal period

Amanda Bye[1,2,3*], Jill Shawe[4], Debra Bick[7], Abigail Easter[2], Megan Kash-Macdonald[1] and Nadia Micali[1,5,6]

Abstract

Background: Eating Disorders (ED) are mental health disorders that typically effect women of childbearing age and are associated with adverse maternal and infant outcomes. UK healthcare guidance recommends routine enquiry for current and past mental illness in antenatal and postnatal care for all women, and that pregnant women with a known ED are offered enhanced monitoring and support. Midwives and health visitors are ideally placed to identify and support women with ED as they are often the primary point of contact during the antenatal and postnatal periods. However, research on the barriers to identifying ED in the perinatal period is limited. This study aimed to understand the barriers to disclosure and identification of ED in pregnancy and postnatally as perceived by women with past or current ED, and midwives and health visitors working in the UK National Health Service.

Methods: Two studies were undertaken: mixed-measures survey of pregnant and postnatal women with current or past ED; focus groups with student and qualified midwives and health visitors.

Results: Five themes emerged on the barriers to disclosure in pregnancy as perceived by women: stigma, lack of opportunity, preference for self-management, current ED symptomatology and illness awareness. Four themes were identified on the barriers to identification of ED in pregnancy and in the postnatal period as perceived by health professionals: system constraints, recognition of role, personal attitudes, and stigma and taboo.

Conclusions: Several barriers to the identification of ED during and after pregnancy were described, the main factors were stigma and poor professional training. Perinatal mental health is becoming increasingly prioritised within national policy initiatives; however, ED continue to be neglected and increased awareness is needed. Similarly, clinical guidance aimed at responding to the rising prevalence of obesity focus on changing nutrition but not on assessing for the presence of ED behaviours that might be affecting nutrition. Improving education and training for health professionals may contribute to reducing stigma and increase confidence in identifying ED. The barriers identified in this research need to be addressed if recognition and response to women with ED during the perinatal period is to improve.

Keywords: Eating Disorders, Pregnancy, Barriers, Disclosure, Identification, Qualitative research

Background

Eating Disorders (ED) are a group of mental health disorders characterised by severe disturbances in eating behaviour that significantly impair health and psychosocial functioning, including Anorexia Nervosa (AN), Bulimia Nervosa (BN) and Binge-Eating Disorder (BED) [1]. ED typically affect women of reproductive age [2] and may affect between 5.1-7.5% of women during pregnancy, if subthreshold disorders are included [3–5]. Women with ED tend to experience a decrease in ED symptoms during pregnancy [6–9]. However, there is evidence that symptoms persist [7, 8] and of postnatal relapse [6, 8, 9]. Furthermore, depression and anxiety symptoms are common during pregnancy and postnatally for women with current and past ED [10, 11].

* Correspondence: a.bye@ucl.ac.uk
[1]Population, Policy and Practice, UCL Great Ormond Street Institute of Child Health, 30 Guilford Street, WC1N 1EH, London, UK
[2]Centre for Implementation Science, Health Service and Population Research, Institute of Psychiatry, Psychology & Neuroscience, King's College London, London, UK
Full list of author information is available at the end of the article

ED have been associated with various adverse pregnancy outcomes, for instance women with AN have higher risk of infertility, unplanned pregnancies, miscarriage, prematurity and low birth weight babies while women with BED have increased risk of higher birth weight babies [12–17]. There is growing evidence of the postnatal impact of maternal ED, such as difficulties with infant feeding [18–20], and behavioural and emotional problems in the infant [21–23].

Given the evidence of adverse outcomes for women and their infants, early identification of ED and appropriate antenatal and postnatal care are highly important. In the UK, National Health Service (NHS) maternity care is informed by a suite of guidance from the National Institute for Health and Care Excellence (NICE). NICE antenatal and postnatal mental health guidance [24] recommends routine enquiry about current and past severe mental illness with all women, and women with ED should be offered enhanced support and monitoring, and referred to specialist care if needed. Midwives and health visitors are ideally placed to identify and support women with ED as they are the primary point of contact delivering routine care for all women from pregnancy until the child is aged five. In a universal healthcare system such as the NHS where these regular routine appointments are provided, guidelines to support effective identification and management of women with ED should be implemented to reduce risk of poor pregnancy and birth outcomes, however evidence on uptake and use of guidance is limited.

To our knowledge, no previous studies have specifically investigated the barriers to identifying ED in the perinatal period. Evidence suggests that women with ED are often reluctant to disclose their ED to a health professional [25] and are unlikely to seek treatment [26], which may be due to feelings of stigma and shame [27, 28]. One UK-based qualitative study investigating women's views of antenatal care found that women were reluctant to disclose their ED because they felt health professionals lacked ED knowledge and sensitivity in dealing with the disorder [29]. A few studies in the US have found poor routine enquiry and knowledge about ED behaviours and symptoms among clinicians, including obstetricians [30–32].

Subsequently, women with ED may go undetected during pregnancy and postnatally, with potential implications for adverse maternal and infant health outcomes if disorders are not managed appropriately. An in-depth understanding of barriers to the identification of ED during and after pregnancy which reflects the perspectives of women and health professionals is needed to assess and inform practice, including implementation of relevant guidelines in to practice.

Objectives

To understand the barriers to disclosure and identification of ED in pregnancy and postnatally as perceived by women with past or current ED, and midwives and health visitors working in the UK NHS.

Methods

Two studies were undertaken:

Study 1

Design and setting

A mixed-measures survey of pregnant and postnatal women with current or past ED was conducted over a seven-month period. Women were recruited via a national parenting website, Netmums, which is a UK-based online parenting organisation with over 1.7 million members. Ethical approval was granted by the University College London's Research Ethics Committee (Ref. 3735/002).

Recruitment and procedure

The study employed convenience sampling by inviting women to voluntarily take part in an online survey via a study advertisement on the organisation website. Before commencing the survey, women were asked to read the information about the study displayed on the website. To be eligible, women had to answer yes to "Do you have, or have you had an eating disorder?", and respond to "How many children do you have?" with either the number of children or that they are currently pregnant. For women who were eligible and willing to take part, consent to participate was implied by virtue of survey completion. The survey was developed specifically for this study, and questions of interest were a combination of seven Likert-type scale questions and an open-ended question (see Additional file 1).

Participants

A total of 101 women completed the mixed-measures survey, the majority of whom were not currently pregnant and already had children and had experienced an ED in the past or currently ($n = 92$; see Table 1). The sample consisted of women from across the UK, with a range of age and educational attainment reflected.

Analysis

Data were analysed using the thematic analysis approach described by Braun and Clark [33]. This approach is an inductive and iterative process involving six phases of analysis: familiarisation with data, generation of initial codes, searching for themes among codes, reviewing themes, defining and naming themes, and producing the final report. Data were independently coded by two researchers (AB and KT), both of whom were trained in qualitative research methods and analysis. The rating-

Table 1 Study 1: Sample characteristics

Characteristics N (%)	*N* = 101
Age	
≦24	21 (21%)
25-35	55 (55%)
≧36	24 (24%)
Missing	*1*
Parity	
Currently pregnant	9 (9%)
1 child	39 (39%)
2 children	37 (37%)
≧3 children	16 (16%)
Missing	–
Location	
England	
London	16 (16%)
Midlands and East of England	18 (18%)
North England	26 (26%)
South England	24 (24%)
Wales	6 (6%)
Scotland	5 (5%)
Northern Ireland	3 (3%)
Missing	*3*
Education	
GCSE or equivalent	27 (27%)
A level or equivalent	28 (28%)
Degree or above	44 (44%)
Missing	*2*
Type of eating disorder	
Anorexia Nervosa	34 (34%)
Bulimia Nervosa	16 (16%)
Binge Eating Disorder	24 (24%)
Eating Disorder Not Otherwise Specified	25 (25%)
Missing	*2*
Any eating disorder symptoms experienced during pregnancy	
No	36 (36%)
Yes	64 (63%)
Missing	*1*
Eating disorder symptoms experienced during pregnancy	
Purging	12 (12%)
Binge eating	29 (29%)
Calorie restriction	31 (31%)
Excessive exercise	14 (14%)
Low weight	17 (17%)
Eating disorder symptoms that improved during pregnancy	
Purging	16 (16%)
Binge eating	21 (21%)
Calorie restriction	27 (27%)
Excessive exercise	12 (12%)
Low weight	15 (15%)
Health professional aware of eating disorder	
Yes	22 (22%)
No	62 (61%)
Unsure	16 (16%)
Missing	*1*
Informed health professional about eating disorder	
Yes	26 (26%)
No	72 (71%)
Missing	*3*

pair familiarised themselves with the data and independently coded the complete data set to ensure reliability and thoroughness, ensuring full consideration could be given to patterns within the data. The pair discussed their codes together, with an 89% agreement being achieved by the rating-pair. At this stage, codes with similar information were grouped, discrepancies discussed, and agreement sought before amendments were made and emerging themes sought. The process was iterative throughout, with continual reference to the original data to validate and refine emerging themes. The themes were then clustered into subordinate themes, and finally superordinate themes. The research team contributed to the refining, naming and interpretation of the themes. Quotes that were illustrative of the themes and subthemes are presented in the results and additional files.

Study 2

Design and setting

Focus groups with student and qualified midwives and health visitors were conducted over a seven-month period at participating universities and NHS hospital and community services in the South of England. Ethical approval was granted by the University College London's Research Ethics Committee (Ref. 3735/001) and the Joint Research and Development Office for Great Ormond Street Hospital for Children NHS Foundation Trust & The UCL Institute of Child Health (Ref. 11BS33).

Recruitment and procedure

A convenience sampling strategy was employed to recruit participants to the focus groups. Student midwives were recruited from across three universities, and student health visitors from one university. Qualified midwives were recruited from two hospital and community services, and qualified health visitors from one community service. Five focus groups were conducted, with one group per professional group, except for qualified midwives who required two separate groups to be conducted as staff were unable to travel between the two locations due to time and resource constraints. Participants provided written informed consent prior to taking part in the focus group. The focus groups were facilitated by AB.

The focus group topic guide was developed specifically for this study and refined by the research team and other experts, including researchers with qualitative research experience and training and clinical specialists in ED, midwifery and health visiting. The guide facilitated an informal discussion in each focus group on attitudes, knowledge, and clinical practice on identifying ED in pregnancy and in the postnatal period, focusing on the role of midwives and health visitors (see Additional file 2). Health professionals were not asked directly if they had a personal experience of ED.

Participants

Thirty-three health professionals took part in the focus groups, the majority of whom were qualified health professionals (see Table 2). The sample was predominately white, female and over twenty-five years of age. The majority had trained in the UK and as part of that training had been educated in perinatal mental health, however only a small proportion had received training specifically in ED ($n = 10$; 29%).

Analysis

The focus group discussions were recorded and transcribed verbatim with identifying material removed. Data were analysed following the same procedure as detailed for Study 1 using a thematic analysis approach [33] to refine the emerging themes. The data were independently coded by two trained researchers (AB and MKM) and a percentage agreement of 79% was achieved by the rating-pair, with discrepancies resolved in the same manner as detailed for Study 1.

Table 2 Study 2: Sample characteristics

Characteristics N (%)	$N = 33$
Age	
≤ 24	4 (12%)
25-35	11 (32%)
≧36	12 (35%)
Missing	*7*
Gender	
Female	32 (97%)
Male	1 (3%)
Ethnicity	
White	24 (73%)
Black	5 (15%)
Asian Indian	1 (3%)
Mixed ethnicity	1 (3%)
Missing	*2*
Professional category	
Student	
Midwife	5 (15%)
Health Visitor	5 (15%)
Qualified	
Midwife	14 (42%)
Health Visitor	9 (27%)
Training for current post in the UK	
Yes	28 (82%)
No	3 (9%)
Missing	*3*
Previous nurse training	
Yes	19 (56%)
No	12 (35%)
Missing	*2*
Received training in perinatal mental health	
Yes	24 (71%)
No	5 (15%)
Missing	*5*
Received training specifically in ED	
Yes	10 (29%)
No	21 (62%)
Missing	*3*

Results

Study 1

Women reported experiencing some improvements in ED symptoms during pregnancy, however over half of the sample reported experiencing any ED symptoms during pregnancy ($n = 64$; 63%), most common was calorie restriction and binge eating. Only a quarter ($n = 26$; 26%) of the sample reported disclosing their ED to a health professional involved in their antenatal care, and of the seventy-two (71%) women who did not disclose, seventy-one (70%) explained their reasons for not doing so (see Table 1). The findings generated five themes on the barriers to disclosure of ED in pregnancy as perceived by women: stigma, lack of opportunity, preference for self-management, current ED symptomatology and illness awareness (see Additional file 3).

Stigma

Stigma of ED was an important theme for women's non-disclosure to a health professional. Many women reported that they felt shameful and embarrassed and feared judgement. Some women described feeling judged by health professionals based on their physical appearance, as illustrated by one woman who stated: *"I was overweight according to my BMI. I didn't think they would believe me to tell them I had an actual problem. I was patronised by more than one healthcare professional who tried to educate me on nutrition. I got the impression they thought I was just lazy and ate junk food all of the time when this wasn't the case. I felt they were too judgemental to approach"* (W42). A few women expressed concern that a disclosure would lead to unwanted referrals to social services and other services: *"I would have been to worried to discuss with my midwife etc. for fear of being reprimanded for it (i.e. referred to social services"* (W49).

Lack of opportunity

Several women expressed a lack of opportunity to disclose and discuss an ED with a health professional. It was felt there was limited and insufficient enquiry by health professionals as *"they didn't ask and it wasn't raised as a concern"* (W67). One woman expressed difficulties in establishing a rapport with a midwife that may have facilitated a disclosure: *"I didn't have the same midwife for long enough to speak to them, it was rather stressful and upsetting"* (W21).

Preference for self-management

Some women reported not disclosing their ED to a health professional as they did not need or want specialist care and preferred to self-manage their disorder: *"I don't like to talk about it and think I can manage on my own"* (W26), and *"I just wanted to deal with it myself"* (W36). In some cases, this feeling appeared to relate to how long their ED had been undetected for: *"I don't really like to talk about it I have had some sort of disordered eating for a very long time it is very much part of me and no one else's business"* (W27).

Current ED symptomatology

For some women disclosure was dependent on their current mental health status and perceived need to disclose a history of an ED to a health professional. A few women who experienced ED prior to becoming pregnant did not think it necessary to raise this with a healthcare professional: *"I didn't think it was relevant as I have been OK for a few years now"* (W23). Other women reported improvements in ED symptoms during pregnancy so similarly did not feel it relevant to disclose: *"It wasn't affecting me during my pregnancy, it helped"* (W50) and *"I felt like I was a lot better when I fell pregnant"* (W30).

Illness awareness

For several women, disclosure of an ED was dependent on their awareness of ED and acknowledging that their symptoms were that of an ED. This was particularly notable in women with BED as retrospectively some considered that they had dismissed their binge eating behaviours as general over eating:

"Binge eating doesn't seem like that big of an issue and I've never seen it as an eating disorder before" W4.

"I have only really just recognised that I have an issue & at the time I was pregnant did not realise. I just thought I was a greedy person" W34.

Study 2

Four main themes emerged on the barriers to identification of ED in the perinatal period as perceived by health professionals: system constraints, recognition of role, personal attitudes, and stigma and taboo (see Additional file 4).

System constraints

System constraints and associated sub-themes were the dominant theme affecting the identification of ED among health professionals. All the professionals reported receiving minimal, if any training on ED as part of their pre or post-registration clinical education, as one participant described: *"I know what an eating disorder is but I've not come across it through my health visitor training"* (P7). Some health professionals felt knowledge had to be inferred from other taught topics as ED were not specifically addressed, as illustrated by one qualified midwife involved in midwifery education: *"it wouldn't be a module...it would be linked into mental ill health or BMI"* (P22). Several qualified and student participants reported receiving training, but considered that this was a general introduction to ED which was not specific to women during or after pregnancy and did not clarify their clinical role in identifying or managing ED: *"I don't know whether it was actually mentioned apart from refer to a dietician, there wasn't really any practical advice of what we need to do"* (P17). Some student midwives felt that module and programme leads expected knowledge of ED to be gained from self-directed learning or 'learning' in clinical practice: *"I think university often relies on us learning this kind of thing in practice that obviously we've got so much learning in the three years"* (P4).

Across all groups, most participants felt that the media was their main source of ED knowledge, with personal and previous clinical experience and training less likely to be described as a source. Most participants expressed limited understanding of ED beyond food-restriction associated with AN and self-induced vomiting associated with BN, and were not aware of implications for maternal and infant health. Some reported a lack of awareness that ED was classed as a mental health disorder, as one qualified health visitor explained: *"I have a very limited knowledge about the, those terms as in Bulimia and Anorexia, I've heard the words being thrown round quite a lot...but what I know as well is that it's kind of linked...to mental health issues"* (P30). Consequently, many health professionals lacked evidence-based knowledge on ED which impacted on their confidence in enquiring and identifying ED. One qualified midwife described: *"it's really hard when you've, when people give you information but you don't know anything about it or there's nothing much you can do"* (P17), and likewise this feeling was expected to affect disclosure by women: *"It's that kind of feeling that, like a bit awkward and stuff like you don't really know what to say and then it's not going to help the women open up and discuss anymore with you"* (P4).

Health professionals related their poor awareness of relevant policies, guidance, care management plans and referral pathways to their lack of relevant training on ED: *"If it's in the trust policy and guidelines I haven't found it yet because I haven't sort of come across it or it hasn't been emphasised in the training"* (P3). Several qualified and student professionals reported not routinely including ED when asking women about their history of mental health problems: *"I never mention those words, I don't think I ever ask a question that you know"* (P11). However, several midwives that had asked women felt *"there's no point in asking the question if you don't know what to say next"* (P13) referring to the lack of awareness on care pathways.

Midwives reported that time constraints in antenatal clinics would be likely to impact on their ability to enquire effectively about ED, with opportunities to screen for physical and mental health risk often limited to the initial pregnancy 'booking' appointment: *"these really big questions you know which can't just be rushed over"* (P15). Some health visitors reported they would ask about women's mental health at a 'new baby' visit which was usually allocated more time than other routine clinic appointments, but there was less focus on this being the main opportunity as *"when you see them for the first visit...you know the chances are you won't see that person again...I've got someone who comes to clinic...the health visitor probably never saw her again anyway, whereas now it would be much more appropriate for me to say to her"* (P31).

In all groups, poor sharing of information about a woman's physical and mental health was reported to be problematic. Qualified and student midwives reported limited means of relaying sensitive information or raising concerns about a woman's mental health between colleagues. A woman's pregnancy and medical history was expected to be documented in the woman's handheld maternity notes, with concerns about confidentiality if a woman's history of ED was included. Several midwives used domestic violence as an example of the limitations of using women's handheld notes: *"obviously because they are handheld notes we're very careful of what we write in them"* (P3). Communication between services particularly within primary care, for instance between the family doctor (GP), midwives and health visitors, was described by some qualified health visitors as limited, with services increasingly fragmented across acute and primary healthcare sectors: *"there was one midwife in every Sure Start and we were all attached so we would always be able to liaise with that midwife and they would liaise with us...now it's like five midwives, like different midwives' every time and they, they don't build up that kind of rapport"* (P26). Sure Start is a UK parenting support programme, with centres primarily across England with slightly different versions in Wales, Scotland and Northern Ireland, but funding cuts have led to many of these centres closing in recent years [34]. Clinicians felt there were few opportunities to be involved in shared care as part of a multidisciplinary team, resulting in limited access to mental health expertise within or between services, particularly within health visiting: *"if you had some supervision around those sorts of issues, any sorts of issue where you're just feeling like you're holding something but you haven't necessarily got the skills"* (P26). Furthermore, a few health visitors described poor awareness about ED generally among health professionals and not isolated to health visiting: *"I do really think that if we had it everybody else in the community teams would need it too because there would be no point in just training us if it then stopped with us"* (P27).

Recognition of role

Many clinicians were in favour of enquiring about ED but several considered their confidence and competence to identify complex mental health problems was limited, and their role should be more advisory and supportive. This was illustrated by one student midwife who described: *"we tell people what not to eat but not how do you eat"* (P3). Some qualified midwives felt that the primary focus in antenatal care was physical wellbeing of the woman and the fetus rather than the woman's mental health: *"We would be just making sure that the baby was growing adequately... and then leaving the woman well alone in a way just focusing on the wellbeing of the baby"* (P11). The focus on the infant after the birth was similarly expressed by some of the qualified health visitors. A few student midwives considered whether women's perceptions of their clinical roles could support or hinder a discussion about ED as *"a midwife...usually it's for normal pregnancies, normality, and also is a figure that only she's for the women and babies and the doctors maybe they seem, or the mental health services don't sound probably very nice...maybe it's easier because they know that this, the midwife is gonna follow them through the pregnancy"* (P2), whereas *"the health visitors kind of some were viewed for the baby and kind of for the child's sake not someone to support the mum"* (P4).

Personal attitudes

The majority felt that health professionals needed to be empathic and positive so that women felt comfortable to raise and discuss their mental health problems: *"there is no room for negativity in midwifery"* (P12). However, one health visitor did express that she would feel uncomfortable to enquire about ED with women who were overweight compared to women who were underweight. One midwife discussed the need to recognise the health professional as an individual: *"we make assumptions that we all will deliver that health promotion message when actually attitudes and beliefs are integral to who we are, influence how we ask the question"* (P22).

Stigma and taboo

Health professionals in all groups discussed the stigma of ED, with some referring to it as a 'taboo' subject for women and clinicians, with less experienced midwives and health visitors describing greater anxiety about asking women. As one student midwife said: *"it does feel kind of sometimes like it's one of those taboo questions a bit like domestic violence...but you kind of like skirt over like 'you haven't ever had any eating disorders, have you? No right moving on"* (P4). One qualified midwife explained: *"one needs to be sensitive about these things, mental health issues equals social services take away baby"* (P15).

Discussion

This is the first research to specifically explore the perspectives of women and health professionals on the barriers to identifying ED during and after pregnancy. Our main findings were that perceived stigma had a major impact on women's disclosure of their illness, and health professionals had low confidence in identifying ED as they lacked evidence-based knowledge and training. The discussion will mainly focus on these outcomes as they were the most prominent, and have direct implications to support effective identification of ED during and after pregnancy.

Consistent with general and pregnancy ED research, women were often reluctant to disclose their ED to a health professional [25, 29]. Stigma was a key barrier reported by the women in this research, and health professionals similarly felt it hindered discussion and enquiry about ED. Stigma is consistently implicated as a barrier to disclosure and treatment-seeking in the ED and wider mental health literature [27, 28, 35]. The term stigma involves perceived and experienced stereotyping, prejudice and discrimination to the detriment of the targeted group [36]. The stigma of mental health is widely recognised, but it can be greater for ED as sufferers are perceived as more responsible and in control of their ED behaviours [37, 38]. The stigmatising attitudes towards BED specifically are comparable to attitudes towards obesity and overweight status [39]. Weight stigma is well recognised and reinforced by some of the more pervasive anti-obesity campaigns [39]. Given the association between BED and obesity [40], the stigma women with BED experience may be compounded by their weight status. Stigmatising attitudes can contribute to feelings of shame and guilt, which cause an individual to feel personal responsibility for their behaviours. As a consequence, an individual may want to hide their disorder [41], avoid disclosure and show reluctance to seek help for their ED [27–29].

In the UK, several campaigns have been launched to raise public awareness and reduce stigma about mental health, such as the 'Time to Change' campaign [42], and several initiatives have been launched to address perinatal mental health awareness specifically, such as the 'Better Births' initiative [43]. Similar anti-stigma programmes exist in other countries, such as 'Beyond Blue' in Australia [44], 'Mental Health Commission of Canada' [45], and 'Bring Change 2 Mind' in the US [46], and these, along with other campaigns, have formed a global alliance to reduce mental health stigma [47]. However, ED continue to be largely neglected in these mental health awareness campaigns. BED is also not considered and neither is the broader issue of weight stigma within the anti-obesity and healthy eating campaigns and clinical guidance [48–50]. The campaigns and clinical guidance [48–50] aimed at addressing the rising prevalence of obesity focus on changing nutrition but not on eating disorder behaviours that might affect nutrition. Considering the high level of comorbidity [40], the identification of ED perinatally may subsequently support obesity prevention in pregnancy and postnatally. Initiatives are needed to specifically target and address the broad range of ED to reduce stigma, prevent discrimination and raise awareness. Only by raising the profile of ED and reducing stigma will disclosure and open discussion with health professionals be encouraged among women during and after pregnancy who suffer these mental health disorders.

Health professionals considered an important barrier to identifying ED was their lack of evidence-based knowledge and training, which subsequently impacted on their confidence. This finding was not unexpected as ED are not currently specified in the core clinical competencies required as part of pre-registration training of midwives and health visitors in the UK [51, 52]. This reflects poor integration of available guidance in to pre and post-registration training [24]. Future curriculum revisions need to educate about the complexity and range of ED and ED behaviours, and include the changes in symptoms that may be experienced during and after pregnancy [3, 6–9]. Research is needed to explore facilitators to disclosure to identify acceptable means of enquiry and management that are sensitive and responsive to the needs of women, and findings need to be incorporated in to future training. Training also needs to address individual attitudes about ED given the expectation for health professionals to deliver care in a consistent manner.

Other system level barriers to identifying ED in pregnancy and postnatally were identified, specifically poor continuity of care and poor communication between health professionals and women, and between health professionals. Women and health professionals described the lack of opportunity and time within routine antenatal and postnatal care contacts to discuss ED in a comfortable way to encourage disclosure, with midwives advocating the potential benefit of a 'case loading' model of midwifery care. This model of midwifery care is considered to promote better continuity of care in pregnancy and is advocated in UK policy and guidance [53, 54] and other countries with similar healthcare systems such as Australia [55]. Case loading models of midwifery care have been associated with better maternal and infant outcomes, patient satisfaction, and cost effectiveness in comparison to other models of maternity care [56–58], yet provision remains variable [59, 60]. Poor communication between health professionals was similarly an important barrier as methods of relaying concern about women were complicated by the need to balance communication of crucial information with respecting the sensitive and confidential nature of disclosure. The issue of communication of risk between acute and primary care services is increasingly affected by fragmented and poorly integrated maternity services, particularly in primary care settings with services central to coordinating healthcare [61]. Addressing these system level barriers could promote an environment conducive to open discussion and support the role of the health professionals in the identification of ED in the perinatal period.

Strengths and limitations

Strengths of this research include the exploration of experiences from both women and health professionals, with consistency in the findings between the two groups. Research findings are likely to be relevant for women who have ED regardless of place of birth, with issues for health professional training likely to be relevant in settings where women can access care from midwives and health visitors or an equivalent health professional.

There are several limitations to the research to be taken in to account when considering the implications of the findings. Convenience sampling was necessary for logistical reasons however, it limits the representativeness of the sample and generalisability of the findings. There may have been recall bias as most women were reflecting on past experiences of antenatal care. The single eligibility question may have been ambiguous in the absence of a clinical diagnosis and did not distinguish between past or current ED. However this type of self-report indicator was used primarily for practical reasons, further it has been validated in an antenatal sample [62] and no ED screening measures have been validated in pregnancy. Future research could focus on women who have been clinically diagnosed with ED.

Conclusions

There are several important barriers to the identification of ED in pregnancy and the postnatal period. Stigma had a major impact on women's disclosure of their illness, whilst health professionals had poor confidence in identifying ED as they lacked evidence-based knowledge and training. The need to identify perinatal mental health problems has been increasingly recognised, however ED continue to be neglected and it is important to raise awareness with health professionals. Similarly, clinical guidance aimed at responding to the rising prevalence of obesity focus on changing nutrition but not on ED behaviours that might affect nutrition. Improving ED education and training for health professionals may contribute to reducing stigma and increase confidence in identifying ED. The barriers identified in this research need to be addressed if recognition and response to women with ED during the perinatal period is to improve.

Additional file

Additional file 1: Study 1: Mixed-measures survey.
Additional file 2: Study 2: Focus group topic guide.
Additional file 3: Study 1: Themes with illustrative quotations.
Additional file 4: Study 2: Themes with illustrative quotations.

Abbreviations

AN: Anorexia Nervosa; BED: Binge Eating Disorder; BN: Bulimia Nervosa; ED: Eating Disorders; NHS: National Health Service; NICE: National Institute for Health and Care Excellence

Acknowledgements

We are extremely grateful to the women, students, staff, NHS Trusts and Universities that have contributed to this research. We would like to thank NetMums for their support in administering the survey. We would like to thank Dr. Kylee Trevillion for contributions to the data analysis, and Jennifer Elglumati for assistance with data collection. Finally, we are grateful for the support received from the Open Access Funding Team at the University College London Library Services towards publishing this manuscript as an open access publication.

Funding
DB is supported by the National Institute for Health Research (NIHR) Collaboration for Leadership in Applied Health Research and Care South London at King's College Hospital NHS Foundation Trust (NIHR, CLAHRC-2013-10022). AE is funded through a King's Improvement Science Fellowship award. King's Improvement Science is part of the NIHR CLAHRC South London and comprises a specialist team of improvement scientists and senior researchers based at King's College London. Its work is funded by King's Health Partners (Guy's and St Thomas' NHS Foundation Trust, King's College Hospital NHS Foundation Trust, King's College London and South London and Maudsley NHS Foundation Trust), Guy's and St Thomas' Charity, the Maudsley Charity and the Health Foundation. NM was funded by a National Institute of Health Research (NIHR) clinician scientist award (DHCS/08/08/012). The views expressed in this publication are those of the authors and not necessarily those of the NHS, the NIHR or the Department of Health.

Authors' contributions
All authors contributed significantly to this work. AB and NM conceived and designed the studies, with input from JS, DB and AE. AB carried out the data collection. AB and MKM analysed the data. All authors contributed to interpreting the findings. AB drafted the manuscript, and all authors read and approved the final manuscript.

Competing interests
JS is an Associate Editor for BMC Pregnancy and Childbirth. The other authors declare that they have no competing interests.

Author details
[1]Population, Policy and Practice, UCL Great Ormond Street Institute of Child Health, 30 Guilford Street, WC1N 1EH, London, UK. [2]Centre for Implementation Science, Health Service and Population Research, Institute of Psychiatry, Psychology & Neuroscience, King's College London, London, UK. [3]Department of Midwifery, Florence Nightingale Faculty of Nursing, Midwifery & Palliative Care, King's College London, London, UK. [4]Institute of Health and Community, University of Plymouth, Devon, UK. [5]Child and Adolescent Psychiatry Division, Department of Child and Adolescent Health, Geneva University Hospital, Geneva, Switzerland. [6]Department of Psychiatry, Faculty of Medicine, University of Geneva, Geneva, Switzerland. [7]Department of Women and Children's Health, School of Life Course Sciences, Faculty of Life Sciences and Medicine, King's College London, London, UK.

References
1. American Psychiatric Association. Diagnostic and statistical manual of mental disorders, fifth edition (DSM-5TM) 5Washington, D.C.;American Psychiatric Association 2013.
2. Micali N, Hagberg KW, Petersen I, Treasure JL. The incidence of eating disorders in the UK in 2000–2009: findings from the general practice research database. BMJ Open. 2013;3:e002646. https://doi.org/10.1136/bmjopen-2013-002646.
3. Easter A, Bye A, Taborelli E, Corfield F, Schmidt U, Treasure J, et al. Recognising the symptoms: how common are eating disorders in pregnancy? Eur Eat Disord Rev. 2013;21:340–4. https://doi.org/10.1002/erv.2229.
4. Pettersson CB, Zandian M, Clinton D. Eating disorder symptoms pre- and postpartum. Arch Womens Ment Health. 2016; https://doi.org/10.1007/s00737-016-0619-3.
5. Turton P, Hughes P, Bolton H, Sedgwick P. Incidence and demographic correlates of eating disorder symptoms in a pregnant population. Int J Eat Disord. 1999;26:448–52.
6. Blais MA, Becker AE, Burwell RA, Flores AT, Nussbaum KM, Greenwood DN, et al. Pregnancy: outcome and impact on symptomatology in a cohort of eating-disordered women. Int J Eat Disord. 2000;27:140–9.
7. Crow SJ, Keel PK, Thuras P, Mitchell JE. Bulimia symptoms and other risk behaviors during pregnancy in women with bulimia nervosa. Int J Eat Disord. 2004;36:220–3. https://doi.org/10.1002/eat.20031.
8. Micali N, Treasure J, Simonoff E. Eating disorders symptoms in pregnancy: a longitudinal study of women with recent and past eating disorders and obesity. J Psychosom Res. 2007;63:297–303. https://doi.org/10.1016/j.jpsychores.2007.05.003.
9. Crow SJ, Agras WS, Crosby R, Halmi K, Mitchell JE. Eating disorder symptoms in pregnancy: a prospective study. Int J Eat Disord. 2008;41:277–9. https://doi.org/10.1002/eat.20496.
10. Easter A, Solmi F, Bye A, Taborelli E, Corfield F, Schmidt U, et al. Antenatal and postnatal psychopathology among women with current and past eating disorders: longitudinal patterns. Eur Eat Disord Rev. 2015;23:19–27. https://doi.org/10.1002/erv.2328.
11. Micali N, Simonoff E, Treasure J. Pregnancy and post-partum depression and anxiety in a longitudinal general population cohort: the effect of eating disorders and past depression. J Affect Disord. 2011;131:150–7. https://doi.org/10.1016/j.jad.2010.09.034.
12. Bulik CM, Von Holle A, Siega-Riz AM, Torgersen L, Lie KK, Hamer RM, et al. Birth outcomes in women with eating disorders in the Norwegian mother and child cohort study (MoBa). Int J Eat Disord. 2009;42:9–18. https://doi.org/10.1002/eat.20578.
13. Easter A, Treasure J, Micali N. Fertility and prenatal attitudes towards pregnancy in women with eating disorders: results from the Avon longitudinal study of parents and children. BJOG. 2011;118:1491–8. https://doi.org/10.1111/j.1471-0528.2011.03077.x.
14. Linna MS, Raevuori A, Haukka J, Suvisaari JM, Suokas JT, Gissler M. Pregnancy, obstetric, and perinatal health outcomes in eating disorders. Am J Obstet Gynecol. 2014;211:392.e1–8. https://doi.org/10.1016/j.ajog.2014.03.067.
15. Micali N, Simonoff E, Treasure J. Risk of major adverse perinatal outcomes in women with eating disorders. Br J Psychiatry. 2007;190:255–9. https://doi.org/10.1192/bjp.bp.106.020768.
16. Micali N, Stemann Larsen P, Strandberg-Larsen K, Nybo Andersen A-M. Size at birth and preterm birth in women with lifetime eating disorders: a prospective population-based study. BJOG An Int J Obstet Gynaecol. 2016; 123:1301–10. https://doi.org/10.1111/1471-0528.13825.
17. Solmi F, Sallis H, Stahl D, Treasure J, Micali N. Low birth weight in the offspring of women with anorexia nervosa. Epidemiol Rev. 2014;36:49–56. https://doi.org/10.1093/epirev/mxt004.
18. Larsson G, Andersson-Ellstrom A. Experiences of pregnancy-related body shape changes and of breast-feeding in women with a history of eating disorders. Eur Eat Disord Rev. 2003;11:116–24. https://doi.org/10.1002/erv.497.
19. Micali N, Simonoff E, Treasure J. Infant feeding and weight in the first year of life in babies of women with eating disorders. J Pediatr. 2009;154:55–60.e1.
20. Reba-Harrelson L, Von Holle A, Hamer RM, Torgersen L, Reichborn-Kjennerud T, Bulik CM. Patterns of maternal feeding and child eating associated with eating disorders in the Norwegian mother and child cohort study (MoBa). Eat Behav. 2010;11:54–61. https://doi.org/10.1016/j.eatbeh.2009.09.004.
21. Henrichs J, Schenk JJ, Schmidt HG. Maternal pre- and postnatal anxiety and infant temperament. Generation R Study. 2009;572:556–72.
22. Patel P, Wheatcroft R, Park RJ, Stein A. The children of mothers with eating disorders. Clin Child Fam Psychol Rev. 2002;5:1–19.
23. Zerwas S, Von Holle A, Torgersen L, Reichborn-Kjennerud T, Stoltenberg C, Bulik CM. Maternal eating disorders and infant temperament: findings from the Norwegian mother and child cohort study. Int J Eat Disord. 2012;45:546–55. https://doi.org/10.1002/eat.20983.
24. National Institute for Health and Care Excellence. Antenatal and postnatal mental health: clinical management and service guidance. Clinical guideline CG192; 2014.
25. Becker AE, Thomas JJ, Franko DL, Herzog DB. Disclosure patterns of eating and weight concerns to clinicians, educational professionals, family, and peers. Int J Eat Disord. 2005;38:18–23. https://doi.org/10.1002/eat.20141.
26. Hudson JI, Hiripi E, Pope HG, Kessler RC. The prevalence and correlates of eating disorders in the National Comorbidity Survey Replication. Biol Psychiatry. 2007;61:348–58. https://doi.org/10.1016/j.biopsych.2006.03.040.
27. Swan S, Andrews B. The relationship between shame, eating disorders and disclosure in treatment. Br J Clin Psychol. 2003;42(Pt 4):367–78. https://doi.org/10.1348/014466503322528919.
28. Hepworth N, Paxton SJ. Pathways to help-seeking in bulimia nervosa and binge eating problems: a concept mapping approach. Int J Eat Disord. 2007;40:493–504. https://doi.org/10.1002/eat.20402.
29. Stringer E, Tierney S, Fox J, Butterfield C, Furber C. Pregnancy, motherhood

and eating disorders: a qualitative study describing women's views of maternity care. Evid Based Midwifery. 2010;8:112–21.
30. Abraham S. Obstetricians and maternal body weight and eating disorders during pregnancy. J Psychosom Obstet Gynaecol. 2001;22:159–63.
31. Supina D, Herman BK, Frye CB, Shillington AC. Knowledge of binge eating disorder: a cross-sectional survey of physicians in the United States. Postgrad Med. 2016;128:311–6. https://doi.org/10.1080/00325481.2016.1157441.
32. Banas DA, Redfern R, Wanjiku S, Lazebnik R, Rome ES. Eating disorder training and attitudes among primary care residents. Clin Pediatr (Phila). 2013;52:355–61. https://doi.org/10.1177/0009922813479157.
33. Braun V, Clarke V. Using thematic analysis in psychology. Qual Res Psychol. 2006;3:77–101. https://doi.org/10.1191/1478088706qp063oa.
34. Bate A, Foster D. Sure start (England). Briefing paper number 7257. London: House of Commons Library; 2017.
35. Clement S, Schauman O, Graham T, Maggioni F, Evans-Lacko S, Bezborodovs N, et al. What is the impact of mental health-related stigma on help-seeking? A systematic review of quantitative and qualitative studies. Psychol Med. 2015;45:11–27. https://doi.org/10.1017/S0033291714000129.
36. Link BG, Phelan JC. Conceptualizing Stigma. Annu Rev Sociol. 2001;27:363–85. https://doi.org/10.1146/annurev.soc.27.1.363.
37. Ebneter DS, Latner JD. Stigmatizing attitudes differ across mental health disorders: a comparison of stigma across eating disorders, obesity, and major depressive disorder. J Nerv Ment Dis. 2013;201:281–5. https://doi.org/10.1097/NMD.0b013e318288e23f.
38. Roehrig JP, CP ML. A comparison of stigma toward eating disorders versus depression. Int J Eat Disord. 2010;43:671–4. https://doi.org/10.1002/eat.20760.
39. Puhl R, Peterson JL, Luedicke J, Keranen L, Komesaroff P, Komesaroff PA. Motivating or stigmatizing? Public perceptions of weight-related language used by health providers. Int J Obes. 2013;37:623. https://doi.org/10.1038/ijo.2013.17.
40. de Zwaan M. Binge eating disorder and obesity. Int J Obes Relat Metab Disord. 2001;25(Suppl 1):S51–5. https://doi.org/10.1038/sj.ijo.0801699.
41. Tangney JP, Miller RS, Flicker L, Barlow DH. Are shame, guilt, and embarrassment distinct emotions? J Pers Soc Psychol. 1996;70:1256–69.
42. Time To Change. 2007. http://www.time-to-change.org.uk/. Accessed 31 Mar 2017.
43. Royal College of Midwives. Better births initiative. 2016. https://www.rcm.org.uk/better-births-initiative. Accessed 30 Mar 2017.
44. Beyond Blue. https://www.beyondblue.org.au/. Accessed 9 Apr 2018.
45. Mental Health Commission of Canada. Mental Health Commission of Canada - strategic plan 2017-2022. 2016.
46. Bring Change To Mind. https://bringchange2mind.org/. Accessed 21 Apr 2017.
47. Global anti-stigma campaigns | Time To Change. https://www.time-to-change.org.uk/about-us/what-we-do/global-anti-stigma-alliance/global-campaigns. Accessed 21 Apr 2017.
48. National Institute for Health and Care Excellence. Obesity prevention. Clinical guideline (CG43); 2006.
49. Public Health England. Change4Life - Be Food Smart. https://www.nhs.uk/change4life-beta/be-food-smart#bRG6l1Y9HOKh4u8b.97. Accessed 26 Apr 2017.
50. National Institute for Health and Care Excellence. Weight management before, during and after pregnancy. Clinical guideline (PH27); 2010.
51. Nursing & Midwifery Council. Standards for pre-registration midwifery education. London: Nursing & Midwifery Council; 2009.
52. Nursing & Midwifery Council. Standards of proficiency for specialist community public health nurses. London: Nursing & Midwifery Council; 2004.
53. Department of Health. Maternity matters: choice, access and continuity of care in a safe service. London: Department of Health; 2007.
54. National Institute of Health and Care Excellence. Antenatal care. Clinical Guideline (QS22); 2012.
55. Commonwealth of Australia. Improving maternity Services in Australia: the report of the maternity services review. Canberra: Commonwealth of Australia; 2009.
56. Sandall J, Soltani H, Gates S, Shennan A, Devane D. Midwife-led continuity models versus other models of care for childbearing women. Cochrane Database Syst Rev. 2013;8:CD004667. https://doi.org/10.1002/14651858.CD004667.pub3.
57. Tracy SK, Hartz DL, Tracy MB, Allen J, Forti A, Hall B, et al. Caseload midwifery care versus standard maternity care for women of any risk: M@NGO, a randomised controlled trial. Lancet. 2013;382:1723–32. https://doi.org/10.1016/S0140-6736(13)61406-3.
58. Forster DA, McLachlan HL, Davey M-A, Biro MA, Farrell T, Gold L, et al. Continuity of care by a primary midwife (caseload midwifery) increases women's satisfaction with antenatal, intrapartum and postpartum care: results from the COSMOS randomised controlled trial. BMC Pregnancy Childbirth. 2016;16:28. https://doi.org/10.1186/s12884-016-0798-y.
59. Care Quality Commission. CQC's response to the 2015 survey of women's experiences of maternity care. London: Care Quality Commission; 2016.
60. Commonwealth of Australia. National Maternity Services Plan 2010. Canberra: Commonwealth of Australia; 2011.
61. Watton R. The loss of multidisciplinary primary healthcare teams is bad for patient care. BMJ. 2013;347:f5450. https://doi.org/10.1136/bmj.f5450.
62. Micali N, De Stavola B, dos-Santos-Silva I, Steenweg-de Graaff J, Jansen PW, Jaddoe VWV, et al. Perinatal outcomes and gestational weight gain in women with eating disorders: a population-based cohort study. BJOG. 2012;119:1493–502. https://doi.org/10.1111/j.1471-0528.2012.03467.x.

3

They receive antenatal care in health facilities, yet do not deliver there: predictors of health facility delivery by women in rural Ghana

Michael Boah[1*], Abraham B. Mahama[2] and Emmanuel A. Ayamga[1]

Abstract

Background: Research has shown that use of antenatal services by pregnant women and delivery in health facilities with skilled birth attendants contribute to better delivery outcomes. However, a gap exists in Ghana between the use of antenatal care provided by health facilities and delivery in health facilities with skilled birth attendants by pregnant women. This study sought to identify the predictors of health facility delivery by women in a rural district in Ghana.

Methods: This was a cross-sectional study conducted in June 2016. Women who delivered in the past 6 months preceding the study were interviewed. Data on socio-demographic characteristics, use of antenatal care, place of delivery and reasons for home delivery were collected from study participants. Chi-square test and multiple logistic regression analysis were used to assess an association between women's socio-demographic and obstetric characteristics and place of delivery at 95% confidence interval.

Results: The study found that 98.8% of women received antenatal care services at least once during their recent pregnancy, and 67.9% attended antenatal care at least four times before delivery. However, 61.9% of the women delivered in a health facility with a skilled attendant. The frequently mentioned reason for home delivery was "unaware of onset of labour and delivery". The odds for delivery at a health facility were reduced among women with four living children [(AOR = 0.07, CI = 0.15–0.36, p = 0.001)], with no exposure to delivery care information [(AOR = 0.06, CI = 0.01–0.34, p = 0.002), who started their first ANC visit from the second trimester of pregnancy[(AOR = 0.003, CI = 0.01–0.15, $p < 0.001$)] and increased among women who made at least four ANC visits before delivery [(AOR = 17.53, CI = 6.89–44.61, $p < 0.001$)].

Conclusion: Findings from this study revealed a low rate of delivery at health facilities although visits to antenatal care sessions were high, an indication that there was the need to intensify health education on early initiation of antenatal care, signs of labour and delivery, and importance of health facility delivery.

Keywords: Predictors, Ghana, Health facility, Delivery place, Skilled attendant

* Correspondence: boahmichael@gmail.com
[1]Ghana Health Service, Kassena Nankana West District Health Directorate, P. O. Box 21, Paga, Upper East Region, Ghana
Full list of author information is available at the end of the article

Background

Low-and middle-income countries (LMIC) contribute about 99% of the maternal deaths that occur worldwide [1]. An analysis of the causes of maternal deaths in Africa shows that most of these deaths are as a result of direct obstetric complications notably, haemorrhage, hypertension, sepsis and obstructed labour that emerge around the time of labour and delivery [2]. However, deaths from these complications can be prevented. In Ghana, though there has been a decline in maternal mortality from 760 deaths per 100,00 live births in 1990 to 319 deaths per 100,000 live births in 2015, it is still very high [1].

Complications that may arise from pregnancy are impossible to predict. The World Health Organization (WHO) therefore recommends delivery by a skilled birth attendant (SBA) [3]. The presence of an SBA at delivery has also been stressed in many summits and international conferences worldwide [4]. The contribution of skilled delivery in the reduction of deaths among pregnant women and neonates has been highlighted by several studies [5–7].

A high proportion of women in developing countries are reported to have received antenatal care (ANC) at least once from a qualified health provider during pregnancy [8–12]. However, in spite of the importance placed on the use of an SBA by women during delivery to prevent complications, it is not uncommon to find one in three women using an SBA during delivery, especially in sub-Sahara Africa [13]. Cost, number of ANC visits made by a woman before delivery, maternal education, poor attitude of health care providers, parity and distance, the effect of which is compounded by the lack of transport, have been identified as some barriers to the use of health facility by pregnant women for delivery in developing countries [14–17].

To improve geographic access to health services by all, the Community-based Health Planning and Services (CHPS) initiative was implemented by the Ghana Health Service (GHS) in 2002 and covered all the regions in Ghana. This was followed by the implementation of the free maternal health care policy in 2003 under which pregnant women do not pay user fees to receive health services from the time of pregnancy to 3 months postpartum. Additionally, routine health education and promotion activities on the benefits of delivery with a SBA are carried out [18, 19]. Consequently, nine out of ten women in Ghana have utilized ANC services from health professionals during their recent pregnancy [20–23]. However, the high prevalence of ANC usage does not translate into the use of health facility for delivery. The 2014 Ghana Demographic and Health Survey (GDHS) report revealed that an overwhelming 97% of women received ANC at least once during their recent pregnancy, but 73% went on to deliver in a health facility where SBAs are available [24].

With these strategies in place, it is expected that the high prevalence of ANC utilization should correspond to an increase in health facility delivery. This is however not the case. The question is why? The reasons for this phenomenon needed to be ascertained.

Skilled delivery in the Upper East Region of northern Ghana is high (84.1%), though there are variations across the thirteen districts in the region [24, 25]. The 2014 annual report of the Builsa district showed that an appreciable 71.5% of pregnant women received ANC services once during pregnancy, 90.7% made at least four follow up visits before delivery while only 46.2% delivered in a health facility [25, 26]. These findings on ANC utilization and health facility delivery put together demonstrate that a gap exists between receiving ANC services from health facilities and delivery in health facilities.

Studies conducted in Ghana [23, 27, 28] have identified factors such as maternal age, religion, household income and maternal occupation to predict health facility delivery. However, the focus of these studies still presents gaps in the literature. For instance, two of the studies did not assess the effect of the gestation of pregnancy at the onset of ANC on the place of delivery [23, 27]. Furthermore, the study by Esena & Sappor [28] was carried out in an urban setting, hence the results may not be wholly applicable in a rural setting. The gestation of pregnancy at the onset of ANC and place of residence (rural or urban) have been reported to influence the use of health facility for delivery services elsewhere [15, 20]. Therefore, results of this present study will inform policy and add to existing literature by examining the factors behind the existing gap between the use of ANC and health facility delivery by women.

The aim of this study was to explore socio-demographic and obstetric factors such as maternal age, education, ethnicity, religion, occupation, health insurance status, the gestation of pregnancy at first ANC attendance, and parity as predictors of health facility delivery by women in a rural district in northern Ghana.

Methods

Study setting

This study was cross-sectional by design. It was carried out in June 2016 in the Builsa South District, a predominantly rural district located in the Upper East Region of northern Ghana. The district comprises of six sub-districts. The district has 3 health centres and 14 CHPS zones serving a population of 38, 298 (projected from the 2010 population and housing census). Women in reproductive age form 24% (9192) of the total population of the district. There are no private maternity homes [26].

Study population and sampling

Women included in this study were all women aged 15–49 years resident in the district who delivered in the past 6 months preceding the survey. Antenatal care record book of each study participant was used to confirm obstetric information given. Women not resident in the study district, who delivered more than 6 months preceding the survey were excluded.

A sample size of 423 women was computed using the formula, z^2pq/d^2: p, the proportion of first trimester ANC registrants was estimated as 49% from a previous study in Ghana [29] with 5% error margin at 95% confidence interval and 10% non-response rate.

A multi-stage sampling technique was used in the selection of study communities and participants. First, simple random sampling by lottery was used to select six communities, one in each of the six sub-districts. The total sample size was then allocated proportionally to the selected communities.

Second, a sampling frame of eligible women was developed with the aid of existing community filariasis and child welfare clinic registers in the health facilities serving the selected communities. The two registers were used in order to have an up-to-date information about the women in the various households. A systematic random sampling method was employed to select a participating household. Only one woman in participating household was interviewed. A lottery was used to select one woman for the interview whenever a selected household had more than one eligible woman.

Variables

The delivery place was selected as the main outcome variable. It was dichotomized as 0 "Home" for all deliveries occurring outside the health facility and 1 "Health facility" for deliveries occurring in the health facility. This information was obtained by asking the question "Where did you deliver [name of child]?" Based on available literature, predictor variables included were age, marital status, occupation, highest educational level, religion, parity, ethnicity, health insurance validity status, exposure to information on delivery care (irrespective of source), the gestation of pregnancy at the onset of ANC and the number of ANC visits made before delivery.

Data collection

Data on socio-demographic characteristics of respondents, place of delivery and reasons for home delivery were gathered using a structured questionnaire. The questionnaires were administered mainly in the local language (Buili).

Ten data collectors with at least secondary education and familiar with the customs and traditions of the area were recruited to assist in data collection. Six supervisors with previous experience in data collection supervised the data collection process. Data collectors and supervisors were trained together in a two-day training session. Training for the first day covered translation of the questionnaire from English to Buili and the interview process. A pre-test was carried out the second day in a neighbouring district with similar characteristics as the study district. Data collected in pre-test were excluded in the final analysis. Woman's ANC card and index child's road to health record booklet were used to confirm information given by mother where applicable.

Data analysis

Administered questionnaires were checked daily for completeness and consistency. Data were entered in EpiData Entry Client version 2.06.20 (EpiData Association, Denmark), and the dataset exported to STATA 13 Special Edition (StataCorp, College Station Taxes, USA LP) for cleaning and analysis.

Pearson chi-square (χ^2) and Fisher's exact tests were used, where appropriate to identify associations between the predictor variables and the outcome variable. Tests were two-tailed and a $p < 0.05$ was considered statistically significant. A possible correlation between statistically significant variables was checked using the Pearson Correlation Matrix before they were put in a multiple logistic regression model. None was found to be collinear.

Ethical considerations

Approval to carry out this study was obtained from the Ethics Review Committee of the Ghana Health Service (ID No. GHS-ERC 31/12/15). Participants consented by signing or thumb printing the consent form after the purpose and benefits of participating in the study were explained to them. Approval was obtained from parents of participants younger than 18 years before the interview. Anonymity and safety of participants were ensured.

Results

Socio-demographic characteristics of study participants

The mean age of participants was 29.2 ± 7.4 SD (range 15–49 years). The majority were married 402 (95.0%), were farmers 274 (64.8%) and belonged to the Christian religion 263 (62.2%). Of the 423 respondents, 172 (40.7%) had no formal education, 101 (23.9%) had two living children, 351 (83%) had ever enrolled onto the national health insurance scheme, and 254 (72.0%) had valid insurance during their recent pregnancy (see Table 1).

Obstetric characteristics of study participants

The obstetric characteristics of the study participants are presented in Table 2. Of the 423 women interviewed, 98.8% had attended antenatal care at least once during their recent pregnancy, and the majority (67.9%) made at least

Table 1 Socio-demographic characteristics of the study participants ($N = 423$ unless stated)

Variable	Number	Percent
Age group (years)		
15–19	32	7.6
20–24	99	23.4
25–29	100	23.6
30–34	79	18.7
35–39	67	15.8
40 and above	46	10.9
Marital status		
Single	8	1.9
Married	402	95.0
Cohabiting	4	0.9
Separated	5	1.2
Widow	4	0.9
Highest educational level attained		
No education	172	40.7
Primary	137	32.4
Middle/Junior High School	67	15.8
Secondary and above	47	11.1
Occupation		
Unemployed	79	18.7
Famer	274	64.8
Self-employed	62	14.7
Formal sector employee	8	1.9
Religion		
Traditional	115	27.2
Christian	263	62.2
Muslim	45	10.6
Parity (Birth order)		
1	87	20.6
2	101	23.9
3	73	17.3
4	86	20.3
5+	76	18.0
Ethnic group		
Builsa	413	97.6
Mamprusi	4	0.9
Kassena	4	0.9
Sissala	2	0.5
Health insurance enrolment status		
Enrolled	351	83.0
Never enrolled	72	17.0
Health insurance status during recent pregnancy ($N = 356$)		
Valid	254	72.0
Not valid	97	28.0
Exposure to information on delivery care		
Yes	387	91.5
No	36	8.5
Type of information received (multiple responses allowed) ($N = 387$)		
Sleep under an insecticide-treated bed net	194	49.6
Observe personal and environmental hygiene	134	34.6
Deliver in health facilities	132	34.1
Practice exclusive breastfeeding for first 6 months	121	31.3
Send children for monthly growth monitoring and promotion	64	16.5
Signs of labour and delivery	35	9.0

four visits before delivery. However, less than half (43.1%) started ANC in the first 3 months of their pregnancy. Many of the women received ANC services from the CHPS facility (60.3%) and health centres (38.5%). Regarding the place of delivery, 61.9% of respondents reported delivering in a health facility, of which the majority (84.4%) were assisted by the Midwife. The most frequently mentioned reasons for home delivery were unaware of onset of labour and delivery (68.0%), and no previous complications with delivery from previous pregnancies (19.6%).

Factors associated with place of delivery

A bivariate analysis was done to assess the association between individual socio-demographic and obstetric characteristics and the place of delivery. The results showed that nine of the eleven selected variables had a significant ($p < 0.05$) association with place of delivery. These variables included age, occupation, highest educational level attained, religion, parity, having a valid insurance during pregnancy, gestational age of pregnancy at the onset of ANC attendance, number of ANC visits made before delivery, and exposure to information on delivery care during the recent pregnancy (see Table 3).

Predictors of health facility delivery

Factors that were significantly associated with place of delivery in the bivariate analysis were put into a multiple logistic regression model to measure their strength of association. Parity, exposure to information on delivery care, the gestation of pregnancy at the onset of ANC, and the number of ANC visits made before delivery were strong predictors of delivery in a health facility (see Table 4). The odds of delivering in a health facility decreased with increasing parity from two children to four

Table 2 Obstetric characteristics of study participants ($N = 423$ unless stated)

Variable	Number	Percent
ANC use during recent pregnancy		
Yes	418	98.8
No	5	1.2
Gestation of pregnancy at first ANC visit ($N = 418$)		
First trimester	180	43.1
Second trimester	235	56.2
Third trimester	3	0.7
Source of ANC services for last pregnancy (N = 418)		
Hospital	1	0.2
Health centre/clinic	161	38.5
CHPS only	252	60.3
TBA only	1	0.2
CHPS & TBA	1	0.2
Number of ANC visits made before delivery (N = 418)		
1	1	0.2
2	14	3.3
3	119	28.5
4 and more visits	284	67.9
Place of delivery		
Health facility	262	61.9
Home	161	38.1
Assistance at health facility delivery ($N = 262$)		
Doctor	25	9.5
Midwife	220	84.0
CHN	17	6.5
[a]Reasons for home delivery ($N = 161$)		
Unaware of onset of labour and delivery	109	67.7
No complications with delivery from previous pregnancies	32	19.9
The home was the only delivery place available	18	11.2
Better care outside the health facility	8	5.0
Husband's decision	6	3.7
Cheaper cost of delivery	4	2.5
Advice from mother-in-law	3	1.9
Health facility too far	2	1.2
No means of transport	1	0.6

[a]Multiple responses allowed

living children. Compared to women with one living child, women with two, three or four living children had 77.0%, 80.0% and 93.0% less the chances of delivering in health facility respectively [(AOR = 0.23, CI = 0.06–0.90, $p = 0.034$), (AOR = 0.20, CI = 0.04–0.99, $p = 0.048$), and (AOR = 0.07, CI = 0.15–0.36, $p = 0.001$) respectively]. However, women with at least five living children had increased odds of delivering in a health facility compared with women with four living children [(AOR = 0.11, CI = 0.02–0.67, $P = 0.017$)]. Also, women without exposure to information on delivery during their recent pregnancy were 94% less likely to deliver in a health facility [(AOR = 0.06, CI = 0.01–0.34, $p = 0.001$)]. Additionally, women who started their first ANC visit from the fourth month of pregnancy had 97.0% fewer chances of delivering in a health facility compared to women who started ANC in the first 3 months of pregnancy [(AOR = 0.03, CI = 0.01–0.15, $p < 0.001$)]. Furthermore, the odds of using a health facility for delivery were about 18 times more among women who attended ANC for at least four times before delivery compared to women who made less than four ANC visits before delivery [(AOR = 17.53, CI = 6.89–44.611, $p < 0.001$)].

Discussion

The results from this study aimed at identifying the predictors of health facility delivery in a rural district in Ghana showed that ANC utilization is high in the study area, as 98.8% of women reported using ANC at least once during their recent pregnancy and about 68.0% made four and more visits before delivery. However, the proportion of women who delivered in a health facility was 61.9% which was not very different from the proportion of women who made at least four follow up visits before delivery (67.9%). The high ANC utilization and low health facility delivery in this study conform to findings from other studies conducted in Ghana [20, 22, 23, 30] and other parts of sub-Saharan Africa [31–33]. The "unaware of onset of labour and delivery" mentioned as the main reason for home delivery in this study possibly explains the gap that exists between ANC utilization and health facility delivery. Women may be more vulnerable during labour than during ANC. Therefore, in the case of ANC utilization, they may have the privilege of time in deciding when, how and where they want to use ANC service but the situation is different when labour starts. The situation may be exacerbated when the woman does not know or recognize early the signs of labour and delivery.

Factors such as age, occupation, maternal education, religion, parity, having a health insurance during pregnancy, exposure to information on delivery care during the recent pregnancy, gestational age of pregnancy at onset of ANC attendance and the number of ANC visits made before delivery were significantly associated with the place of delivery in the bivariate analysis. Older women (35 years and above) were more likely than younger women to deliver at home in this study. This may be because, after many previous deliveries, older women may build more self-confidence and experience in the childbearing process than younger women especially in the absence of any previous birth complications

Table 3 Factors associated with place of delivery in rural Ghana (*N* = 431 unless stated)

Exposure variable	n	Place of delivery		*P*-value
		Home	Health facility	
		n (%)	n (%)	
Age (years)				< 0.001
15–19	32	5 (15.6)	27 (84.4)	
20–24	99	20 (20.2)	79 (79.0)	
25–29	100	37 (37.0)	63 (63.0)	
30–34	79	33 (41.8	46 (58.2)	
35–39	67	36 (53.7)	31 (46.3)	
40 and above	46	30 (65.2)	16 (34.8)	
Marital status				0.921[a]
Single	8	2 (25.0)	6 (75.0)	
Married	402	154 (38.3)	248 (61.7)	
Cohabiting	4	1 (25.0)	3 (75.0)	
Separated	5	2 (40.0)	3 (60.0)	
Widow	4	2 (50.0)	2 (50.0)	
Occupation				< 0.001
Unemployed	79	49 (62.0)	30 (38.0)	
Farmer	274	90 (32.9)	184 (67.1)	
Self-employed	62	21 (33.9)	41 (66.1)	
Formal sector employee	8	1 (12.5)	7 (87.5)	
Highest educational level attained				< 0.001
No education	172	107 (62.2)	65 (37.8)	
Primary	137	42 (30.7)	95 (69.3)	
Middle/Junior High	67	8 (11.9)	59 (88.1)	
Secondary and above	47	4 (8.5)	43 (91.5)	
Religion				< 0.001
Traditional	115	70 (60.9)	45 (39.1)	
Christian	263	76 (28.9)	187 (71.1)	
Moslem	45	15 (33.3)	30 (66.7)	
Ethnicity				0.487[a]
Builsa	413	158 (38.3)	255 (61.7)	
Mamprusi	4	0 (0.0)	4 (100.0)	
Kassena	4	2 (50.0)	2 (50.0)	
Sissala	2	1 (50.0)	1 (50.0)	
Parity				< 0.001
1	87	12 (13.8)	75 (86.2)	
2	101	32 (31.7)	69 (68.3)	
3	73	23 (31.5)	50 (68.49)	
4	86	40 (46.5)	46 (53.5)	
5+	76	54 (71.1)	22 (28.9)	
Health insurance status during recent pregnancy (*N* = 351)				< 0.001
Invalid insurance	97	51 (52.6)	46 (47.4)	
Valid insurance	254	65 (25.6)	189 (74.4)	
Exposure to information on delivery care				0.001
Yes	387	138 (35.7)	249 (64.3)	
No	36	23 (63.9)	13 (36.1)	
Gestation of pregnancy at the onset of ANC (N = 418)				< 0.001
First trimester	180	7 (3.9)	173 (96.1)	
Second trimester and beyond	238	149 (62.6)	89 (37.4)	
Number of ANC visit made before delivery (*N* = 418)				< 0.001
Less than 4 visits	134	115 (85.8)	19 (14.2)	
4 and more visits	284	41 (14.4)	243 (85.6)	

[a]Fisher's exact test

and may not see the relevance to deliver in the presence of a SBA. Also, older women may be deeply buried in traditional beliefs and practices that prohibit the uptake of modern medicine [34]. This could possibly explain the reason why women belonging to the traditional religious group were less likely than their counterparts to use a health facility for delivery as revealed in this study. Age and religion were positively associated with health facility delivery in a different district in the same region [34]. Having some source of income could imply an improvement in household socioeconomic status. Though delivery services are free in public health facilities in Ghana, there may be some indirect costs involved with the use of a health facility for delivery services such as the cost of transportation which is a barrier to the use of health facility for delivery by especially rural women [35] and other materials that may be required for delivery. An employed woman may be able to overcome this barrier easily relative to an unemployed woman. An educated woman relative to a woman with no formal education may have a better access to health-related information and be more concerned about her health and the health of her unborn baby thereby choosing to deliver in a health facility. High maternal education has been associated with increased use of maternal health services in Uganda [33] and Ethiopia [36]. The health insurance scheme in Ghana aims at removing out-of-pocket user fees as barriers to accessing health services [19]. In this study, having a valid health insurance was associated with health facility delivery. This finding supports the findings of another study in Ghana that

Table 4 Predictors of health facility delivery in rural Ghana

Exposure variable	AOR(95% CI)	P-value
Age (years)		
15–19	1.00	
20–24	1.67 (0.26–10.60)	0.586
25–29	1.34 (0.20–8.83)	0.76
30–34	1.64 (0.22–12.42)	0.631
35–39	0.95 (0.11–7.90)	0.959
40 and above	0.58 (0.06–6.08)	0.654
Occupation		
Unemployed	1.00	
Farmer	7.88 (2.45–25.33)	0.001
Self-employed	5.13 (1.39–18.87)	0.014
Formal sector employee	5.97 (0.44–80.94)	0.178
Highest educational level attained		
No education	1.00	
Primary	1.10 (0.42–2.84)	0.848
Middle/Junior High	0.44 (0.09–2.21)	0.318
Secondary and above	0.32 (0.04–2.56)	0.284
Religion		
Traditional	1.00	
Christian	0.80 (0.31–2.07)	0.651
Moslem	5.96 (1.59–22.41)	0.008
Parity		
1	1.00	
2	0.23 (0.06–0.90)	0.034
3	0.20 (0.04–0.99)	0.048
4	0.07 (0.15–0.36)	0.001
5+	0.11 (0.02–0.67)	0.017
Health insurance status		
Invalid insurance	1.00	
Valid insurance	1.50 (0.63–3.58)	0.363
Exposure to information on delivery care		
Yes	1	
No	0.06 (0.01–0.34)	0.002
Gestation of pregnancy at the onset of ANC		
First trimester	1.00	
Second trimester and beyond	0.03 (0.01–0.15)	< 0.001
Number of ANC visit made before delivery		
Less than 4 visits	1.00	
4 and more visits	17.53 (6.89–44.61)	< 0.001

reported high utilization of health facility delivery with the possession of a health insurance [37].

Findings from the study revealed that a woman with one child was more likely to use a health facility for delivery compared to a woman with two to four children. Also, a woman with five or more children was likely to deliver in a health facility compared with a woman with four children. It can be explained that a woman delivering for the first time does not have prior experience with childbirth, may lack self-confidence and consider the delivery very challenging and anticipate unforeseen complications. These may compel her to use a skilled attendant for a safer delivery. However, a woman delivering for the second, third or fourth time has had an experience with childbirth from her previous delivery. This may contribute significantly to her decision-making process as to whether to deliver at home or at a health facility, especially if she did not experience any complications with her previous delivery (ies). A study in Nigeria [38] reported that women were more likely to use maternal health services if they had a previous complication with delivery (e.g. stillbirth). Similar to a woman with one child, a woman with five and more children may consider herself at high risk of birth complications due to the many deliveries and thus recourse to a health facility for delivery where she is sure skilled attendants can manage any resulting complication. She may also be advised by health workers to deliver in a health facility because of the high risk involved [39]. A qualitative study in Africa reported that women perceived themselves to be at risk of adverse pregnancy outcomes after five pregnancies [40]. The positive association between parity one and health facility delivery has also been reported by studies conducted in Senegal, Zambia and Kenya [41–43]. However, a study in Nigeria did not report any association between parity and delivery in a health facility [8].

This study identified that women who were not exposed to information on delivery care during their recent pregnancy were less likely to use the health facility for delivery when compared to women who were exposed to information on delivery during their recent pregnancy. The knowledge of women regarding the benefits of health facility delivery and the opportunities available for life-saving in case of any negative outcomes may be enhanced through exposure to information on delivery care. As explained, the perceived benefits of delivery in a health facility may be decided by the knowledge of the mother on the dangers associated with home delivery and life-saving opportunities available in health facilities [44]. Another study in northern Ghana also reported a positive association between media exposure and health facility delivery [30]. A study in Ethiopia reported that women who were exposed to information on maternal health relative to women who did not receive information were over eight times more likely to give birth in a health facility [45]. Though exposure to maternal health information is very instrumental in promoting health-seeking behaviour, the type of information received should also be taken into serious consideration. Although 91.5% of the women in this study received maternal health information during their recent pregnancy, the frequently mentioned (49.6%) health information received by women was about sleeping under insecticide-treated bed net while 9.0% of the women mentioned that they received information on signs of labour and delivery. This might have contributed to the reason (unaware of onset of labour and delivery) for home deliveries in this study mentioned earlier.

Furthermore, this study found that women who initiated ANC in the first trimester of pregnancy and women who made at least four ANC follow up visits before delivery had increased odds of using a health facility for delivery. Starting ANC in within the first 3 months may offer the woman the opportunity to attend many times and have more contact with health professionals before delivery. These contacts, first of all, serve as a window of opportunity for health professionals to provide the woman with adequate information on the benefits derived from delivering in a health facility and the dangers associated with home delivery. This might enhance the woman's knowledge on maternal health and promote delivery in a health facility. A study in Kenya concluded that starting ANC in the first trimester was a precursor for delivery in a health facility [46]. Similarly, a study in Mali reported that women whose knowledge on maternal health was enhanced through contacts with health staff during ANC were more likely to deliver in health facilities [47]. Secondly, a woman may build confidence and trust in health professionals from continuous visits to the health facility for ANC during pregnancy. She may also listen to encouragement and advice from these health workers to deliver in the health facility. Other studies have also reported that at least four ANC visits before delivery increases the woman's chances of using the health facility for delivery [34, 43, 48, 49].

This study, like many other studies, has strengths and limitations. The major strength of this study was that it limited respondents to women who delivered in the past 6 months, thereby minimizing the tendency of recall bias. Also, obstetric history of the woman was confirmed from the woman's ANC card to ensure the credibility of obstetric information obtained. However, a limitation of this study was its design as cross-sectional. A cross-sectional study only assesses association and not causality. Additionally, the study did not assess the association between non-use of ANC and delivery place.

However, in spite of these limitations, the findings from this study provide information on predictors of health facility delivery in the study district since it is the first of its kind, and adds to existing literature in Ghana on issues related to maternal health-seeking behaviour.

Conclusions

This study sought to identify the predictors of health facility delivery in a rural district in Ghana. Factors such as maternal age, occupation, the educational level attained, religion, parity, health insurance status, exposure to information on delivery care, the gestation of pregnancy at the start of first ANC visit and the number of ANC visits made before delivery were more likely to influence the choice of delivery place. Additionally, the small proportion of women who received health information on signs of labour and delivery might have contributed to the significant proportion of home deliveries in this study since the common reason cited for home delivery was "unaware of onset of labour and delivery".

In addition to using the socio-demographic and obstetric characteristics of the women by health care professionals (especially midwives) to identify potential women who will attend ANC and still deliver at home, there is an urgent need to intensify health education especially during focused ANC sessions on signs of labour and delivery, and birth preparedness to enhance the knowledge of women to be able to identify early signs of labour and report to the nearest health facility to deliver with SBAs.

Abbreviations

ANC: Antenatal care,; CHPS: Community Health Planning and Services,; DDHS: District Director of Health Service,; GDHS: Ghana Demographic and Health Survey,; GHS: Ghana Health Services,; LMIC: Low and middle-income country,; RDHS: Regional Director of Health Service,; SBA: Skilled birth attendant,; WHO: World Health Organization

Acknowledgements

We acknowledge the support of the Regional Director of Health Services (RDHS) for the Upper East Region and the District Director of Health Services (DDHS) for the Builsa district. We also appreciate the contribution of Dominic Achinkok, Linda Abada, Emmanuel Akanpabadae, Bernard Akubolgo, Drahmani Zuwah and Barnabas Ayaric during the data collection. We thank the data collectors and the participants in this study. The content of this manuscript are the sole responsibility of the authors and do not represent the views of the publisher.

Funding

This study received no funding support from any organization or institution.

Authors' contributions

MB came up with the research idea, was involved in the conceptualization of the study design, reviewed literature, supervised data collection, carried out the data analysis, and wrote the methods and results section. ABM supported in revising the initial research idea, reviewed literature, supervised data collection, wrote the introductory section and reviewed the draft manuscript. EAA was involved in the conceptualization of the study design and implementation of the study, involved in the data analysis, and wrote the discussion and draft manuscript. All authors read and approved the final manuscript.

Authors' information
Michael Boah (MPH—Public Health): Nutrition Officer, Ghana Health Service, PhD candidate in Epidemiology, Harbin Medical University, Harbin—Heilongjiang province, China. Abraham B. Mahama (MPH—Health Promotion): Nutrition officer, UNICEF Ghana country office email: bangamsi@gmail.com, and Emmanuel A. Ayamga (BSc Community Nutrition): Nutrition Officer, Ghana Health Service, Nabdam District Upper East Region; Master of Public Health Student, School of Public Health, University of Ghana, Legon Accra, email: eaayamga@gmail.com

Competing interests
The authors declare that they have no competing interests.

Author details
[1]Ghana Health Service, Kassena Nankana West District Health Directorate, P. O. Box 21, Paga, Upper East Region, Ghana. [2]UNICEF- Ghana Country Office, Accra, Ghana.

References

1. World Health Organization, Unicef, UNFPA, World Bank, United Nations Population Division. Trends in Maternal Mortality: 1990–2015: Estimates by WHO, UNICEF, UNFPA, The World Bank and the United Nations Population Division. Geneva: World Health Organization; 2015.
2. Kinney MV, Kerber KJ, Black RE, Cohen B, Nkrumah F, Coovadia H, et al. Sub-Saharan Africa's mothers, newborns, and children: where and why do they die? PLoS Med. 2010;7(6):1–9.
3. World Health Organization. Making pregnancy safer: the critical role of the skilled attendant. A joint statement by WHO, ICM and FIGO. Geneva: World Health Organization; 2004.
4. Stanton C, Blanc AK, Croft T, Choi Y. Skilled Care at Birth in the Developing World: progress to date and strategies for expanding coverage. J Biosoc Sci. 2007;39:109–20.
5. Abera M, Gebre Mariam A, Belachew T. Predictors of safe delivery service utilization in Arsi zone, south-East Ethiopia. Ethiop J Heal Sci. 2011;21(Special Issue):101–13.
6. Adegoke AA, Van Den Broek N. Skilled birth attendance-lessons learnt. BJOG An Int J Obstet Gynaecol. 2009;116(Supp. 1):33–40.
7. Nieburg P. Improving maternal mortality and other aspects of Women's health: the United States" global role. Washington, DC; 2012.
8. Oguntunde O, Aina O, Ibrahim MS, Umar HS. Antenatal care and skilled birth attendance in three communities in Kaduna state, Nigeria. African Journal Reprod Heal. 2010;14(3):89–96.
9. Tadesse B, Mulat A, Gashaw A. Previous early antenatal service utilization improves timely Booking : cross-sectional study at University of Gondar Hospital, Northwest Ethiopia. J Pregnancy. 2014;2014:1–7.
10. Zeine A, Woldie M, Ololo S. Factors influencing antenatal care utilization in Hadiya zone. Ethiop J Heal Sci. 2010;20(2):75–82.
11. Kawungezi PC, Akiibua D, Aleni C, Chitayi M, Kazibwe A, Sunya E, et al. Attendance and utilization of antenatal care (ANC) services: multi-center study in upcountry areas of Uganda. Open J Prev Med. 2015;5(3):132–42.
12. Simkhada B, Van Teijlingen ER, Porter M, Simkhada P. Factors affecting the utilization of antenatal care in developing countries: systematic review of the literature. J Adv Nurs. 2008;61(3):244–60.
13. Koblinsky M, Matthews Z, Hussein J, Mavalankar D, Mridha MK, Anwar I, et al. Going to scale with professional skilled care. Lancet. 2006;368(9544):1377–86.
14. Kruk ME, Rockers PC, Mbaruku G, Paczkowski MM, Galea S. Community and health system factors associated with facility delivery in rural Tanzania: a multilevel analysis. Health Policy (New York). Elsevier Ireland Ltd. 2010;97(2–3):209–16.
15. Moyer CA, Mustafa A. Drivers and deterrents of facility delivery in sub-Saharan Africa: a systematic review. Reprod Health. 2013;10(1):40.
16. Anastasi E, Borchert M, Campbell OMR, Sondorp E, Kaducu F, Hill O, et al. Losing women along the path to safe motherhood: why is there such a gap between women's use of antenatal care and skilled birth attendance? A mixed methods study in northern Uganda. BMC Pregnancy Childbirth. 2015;15(1):287.
17. Fekadu M, Regassa N. Skilled delivery care service utilization in Ethiopia : analysis of ural-urban differentials based on national demographic and health survey (DHS) data. Afr Health Sci. 2014;14(4): 974–84.
18. Ghana Statistical Service. Ghana multiple Indicator cluster survey with an enhanced malaria module and biomarker. Accra, Ghana; 2011.
19. National Health Insurance Authority. 2010 annual report. Accra, Ghana; 2010.
20. Akazili J, Doctor HV, Abokyi L, Hodgson A, Phillips JF. Is there any relationship between antenatal care and place of delivery ? Findings from rural northern Ghana. Afr J Health Sci. 2011;18(1):62–73.
21. Sakeah E, Doctor HV, McCloskey L, Bernstein J, Yeboah-Antwi K, Mills S. Using the community-based health planning and services program to promote skilled delivery in rural Ghana: socio-demographic factors that influence women utilization of skilled attendants at birth in northern Ghana. BMC Public Health. 2014;14(1):344.
22. Nakua EK, Sevugu JT, Dzomeku VM, Otupiri E, Lipkovich HR, Owusu-Dabo E. Home birth without skilled attendants despite millennium villages project intervention in Ghana: insight from a survey of women's perceptions of skilled obstetric care. BMC Pregnancy Childbirth. 2015;15(1):243.
23. Manyeh AK, Akpakli DE, Kukula V, Ekey RA, Narh-Bana S, Adjei A, et al. Socio-demographic determinants of skilled birth attendant at delivery in rural southern Ghana. BMC Res Notes BioMed Central. 2017;10(1):268.
24. Ghana Statistical Service, Ghana Health Service, ICF International. Ghana Demographic and Health Survey, 2014. Rockville, Maryland, USA; 2015.
25. Awoonor-Williams J. 2014 Annual Report: Upper East Regional Health Services. Bolgatanga. 2015.
26. Builsa South District Health Administration. 2014 Annual Report. Bolgatanga. 2015.
27. Gyimah S, Takyi BK, Addai I. Challenges to the reproductive-health needs of African women : on religion and maternal health utilization in Ghana. Soc Sci Med. 2006;62(2006):2930–44.
28. Esena RK, Sappor M. Factors associated with the utilization of skilled delivery services in the Ga east municipality of Ghana part 2 : barriers to skilled delivery. Int J Sci Technol Res 2013;2 (8):195–207.
29. Abor P, Abekah-Nkrumah G, Sakyi K, Adjasi CKD, Abor J. The Socio-Economic Determinants of Maternal Health Care Utilization in Ghana. Int J Soc Econ. 2011:38(7):628–48.
30. Mills S, Williams ÆJE, Adjuik ÆM. Use of health professionals for delivery following the availability of free obstetric Care in Northern Ghana. Matern Child Heal J. 2007;12:509–18.
31. Stephenson R, Baschieri A, Clements S, Hennink M, Madise N. Contextual influences on the use of health facilities for childbirth in Africa. Am J Public Health. 2006;96(1):84–93.
32. Babalola S, Fatusi A. Determinants of use of maternal health services in Nigeria-looking beyond individual and household factors. BMC Pregnancy Childbirth. 2009;13:1–13.
33. Tann CJ, et al. Use of Antenatal Services and Delivery Care in Entebbe, Uganda: A Community Survey. BMC pregnancy and childbirth. 2007;7:23.
34. Saaka M, Aviisah MA. Promoting skilled institutional deliveries: factors to consider in a free maternal health services policy environment. Med Res Chronicles. 2015;2(3):286–302.
35. Ganle KK, Parker M, Fitzpatrick R, Otupiri E. A qualitative study of health system barriers to accessibility and utilization of maternal and newborn healthcare services in Ghana after user-fee abolition. BMC Pregnancy Childbirth. 2014;14(1):1–17.
36. Wado YD, Afework MF, Hindin MJ. Unintended pregnancies and the use of maternal health services in southwestern Ethiopia. BMC Int Health Hum Rights. 2013;13(1):36.
37. Nketiah-Amponsah E, Arthur E. Choice of delivery facility among expectant mothers in Ghana: does access to health insurance matter? J Health Manag. 2013;15(4):509–24.
38. Oladokun A, Oladokun R, Morhason-Bello I, Bello A, Addokum B. Proximate predictors of early antenatal registration among Nigerian pregnant women. Ann Afr Med. 2010;9(4):222–5.
39. Asundep NN, Carson AP, Turpin CA, Tameru B, Agidi AT, Zhang K, et al. Determinants of access to antenatal care and birth outcomes in Kumasi, Ghana. J Epidemiol Glob Health. Ministry of Health, Saudi Arabia. 2013;3:279–88.

40. Sadiq AA, Poggensee G, Nguku P, Sabitu K, Abubakar A, Puone T. Factors associated with adverse pregnancy outcomes and perceptions of risk factors among reproductive age women in soba LGA, Kaduna state 2013. Pan Afr Med J. 2016;25:1–8.
41. Faye A, Niane M, Ba I. Homebirth in women who have given birth at least once in a health facility : contributory factors in a developing country. Acta Obstet Gynecol Scand. 2011;90(2011):1239–43.
42. Hazemba AN, Siziya S. Choice of place for childbirth : prevalence and correlates of utilization of health facilities in Chongwe district, Zambia. Med Journal Zambia. 2002;35(2):53–7.
43. Fotso J-C, Ezeh A, Madise N, Ziraba A, Ogollah R. What does access to maternal care mean among the urban Poor ? Factors associated with use of appropriate maternal health Services in the Slum Settlements of Nairobi, Kenya. Matern Child Health J. 2009;13:130–7.
44. Gabrysch S, Campbell OM. Still too far to walk: literature review of the determinants of delivery service use. BMC Pregnancy Childbirth. 2009;9(1):34.
45. Hailu D, Berhe H. Determinants of institutional childbirth service utilisation among women of childbearing age in urban and rural areas of Tsegedie district, Ethiopia. Midwifery. Elsevier. 2014;2014(30):1109–17.
46. Ochako R, Fotso J, Ikamari L, Khasakhala A. Utilization of maternal health services among young women in Kenya : insights from the Kenya demographic and health survey, 2003. BMC Pregnancy Childbirth. 2011;11(1):1–9.
47. Gage A. Barriers to the utilization of maternal health care in rural Mali. Social Sci Med. 2007;65(8):1666–82.
48. Kidanu S, Degu G, Tiruye TY. Factors influencing institutional delivery service utilization in Dembecha district, Northwest Ethiopia: a community-based cross-sectional study. Reprod Health. 2017;14(1):98.
49. Shah R, Rehfuess EA, Maskey MK, Fischer R, Bhandari PB, Delius M. Factors affecting institutional delivery in rural Chitwan district of Nepal : a community-based cross-sectional study. BMC Pregnancy Childbirth. 2015;15(27):1–14.

4

Facilitating autonomous, confident and satisfying choices: a mixed-method study of women's choice-making in prenatal screening for common aneuploidies

An Chen[1*], Henni Tenhunen[1], Paulus Torkki[1,4], Antti Peltokorpi[2], Seppo Heinonen[3], Paul Lillrank[1] and Vedran Stefanovic[3]

Abstract

Background: Population-based prenatal screening has become a common and widely available obstetrical practice in majority of developed countries. Under the patient autonomy principle, women should understand the screening options, be able to take their personal preferences and situations into account, and be encouraged to make autonomous and intentional decisions. The majority of the current research focuses on the prenatal screening uptake rate, women's choice on screening tests, and the influential factors. However, little attention has been paid to women's choice-making processes and experiences in prenatal screening and their influences on choice satisfaction. Understanding women's choice-making processes and experiences in pregnancy and childbirth is the prerequisite for designing women-centered choice aids and delivering women-centered maternity care. This paper presents a pilot study that aims to investigate women's experiences when they make choices for screening tests, quantify the choice-making experience, and identify the experiential factors that affect women's satisfaction on choices they made.

Method: We conducted a mixed-method research at Helsinki and Uusimaa Hospital District (HUS) in Finland. First, the women's choice-making experiences were explored by semi-structured interviews. We interviewed 28 women who participated in prenatal screening. The interview data was processed by thematic analysis. Then, a cross-sectional self-completion survey was designed and implemented, assessing women's experiences in choice-making and identifying the experiential factors that influence choice satisfaction. Of 940 distributed questionnaires, 185 responses were received. Multivariable linear regression analysis was used to detect the effects of the variables.

Results: We developed a set of measurements for women's choice-making experiences in prenatal screening with seven variables: activeness, informedness, confidence, social pressure, difficulty, positive emotion and negative emotion. Regression revealed that activeness in choice-making ($\beta = 0.176$; $p = 0.023$), confidence in choice-making ($\beta = 0.388$; $p < 0.001$), perceived social pressure ($\beta = -0.306$; $p < 0.001$) and perceived difficulty ($\beta = -0.274$; $p < 0.001$) significantly influenced women's choice satisfaction in prenatal screening.

Conclusions: This study explores the experiential dimension of women's choice-making in prenatal screening. Our result will be useful for service providers to design women-centered choice environment. Women's willingness and capabilities of making active choices, their preferences, and social reliance should be well considered in order to facilitate autonomous, confident and satisfying choices.

Keywords: Women's choice, Choice-making experience, Choice satisfaction, Prenatal screening

* Correspondence: an.chen@aalto.fi
[1]Institute of Healthcare Engineering, Management and Architecture (HEMA), Department of Industrial Engineering and Management, Aalto University, Maarintie 8, P.O. Box 15500, 00076 Espoo, Finland
Full list of author information is available at the end of the article

Background

As a critical component of the delivery of high-quality and evidence-based prenatal care [1], population-based prenatal screening has become a common and widely available obstetrical practice in majority of developed countries [2–5]. It provides women and families with a risk figure that estimates the chances of having a baby with chromosomal abnormalities and allows them to make decisions and preparations in a timely manner [1, 4, 6]. There are different screening options. For example, all pregnant women in Finland are entitled by law for the voluntary first trimester combined screening (FTS) at $9–13^{+6}$ weeks of pregnancy and second trimester genetic sonogram performed at $18^{+0}–22^{+0}$ weeks of pregnancy. For those who have missed the FTS a second trimester maternal serum screening (STS) is offered at $15–16^{+6}$ gestational weeks. The FTS takes into account the mother's age and weight, fetal crown-rump length and nuchal translucency thickness measured by ultrasound as well as results from maternal serum biomarkers [*free β-human chorionic gonadotropin (β-hCG), pregnancy-associated plasma protein-A (PAPP-A)*]. STS is based on maternal serum β-hCG and alpha fetoprotein (AFP) adjusted for the gestational age determined by ultrasound. This method is suitable those who have missed FTS for any reason. Cell-free fetal DNA screening is offered as the second-tier screening in public sector for those who are screen-positive at FTS or STS.

Because the positive result at prenatal screening for fetal aneuploidies leads frequently to the invasive diagnostic procedures and possible termination of affected pregnancies [7], autonomous choice and decision, i.e. informing women about all existing tests and allowing women to make choices and take actions that are based on their personal willingness, beliefs, values and other considerations without any coercion, have been highly recognized [8, 9]. The assumption of this autonomy principle is that women should be able to understand the screening programs, be clear about their situations, and have the capability to make autonomous and intentional decisions [8]. This is not possible to all women, due to plethora of reasons. It has become a high priority to understand women's choice and choice-making, for the purpose of building appropriate choice platforms, assisting women in making choices, and delivering patient-centered care [10].

A growing body of research focuses on the uptake rate of prenatal screening, women's choice on screening tests, and the influential factors of the choice. Bakker et al. [11] evaluated the factors affecting the low uptake of FTS in the Netherlands and reported that the main reasons for the low uptake were the relatively positive attitude towards Down syndrome and a negative attitude towards pregnancy termination. With the same context, Crombag et al. [12] found that advanced maternal age and age related risk perception were strongly affecting women's participation in prenatal screening. Košec et al. [13] conducted a cross-sectional study on a prospective basis in different districts of Croatia, assessing pregnant women's awareness, motives and preferences about the first and the second trimester screening in early pregnancy before they chose any of the recommended tests. They found that education level and previous information were significant variables predictive for the choice of the tests. Informed choice, a choice that is based on relevant knowledge, consistent with decision-maker's values and behaviorally implemented [14], has been regarded as a central feature of screening and testing [15]. The research on informed choice in prenatal screening has become very popular. For example, Marteau et al. [14] developed a multi-dimensional measure of informed choice for women undergoing prenatal screening; Potter et al. [16] employed the measurement and qualitatively evaluated women's choice in their case; Schoonen et al. [6] analyzed the content of decision-relevant knowledge and produced a knowledge structure that can facilitate the informed choice in prenatal screening.

Patient-centered health services cannot be achieved without understanding patient experience and satisfaction [17]. The experiences of pregnancy and childbirth can have immediate as well as long-term effects on women's life, well-being and health [18, 19]. However, only few studies have estimated women's choice-making processes in prenatal screening [20] or explored the choice-making experiences in order to design women-centered choice aids and deliver women-centered maternity care. From a service perspective, experience can be understood as a product of sense-making, which is subjective, interpretive, and individually, contextually and socially-constructed [21–23]. In health service context, patient as a social actor with subjectivity perceives the phenomena, makes sense of events and constructs the experience. Larkin et al. [19] study the concept of experience in the context of pregnancy and childbirth and broadly define experience as "an individual life event, incorporating interrelated subjective psychological and physiological processes, influenced by social, environmental, organizational and policy contexts." However, the current research on women's choice-making processes and experiences has a narrow set of focuses on choice conflict between wishes, preferences and ethical views [9], anxiety and depression affecting choice-making [24], the difficulty of making choices [25] or information needs [26]. There is no comprehensive study deeply exploring women's choice-making experiences in prenatal screening. The main objective of the study is to explore women's experiences when they make choices for screening tests, quantify the choice-making experience, and identify the experiential factors that affect women's satisfaction on choices they made (choice satisfaction). We hope this study can advance the discussions on how to implement screening program, how to counsel pregnant women and how to assist women in making informed and autonomous choices. The experience of this study could also be shared for other medical contexts (e.g. cancer screening) to explore the experiential dimension of patient choice-making.

Methods

Empirical context

We conduct a pilot study to investigate women's choice-making experiences in population-based prenatal screening within the public maternal service system at the Department of Obstetrics and Gynecology, Helsinki and Uusimaa Hospital District (HUS) Finland, where aforementioned non-invasive screening tests (FTS and STS) are offered free of charge to all women. Finnish community-based maternity care unit (Neuvola), a public sector activity led by general practitioners and providing free maternal care service to all pregnant women, is responsible for informing pregnant women about prenatal screening and testing program and helps to arrange the tests. Every pregnant woman receives a booklet (Additional file 1) of prenatal screening and testing from the nearest maternity care unit. This study was approved by the Ethics Committee for Gynecology and Obstetrics, Pediatrics and Psychiatry, Helsinki University Hospital (permission number: 220/13/03/03/2015).

Study design

We applied a mixed-method approach using qualitative data and quantitative data in one study. This could lead to greater validity and rigor and provide a better understanding of the research problem than either research approach alone [27]. Many researchers have agreed that the mixed methods approach can be particularly useful in healthcare research that requires a broader range of perspectives to view the complexity in this field [28–30]. We followed the sequential exploratory design [31], in which qualitative data are collected and analyzed first, followed by quantitative study [32, 33]. This design is useful for exploring the unknown variables, developing new instruments based on an in-depth qualitative analysis, and confirming or generalizing qualitative findings by quantitative study. This is suitable to our case, where the complex phenomenon of women's choice-making experiences needs structuralization and operationalization. We explore how women experience the choice-making process in prenatal screening (qualitative research question) , and identify what are the experiential factors significantly influencing women's choice satisfaction (quantitative research question).

Qualitative study

The details of women's choice-making experiences were explored by semi-structured interviews. Storytelling or narrative inquiry as a way of investigating the subjective experience and delving into individual's "lifeworld" [34–36] produced remarkable contributions for the qualitative study. The inquired modes of experience were quite broad, including individual's feeling, seeing, hearing, reflecting, expecting, acting, and all other kinds of emotional, mental and physical activities. Interviews, that were conducted after the women had gone through the screening, started with open-ended questions about how the woman made a choice between different screening tests. The concrete questions were developed from Theory of Planned Behavior (TPB) [37, 38], which helps to understand the choice-making process from women's perspective with three main constructs: behavioral beliefs, subjective norms and perceived behavioral control. "Behavioral beliefs" refers to personal evaluation of a behavior (e.g. choosing the FTS) and by this we explored women's reflections on the advantages and disadvantages of the choice consequences (e.g. the consequences of choosing the FTS). "Subjective norms" refers to social influence and by this we investigated how women's choices were socially affected by other people. "Perceived behavioral control" refers to the resources and opportunities available to person to make a certain behavior (choice) possible and in this study it helped to evaluate the ease and difficulty of making the choice. Midwives from the Screening Unit and Fetomaternal Medical Center (FMC) in Helsinki helped to recruit the interviewees who participated in prenatal screening by presenting the information letter explaining our study to women and inviting them to participate in the study on a voluntary basis. All the informants voluntarily participating in the interviews signed a written informed consent. Qualitative data collection were collected in a period of December 2015–May 2016. Interviews were conducted in Finnish (author HT conducted) or English (AC conducted). Interviews were tape recorded, transcribed in English and imported into Atlas.ti qualitative data analysis software. The data were processed by thematic analysis. Author AC and HT independently coded the data, identifying the items that could delineate women's choice-making processes and experiences. Then the two authors discussed, reached an agreement on the items and categorized them into the themes. We enhanced the validity of our findings by organizing discussions in the research team, consulting experts from the Screening Unit, and getting feedbacks from professionals. In total, we interviewed 28 women.

Quantitative study

Following the guidelines of scale development provided by DeVellis [39], we developed a framework of measurements for women's choice-making experiences in prenatal screening and designed a cross-sectional self-completion survey on a retrospective basis to assess women's experiences in choice-making processes. The generation of measurements for choice-making experience was based on the themes of choice-making process and experience uncovered by the qualitative study as well as some current validated measurements. In the questionnaire, we also measure women's satisfaction on the choices they made as the primary outcome measurement. Items for measurements were made in a statement format with 5-point Likert scale from "strongly disagree" to "strongly agree". We asked participants to provide demographics information, including maternal age, education level, marital status, occupation, gravidity and previous experiences of fetal aneuploidy. The questionnaire was critically reviewed and approved by the expert in fetomaternal medicine (VS) who was responsible for the organization of prenatal screening at HUS at the time of commencing this study. In order to test and improve the quality of the measurements, we invited three women to fill in the questionnaire and asked them to report their understandings, confusions and difficulties when responding to each item. Questionnaire was made in English and then translated into Finnish and Swedish. Translation service agency, researchers and medical professionals co-worked in translation and back-translation. Our questionnaires were distributed to the women who participated in prenatal screening. Midwives from delivery hospitals, in which certified midwives perform screenings for pregnant women, helped to disseminate the anonymous questionnaires in the Screening Unit where screening tests and ultrasound are performed. The survey lasted 10 months, from June 2016 to March 2017. Factor analysis was employed to further validate the measurements. Factor analysis empirically determined the number of dimensions/constructs underlying a set of items and refined the inclusion of items for each dimension [39]. Each variable of choice-making experience was produced by summating its measurement items and assessed by one-sample t test, testing whether the variable mean was equal to a neutral value. Multivariable linear regression analysis was used to detect the effects of these variables on choice satisfaction. Quantitative data was managed and analyzed by STATA 13. A p-value of < 0.05 was used to establish statistical significance.

Results

Qualitative study results

We interviewed 28 women who participated in prenatal screening, of which 22 (78.6%) chose FTS and 6 (21,4%) participated in STS. Table 1 displays the six dimensions of women's choice-making processes and experiences in prenatal screening: activeness (attitude and behavior), informedness (information needs and sources), preferences/considerations, social influence (perceived social support and pressure), difficulty (difficulty in making choice) and emotional status. For each item under these dimensions, we counted the number of women mentioning it to evaluate its importance, and pictured the choice-making differences between the two groups of women participating in different screening tests. Sample quotations are shown in Table 1.

Active choice

Our participants had a common understanding on active choice, referring to three major constructs: information collection, autonomy and consciousness. Information collection (mentioned by 21 women) means that the woman reads the information, knows all the options and actively searches information from different sources. Autonomy (mentioned by 18 women) means that the woman can freely decide everything by herself based on individual willingness and that she is not forced to do something or to make the decision. Consciousness (mentioned by 6 women) implies that the woman thinks about the options, questions the options and consciously decides between the alternatives. In our study, most of the women reported that they did not actively choose the screening tests, because they were not aware of the STS, they thought it was the default choice to participate in the FTS, or they felt that there was little risk involved in the process.

Informedness

A key finding from our analysis was that, women had different information needs for choosing screening tests. Most of them were aware of the procedures and possible results of the tests. More than half of the women expressed they would have wanted to know that there was a later screening possibility. Some of them considered the features (e.g. accuracy, risk and timing) or the advantages/disadvantages of the tests. Few of them were concerned about the mechanisms and theories of the tests. Maternity care unit booklet and public health nurse were the two main information sources. Some women had previous experience in screening. Few women sought additional information online or other sources.

Preferences/considerations

In the interviews, we asked women what mattered to them for screening and explored their main preferences and considerations. In the table, we listed the prominent preferences/considerations of each group. For most

Table 1 Six dimensions of women's choice-making processes and experiences in prenatal screening

Choice-making dimensions	First trimester combined screening (22)	Second trimester screening (6)
Active choice	didn't make active choices (16) *"I didn't choose the tests actively. I didn't know much about the second trimester serum screening and I just participated in what was recommended"* made active choices (6) *"I made an active choice. It was my decision to participated in the first trimester combined screening, which is better than the other test"*	didn't make active choices (5) *"I didn't choose the tests actively. The participation in screening is nothing, you just go and do what they (public health nurses) arrange for you."* made active choices (1) *"I made an active choice. I consulted about the different options and I preferred the first trimester combined screening. But since I was traveling during the screening week, so I had to do the second trimester serum screening."*
Informedness	Information needs: the possible results of the tests (16); procedures of different programs (16); different options (10); the features, e.g. accuracy, risk and timing of the tests (7); advantages/disadvantage of tests (5); mechanisms and theories of tests (1) *"I got the main information from Neuvola, including the practical information about the screening and its possible results, what it includes in the program and what the ultrasound means. This information is very important."* Information sources: Booklet in maternity care unit (16); Public health nurse of maternity care unit (10); Previous experience (8); Online information (4); Family members (1); Friends (1); *"Information was given by Neuvola for sure, with the information about what it is and what is the expected outcome. I didn't seek for information from other sources by myself."*	Information needs: different options (6); the possible results of the tests (5); procedures of different programs (4); the features, e.g. accuracy, risk and timing of the tests (3); advantages/disadvantage of tests (3); mechanisms and theories of tests (0) *"I could not take the first trimester screening. The midwife told me about the second trimester screening. The timing and schedule information were very important in my case."* Information sources: Booklet in maternity care unit (6); Public health nurse of maternity care unit (6); Online information (2); Previous experience (2); Family members (1); Friends (0); *"The nurse told me about the second trimester screening. I did check the information about screening from internet after that (after I decided to do it). I didn't ask any friends."*
Main preferences/ considerations	Reliability/Accuracy (19): the result is more reliable; certainty is higher; more information is provided. *"Combined screening can give more information than just doing blood test"* Easiness (18): the procedure is simple *"It is quite easy. Some problems can be directly detected when I take the ultrasound."* Recommendation (17): the test is recommended by trusted persons. *"The Neuvola nurse recommended the ultrasound to check if everything was ok."* Timing (10): the test can be organized in good time or suitable to the client's schedule. *"The nurse of Neuvola helped to book the time of blood testing and ultrasound, which is suitable to my schedule."* Rapidness (8): to get the test and result quickly with a short waiting time *"Combined screening can give earlier information and the ultrasound can detect the problems very quickly, so that we can make preparations or take further steps earlier if there is any problem."*	Timing (6): the test can be organized in good time or suitable to the client's schedule. *"I have scheduled a trip during that week, so I could not participate in the first trimester screening. Only the second trimester works for me. I missed the first trimester screening and I had little time left to do the screening"* Reliability/Accuracy (3): the result is more reliable; certainty is higher; with more information. *"I preferred the first trimester screening at the beginning because it can offer more reliable and early result. But I missed it because of the travelling. So I have to rely on the second trimester screening"* Recommendation (2): the test is recommended by trusted persons. *"The Neuvola nurse suggested that I could do the second trimester screening based on my situation."* Easiness (2): the procedure is simple *"Just taking blood sample is quite easy"* Access (1): the option is available and offered freely *"It is not free to do the screening abroad. We participated in the second trimester screening when we came back to Finland."*
Social influence	Perceived social support (19) *"I agreed with the midwife's arrangement. I also talked with my husband and it was a common decision. My husband supported me"* Perceived social pressure (8) *"Some of my friends experienced difficult pregnancies, so I want to participate in the screening and get the information earlier."* Social influence from who: Medical staff (18); Husband/partner (4); Friends (1); Family (1); *"The Neuvola nurse discussed about prenatal screening and testing with me and provided the information to me. She recommended the first trimester screening."*	Perceived social support (3) *"The Neuvola nurse gave me suggestion and helped to arrange everything"* Perceived social pressure (1) *"Everyone participates in screening. I felt I have to do something for the baby. I missed the first trimester combined screening, and I felt upset and disappointed."* Social influence from who: Medical staff (3); Husband/partner (1); Family (1); Friends (0); *"My husband was with me in the Neuvola visit and we made the decision together."*
Difficulty in making choice	it was not difficult to make a choice (22) *"I didn't have any difficulties. It is a kind of routine. I just followed what the nurse recommended"*	it was not difficult to make a choice (4) *"I was quite clear about choice and just followed the suggestion (given by the Neuvola nurse)"* it was difficult to make a choice (2) *"It was not easy to make decision, because of the information insufficiency. I was traveling in the beginning of the pregnancy. I thought I could do the screening abroad but it was difficult to*

Table 1 Six dimensions of women's choice-making processes and experiences in prenatal screening *(Continued)*

Choice-making dimensions	First trimester combined screening (22)	Second trimester screening (6)
		organize. I didn't get clear instruction from Neuvola for my situation."
Emotional status	Neutral (20) *"It is just something straightforward and obvious to do. I didn't feel there is something wrong."* Positive (3) *"I felt content that I can choose the better one"* Negative (1) *"I was worried about the possible risks and bad results."*	Positive (1) *"I missed the first trimester screening, but I felt relieved the other test was still possible."* Negative (3) *"I was annoyed that I missed the combination screening."*

women participating in the FTS, reliability/accuracy was the most important issue (mentioned by 19 women), referring to the reliable test results, high certainty and extensive information. The second most important factor was easiness (mentioned by 18 women), referring to the simplicity of the test performance. Recommendation (mentioned by 17 women) given by the public health nurses of maternity care unit was the third important issue. Other prominent preferences included timing (mentioned by 10 women), which means the test can be organized in good time or suitable to the client's schedule, and rapidness (mentioned by 8 women), which means to get the test and result quickly with a short waiting time. For women participating in the STS, timing (mentioned by 6 women) was the most important factor. Test accuracy (mentioned by 3 women) and recommendation (mentioned by 2 women) were also considered.

Social influence

Our participants recalled whether their choice-making was influenced by other people (including health professionals, e.g. midwives, as well as other people in the society, e.g. husband/partner), and whether their choice got any support or pressure. Most of women who participated in the FTS followed the suggestions from maternity care units without much doubts or discussing seriously with others. Some of them made the decision with their husband or partner. Generally, women did not feel much pressure from others and they found it easy to follow the arrangement suggested by maternity care units or do as other women do. One woman mentioned that she felt some pressure, because her friends experienced difficult pregnancies. Among the women participating in the STS, three mentioned that the public health nurses of maternity care unit gave advice and helped to arrange the tests. Only one woman said that she felt some pressure of making the choice, thinking about other people and their choices.

Difficulty

All women participating in the FTS reported that it was not difficult to make a choice. Some women said they chose combined screening as the first and best option without any hesitation. In contrast, not all women participating in the STS felt it was easy to make choices. Two women complained that they did not get enough information or instructions for their special situation, traveling aboard at the beginning of the pregnancy.

Emotional status

The interviewed women also reflected on their emotional status when making choices. The majority of women who participated in the FTS described that they felt quite neutral when making choice on screening tests. Many women said it was something very straightforward and obvious to do and nothing seemed to be going wrong. Some women reported positive feelings, e.g. being content for choosing the better screening option. One woman was worried about the possible risks and bad results. Some women who missed the FTS felt upset, disappointed or anxious. One woman said that she felt relieved when she discovered there was a backup option for the screening.

Quantitative study results

Starting from June 2016, 940 questionnaires were distributed, 185 were returned by March 2017 with an overall response rate of 19.7% and 183 were valid. In our sample, 163 (89.1%) women participated in the FTS, 3 (1.6%) participated in the STS and 17 (10.4%) did not know which screening test they participated in. The demographic characteristics of the sample are shown in Table 2.

The design of the choice-making experience measurements was based on the results of the qualitative study, group discussions and validated measurements including Decisional Conflict Scale [40, 41] (Additional file 2) and six-item short-form of the state scale of the Spielberger State-Trait Anxiety Inventory [42] (Additional file 3). Additional file 4 summarizes the initially developed constructs (7 constructs for choice-making experience and one for choice satisfaction) with the meanings, measurement items and score ranges. The constructs created by factor analysis (Additional file 5) for all the items

Table 2 Sample characteristics of the survey

Demographic characteristics	Sample size = 183
Mean age (years) (SD)	32 (4.46)
Education (*n*) (%)	
1. Basic education or less	1 (0.55)
2. Secondary education or vocational qualifications	33 (18.03)
3. Bachelor level	54 (29.51)
4. Master level	82 (44.81)
5. Licentiate or doctor's degree	13 (7.10)
Marital status (*n*) (%)	
1. Single	10 (5.46)
2. Married	101 (55.19)
3. Co-habitation	71 (38.80)
4. Divorced	1 (0.55)
Occupation (*n*) (%)	
1. Student	13 (7.10)
2. Labor worker	79 (43.17)
3. Lower white-collar worker	18 (9.84)
4. Upper white-collar worker	53 (28.96)
5. Entrepreneur	6 (3.28)
6. Unemployed	14 (7.65)
7. Pensioner	0 (0)
Gravidity, including current pregnancy (times) (SD)	1.99 (1.20)
Chromosomal abnormality in previous pregnancy (*n*) (%)	
1. with chromosomal abnormality in previous pregnancy	2 (1.09)
2. no chromosomal abnormality in previous pregnancy	181 (98.91)

measuring the choice-making experience were similar with the original conceptual ones, which means that the original categories have a certain level of validity to account for covariation among the items. One adjustment based on factor analysis was that the item "someone else made the choices for me" that was supposed to measure activeness of choice-making grouped with the measurement of social pressure. The second adjustment was that the items that were planned to measure preference consistency and the items that were planned to measure choice support grouped together as one factor, which was named with "choice-making confidence". The third one was that the items reflecting positive emotional status and those reflecting negative emotional status did not belong to one emotion category, and they were divided into two factors. Thus, based on the factor analysis, a more structured and validated set of instruments measuring choice-making experience (Additional file 6) were generated, which included "active choice", "informedness", "confidence", "social pressure", "difficulty", "positive emotion" and "negative emotion".

Table 3 quantitatively outlines women's choice-making experiences in prenatal screening. In general, the survey respondents did not have negative experiences when making choices for screening tests: they were well informed (mean: 22.41; score range: 7–35); they felt confident (mean: 16.83; score range: 5–25); they did not perceive social pressure (mean: 2.94; score range: 2–10); the perceived difficulty of making choices was very low (mean: 5.50; score range: 3–15); they had positive emotion status when making choices (mean: 9.93; score range: 3–15) and the anxiety level was low (mean: 17.62; score range: 9–45); but they did not actively make choices in prenatal screening (mean: 8.66; score range: 4–20). The choice satisfaction with the mean of 8.86 (score range: 2–10) was high.

Table 4 presents the result of the multiple linear regression identifying the experiential factors that significantly influence women's choice satisfaction in prenatal screening. Demographic factors and screening results (normal, abnormal or do not know yet) at the point of filling in the questionnaire were input as control variables in the regression model. Regression revealed that education ($\beta = -0.136$; $p = 0.047$), gravidity ($\beta = -0.182$; $p = 0.008$), activeness in choice-making ($p = 0.023$), confidence ($\beta = 0.388$; $p < 0.001$), perceived social pressure ($\beta = -0.306$; $p < 0.001$) and perceived difficulty ($\beta = -0.274$; $p < 0.001$) significantly influenced women's choice satisfaction in prenatal screening. Women with higher levels of education were more likely to have lower choice satisfaction. Women had lower choice satisfaction as the pregnancy times increased. If women made more active choices, choice satisfaction would increase. While choice-making confidence had strong positive effects on choice satisfaction, social pressure and perceived difficulty were negatively related to choice satisfaction.

Discussion

"Balancing" recommendation

By integrating qualitative and quantitative analysis, one of our principal observations is that when there is a population risk of aneuploidy but the risk has not been individually revealed, women's activeness in choice-making is not very high. A document with clear information on chromosomal screening, the offered test options and the possible results of the tests may be sufficient for women to read and be informed. Some features of the different methods, including the testing coverage, timing and accuracy should be clearly presented. Another important observation is that although they were offered the booklet shown in Additional file 1, the women in our study were not well informed and many of them were not aware of the STS possibility.

Table 3 Exploring the variables of women's choice-making experiences in prenatal screening

Variables	Score range	Neutral score	Mean score (SD)	*p* value of t test (mean score vs. neutral score)	Reliability (Cronbach's alpha)
Activeness in choice-making	4–20	12	8.66 (3.78)	< 0.001	0.8022
Informedness	7–35	21	22.41 (7.67)	0.012	0.9412
Confidence	5–25	15	16.83 (5.24)	< 0.001	0.8778
Social pressure	2–10	6	2.94 (1.71)	< 0.001	0.6427
Difficulty	3–15	9	5.50 (2.60)	< 0.001	0.8489
Negative emotion	9–45	27	17.62 (7.62)	< 0.001	0.9277
Positive emotion	3–15	9	9.93 (3.03)	< 0.001	0.8681
Choice satisfaction	2–10	6	8.82 (1.58)	< 0.001	0.6673

The possible explanations are that they regarded the firstly presented option as the best option, they relied solely on public health nurses' advice or they thought that in their situation it was not necessary to read the information extensively. The regression result indicates that information and knowledge is not the decisive factor for choice satisfaction in prenatal screening. Gourounti et al. [43] have made a similar observation that knowledge component was not decisive for the calculation of informed choice. In general, women do not spend a lot of time considering the screening options. Making an easy and quick choice is what they appear to expect. Recommendation with backup options given by health professionals may work well in this context.

Our study indicates that the recommendation and advice from health professionals (such as the public health nurse of maternity care unit) is highly important for women to make decisions. It is in line with the finding by Aune and Möller [25]: although women knew the health professionals were neutral in their statements and provided 'balanced' information and non-directive counseling, there was still a request for more advice and suggestions. According to Porter and Macintyre [44], women tend to assume that whatever the service system offers is well thought and likely the best option. However, this creates a danger of viewing everything the system suggests as routine procedures that do not require a decision [26]. Therefore, even though in previous studies it has been suggested that women did not see such system recommendations as being incompatible with making autonomous choices, there is a need for clarification of the nature of the discussion and counseling. Guidelines on how to support women's choice-making based on their capability, willingness and preferences should be clearly defined [8].

Constructing active choice environment

A large body of research indicates that pregnant women want to be part of the decision-making process in prenatal screening and testing and make autonomous choices [25, 45, 46]. In our study, women's activeness in choice-making highly influences choice satisfaction. Increased active choice-making leads to higher choice satisfaction, whereas the women in our study do not make active choices in general. This may reflect that the current choice environment in Finland for prenatal screening program does not provide women with enough opportunities or motivations to make active choices. According to women's accounts, they appreciated the recommendation from maternity care units, but they would have wanted to know the different options. Offered with recommendation together with other options, women would be given better chances to think and make choices by themselves.

Our result of women's preference on the screening tests is consistent with many other studies: women have a strong preference for the combination of first trimester maternal serum screening and ultrasound measurement of the nuchal translucency and fetal crown-rump length, over STS, because of the earlier estimation, higher accuracy and providing more information about the baby [47–50]. However, some women have only the option of STS due to special situations such as traveling abroad occurring at the window of the FTS. Our regression analysis showed that choice-making confidence highly influences women's choice satisfaction and preference consistency partially boosts the confidence. In order to facilitate preference-consistent choices in prenatal screening, women should be offered with opportunities to discuss their wishes and personal situations and clarify their preferences [9].

In general, women did not feel much pressure to participate in the screening tests and most of them reported they received some support from others, mostly from public health nurses of maternity care units and husbands/partners. This empirically supports Lawson and Pierson's [51] conclusion that the women identified their physicians and their husbands as the most important individuals from whom they sought support. We can see from the quantitative

Table 4 Multiple linear regression with choice satisfaction as the dependent variable

						95.0% CI for unstandardized coefficients	
Variables	Unstandardized coefficients	SE	Standardized coefficients	t	*p* value	Lower bound	Upper bound
Age	0.020	0.024	0.058	0.86	0.390	−0.026	0.067
Education	−0.235	0.117	−0.136	−2.00	*0.047**	−0.467	−0.003
Gravidity (the number of times that a woman has been pregnant, including current pregnancy)	−0.234	0.088	−0.182	−2.66	*0.008**	−0.407	− 0.061
Chromosomal abnormality in previous pregnancy	−0.867	1.228	−0.042	− 0.71	0.481	−3.292	1.557
Screening result (normal as the referent)							
Abnormal result	−0.177	1.257	−0.009	−0.14	0.888	−2.659	2.305
Don't know yet	0.131	0.252	0.033	0.52	0.605	−0.367	0.628
Activeness	0.072	0.031	0.176	2.30	*0.023**	0.010	0.134
Informedness	−0.004	0.017	−0.022	− 0.26	0.793	− 0.037	0.029
Confidence	0.115	0.024	0.388	4.74	*< 0.001***	0.067	0.164
Social pressure	−0.277	0.062	−0.306	−4.50	*< 0.001***	− 0.399	−0.155
Difficulty	−0.162	0.043	−0.274	−3.75	*< 0.001***	−0.248	− 0.077
Negative emotion	0.004	0.016	0.020	0.26	0.798	−0.028	0.036
Positive emotion	−0.007	0.040	−0.013	−0.16	0.871	−0.086	0.072

$R^2 = 0.44$; *$p<0.05$; **$p<0.001$

study that while social pressure decreases choice satisfaction, confidence in choice-making that embraces social support can increase choice satisfaction. This is in tune with Lawson and Pierson's [51] argument that women who are making decisions in a socially supportive context have higher decisional competence and lower decisional conflict. Therefore, the service provider should build a socially supportive choice environment and encourage women to seek support and advice not only from healthcare professionals but also from others (e.g. husband/partner and friends).

In our study, education level negatively influences women's choice satisfaction, which means that women with higher education level have lower choice satisfaction. It is possible that more highly educated women have higher expectations and more requirements on choice environment. As the number of women with higher education will continue to increase, improving choice environment for prenatal screening demands swift actions. In addition, gravidity (i.e. the number of times that a woman has been pregnant, including current pregnancy) also strongly affect women's choice satisfaction: the more pregnancies, the lower the choice satisfaction. We can conceive that more experienced women have more critical views about the choices and decisions, which should be taken into account by the choice architects.

Reliability and validity

In the qualitative study, reliability was secured by the fact that two researchers carefully planned the interview protocol together, and they consulted medical and language professionals concerning the translations of the interview questions and terms. The two researchers also analyzed the interview data first separately and then together, and a strong mutual agreement on coding and categorization was reached. In addition, using the computerized data analysis package *Atlas.ti* enhanced the reliability [52]. For the quantitative study, Cronbach's alpha was used to assess the measurements reliability, testing how well the measurement items of one variable measure the same construct or idea [52, 53]. Table 3 includes Cronbach's alpha of each variable and the figures are acceptable, indicating reliable measurements. In this study, deriving the measurements from the interviews established the construct validity that concerns how well the measurements reflect the investigated constructs [54]. The similarity between the findings from the interviews and the survey confirmed a certain level of construct validity [55]. Specifically, the acceptable results of confirmatory factor analysis (CFA) [56] indicate convergent and discriminant validity of this study (Additional file 7).

Limitation and future study

One limitation in our study was the low response rate of the survey. This was probably due to asking the respondents to return the survey by mail (with prepaid envelopes) instead of collecting the survey answers at the Screening Unit. Furthermore, we did not set any deadlines for returning the questionnaires and this could lead to many respondents forgetting to return the survey. The other considered issue was that some results could be biased by the generally high education level of women in our sample, which applied to both the interviews and the survey. The generalization of the results may suffer somewhat due to this, as education level has been found to be a significant variable predictive for the choice of tests [13]. It can also be suspected that the beliefs and values of the women with different education levels differ to a certain extent [11]. However, this sample bias should be considered in the nationwide context. According to reports of Statistics Finland, the women in the district of Helsinki and Uusimaa, i.e. in the capital area, are the most highly educated women in whole of Finland [57]. This demographic composition naturally influences the likelihood of getting more answers from women with higher education. There is also a tendency of people who are academically inclined to be more willing to participate in surveys and other studies.

Despite the rather low response rate and slight education sample bias, we consider that the study sample can well represent the maternity population in the hospital district of Helsinki and Uusimaa. According to the Finnish perinatal statistics report for 2015, the mean age of our sample (32) is very close to the mean age of the parturients in Helsinki and Uusimaa region (31,4) [58]. And in terms of the family status, the study group (Married: 55.19%; Cohabitation: 38.80%) is close to the parturient population of the whole country in 2015 [58].

For further study, we plan to expand the sample to include other groups of women (e.g. women who take invasive tests, or women have a lower education status) or cover other regions or other countries. We will conduct the research in other medical fields (e.g. cancer screening) to test the generalization of our conclusions. Meanwhile, we could further the study by addressing the possible influence of personal beliefs and social values on choice-making experience and choice satisfaction.

Conclusions

This study made contributions in the research field of women's choice and experiences in prenatal screening and testing for common aneuploidies. Our study comprehensively investigated women's choice-making processes from women's perspective, explored women's choice-making experiences and identified the experiential factors that may influence choice satisfaction in prenatal screening. In the qualitative study, we structured women's choice-making processes and experiences in prenatal screening with six blocks: active choice (attitude and behavior), informedness (information needs and sources), preferences/considerations, social influence (perceived social support and pressure), difficulty and emotional status. Seven variables were derived from the six blocks to quantified women's choice-making experiences, named with "activeness", "informedness", "confidence", "social pressure", "difficulty", "positive emotion" and "negative emotion". By regression, we found that after controlling for some demographic factors (age, education, gravidity and chromosomal abnormality in previous pregnancy) and screening results, there were four experiential factors that significantly influenced women's choice satisfaction in prenatal screening, including activeness, confidence, perceived social pressure and perceived difficulty. Activeness in choice-making increased choice satisfaction. Choice satisfaction increased if the women had more confidence when making choices. Perceived social pressure and difficulty in choice-making negatively affected choice satisfaction.

Additional files

Additional file 1: Neuvola booklet of the prenatal screening and testing program in Finland (English).

Additional file 2: Decisional Conflict Scale.

Additional file 3: Short-form of the State Scale of the Spielberger State-Trait Anxiety Inventory.

Additional file 4: Measurements (before factor analysis).

Additional file 5: Factor analysis result.

Additional file 6: Measurements (after factor analysis).

Additional file 7: CFA result.

Abbreviations

CFA: Confirmatory factor analysis; FTS: First trimester combined screening, a screening method that takes into account the mother's age, results of the fetal anatomy and nuchal translucency measurement by ultrasound, and results from maternal serum biomarkers (free β-human chorionic gonadotropin (β-hCG), pregnancy-associated plasma protein-A (PAPP-A);
FMC: Fetomaternal Medical Center of Helsinki University Hospital;
HUS: Helsinki and Uusimaa Hospital District, Finland; Neuvola: Finnish community-based maternity care unit; STS: Second trimester serum screening, a screening method that is based on maternal serum β-hCG and alpha fetoprotein (AFP) adjusted for the gestational age; it does not involve ultrasound; TPB: Theory of Planned Behavior, A theory that links beliefs and behavior and assumes that a choice is consistent with the choice maker's goals, expectations, and values. It analyzes and predicts individual's choice with three constructs: behavioral beliefs, subjective norms and perceived behavioral control

Acknowledgements

The work reported here was highly supported by the staff of Fetomaternal Medical Center and delivery hospitals in Helsinki. Special gratitude is owed to Ms. Satu Leminen, Ms. Minna Richards and Ms. Maaria Puupponen. Ms. Eija.Raussi-Lehto and Mr. Antti Niemi from Helsinki Metropolia University of Applied Sciences made great contributions to the research.

Funding

This paper is financially supported by Aalto University, Helsinki University Hospital and Business Finland G3 project.

Availability of data and materials

Regarding the interview data, due to the ethical and legal restrictions required by HUS Ethical committee (Ethics Committee for Gynecology and Obstetrics, Pediatrics and Psychiatry, Helsinki University Hospital) and the agreement reached with patients that their information will be confidential within the research team and used for this research only, we are unable to publically provide the interview data underlying the findings in our study. But excerpts of the relevant interview transcripts are available on request. The excerpt does not include any personal information about our informants, just reporting briefly how the woman made choices. For requesting the data or concerning other data issues, please contact the following persons:
For requesting the access to qualitative data, please contact with HUS Ethics Committee for gynaecology and obstetrics, pediatrics and psychiatry.
Presenting Official: Heli Nevanlinna, p. + 358 9 4717 1750.
Office Secretary: Piia Paavilainen, p. + 358,504,279,493.
For requesting the excerpts or concerning other data issues, please contact with.
Dr. Vedran Stefanovic (vedran.stefanovic@hus.fi), who is one of the authors of the manuscript.
The dataset generated and analysed for the quantitative study is not publicly available due to the restrictions claimed in the document of the HUS (The Hospital District of Helsinki and Uusimaa) research permission. But the data are available from the HUS Committee for researchers who meet the criteria for access to confidential data.
For requesting the access to quantitative data, please contact with HUS Ethics Committee for gynaecology and obstetrics, pediatrics and psychiatry.
Presenting Official: Heli Nevanlinna, p. + 358 9 4717 1750.
Office Secretary: Piia Paavilainen, p. + 358,504,279,493.
For concerning other issues related to the quantitative data, please contact with.
Dr. Vedran Stefanovic (vedran.stefanovic@hus.fi), who is one of the authors of the manuscript.
We quote some key information from the document of HUS research permission that has been attached in the resubmission:
Quote 1:
"Tutkimuksen henkilörekisterin avainrekisteriä pidetään HUS:ssa ja sen vastuuhenkilönä toimii Vedran Stefanovic. Tässä tutkimuksessa HUS:n avainrekisterin tietoja tai salasia ja arkaluonteisia tietoja sisältäviä asiakirjoja ei luovuteta HUS:n ulkopuolelle."
Translation into English:
"The key code of the personal register of this research is to be kept in HUS and the person in charge is Vedran Stefanovic. Personal data or secret and sensitive information are not to be disposed outside of HUS".
Quote 2:
"..saatuja tietoja ei saa luovuttaa, siirtää taikka myydä kolmannelle osapuolelle Suomeen tai ulkomaille...."
Translation into English:
"...it is forbidden to provide, transfer and/or sell obtained data to any third part in Finland or abroad...".

Authors' contributions

This is a co-authored article. The first author of this paper, AC, was responsible for defining the topic, designing the study, and implementing the research. She designed the interviews and surveys, collected and analysed the data, interpreted the results, and drafted the paper. HT performed most of the interviews for the study, translated the data, and participated in analysing the interview data and interpreting the results; she participated in translating and refining the survey's questionnaire, interpreting the findings, and revising the paper throughout the drafting process. VS guided the empirical research, helped to recruit the interview participants and distribute the questionnaires, provided medical expert comments, revised the paper often throughout the drafting process, and gave the final approval of the version to be published. PT and AP gave advice for the study's design, data analysis, and interpretation of the results. SH provided insights into the research plan and implementation as a medical expert and institution manager. PL supervised the whole research and made substantial contributions to conception and design and revised the manuscript for important intellectual content. All authors participated sufficiently in the work to take public responsibility for appropriate portions of the content, and agreed to be accountable for all aspects of the work in ensuring that questions related to the accuracy or integrity of any part of the work were appropriately investigated and resolved. The development of the paper for publication was the collective effort of all the authors.

Competing interests

The authors declare that they have no competing interests.

Author details

[1]Institute of Healthcare Engineering, Management and Architecture (HEMA), Department of Industrial Engineering and Management, Aalto University, Maarintie 8, P.O. Box 15500, 00076 Espoo, Finland. [2]Department of Civil Engineering, Aalto University, Rakentajanaukio 4, 02150 Espoo, Finland. [3]Department of Obstetrics and Gynaecology, Helsinki University Hospital and University of Helsinki, Haartmaninkatu 2, 00290 Helsinki, Finland. [4]Department of Public Health, Faculty of Medicine, Helsinki University, Biomedicum 1, 00290 Helsinki, Finland.

References

1. Sutherland S, Farrell RM, Lockwood C. Genetic screening and testing in an episode-based payment model: preserving patient autonomy. Obstet Gynecol. 2014;124(5):987–91.
2. Carroll FE, Al-Janabi H, Flynn T, Montgomery AA. Women and their partners' preferences for Down's syndrome screening tests: a discrete choice experiment. Prenat Diagn. 2013;33(5):449–56.
3. García E, Timmermans DR, van Leeuwen E. The impact of ethical beliefs on decisions about prenatal screening tests: searching for justification. Soc Sci Med. 2008;66(3):753–64.
4. Lou S, Mikkelsen L, Hvidman L, Petersen OB, Nielsen CP. Does screening for Down's syndrome cause anxiety in pregnant women? A systematic review. Acta Obstet Gynecol Scand. 2015;94(1):15–27.
5. Santalahti P, Hemminki E, Latikka A-M, Ryynänen M. Women's decision-making in prenatal screening. Soc Sci Med. 1998;46(8):1067–76.
6. Schoonen H, van Agt H, Essink-Bot M-L, Wildschut H, Steegers E, de Koning H. Informed decision-making in prenatal screening for Down's syndrome: what knowledge is relevant? Patient Educ Couns. 2011;84(2):265–70.
7. Dormandy E, Hooper R, Michie S, Marteau T. Informed choice to undergo prenatal screening: a comparison of two hospitals conducting testing either as part of a routine visit or requiring a separate visit. J Med Screen. 2002; 9(3):109–14.
8. Ahmed S, Bryant LD, Tizro Z, Shickle D. Is advice incompatible with autonomous informed choice? Women's perceptions of advice in the context of antenatal screening: a qualitative study. Health Expect. 2014; 17(4):555–64.
9. Garcia E, Timmermans D, van Leeuwen E. Reconsidering prenatal screening: an empirical-ethical approach to understand moral dilemmas as a question of personal preferences. J Med Ethics. 2009;35(7):410–4.
10. Yu J. A systematic review of issues around antenatal screening and prenatal diagnostic testing for genetic disorders: women of Asian origin in western countries. Health Soc Care Community. 2012;20(4):329–46.
11. Bakker M, Birnie E, Pajkrt E, Bilardo CM, Snijders RJM. Low uptake of the combined test in the Netherlands–which factors contribute? Prenat Diagn. 2012;32(13):1305–12.
12. Crombag NM, Schielen PC, Hukkelhoven CW, Iedema R, Bensing JM, Visser GH, Stoutenbeek P, Koster MP. Determinants of first trimester combined test participation within the central region of the Netherlands. Prenat Diagn. 2015;35(5):486–92.
13. Košec V, Zec I, Tišlarić-Medenjak D, Kuna K, Šimundić AM, Lajtman-Križaić M, Lovrić B, Mimica M, Komadina Estatiev Z, Borgudan V. Pregnant women's knowledge and attitudes to prenatal screening for fetal chromosomal abnormalities: croatian multicentric survey. Coll Antropol. 2013;37(2):483–9.
14. Marteau TM, Dormandy E, Michie S. A measure of informed choice. Health Expect. 2001;4(2):99–108.
15. Williams C, Alderson P, Farsides B. What constitutes 'balanced information in the practitioners' portrayals of Down's syndrome? Midwifery. 2002;18(3): 230–7.
16. Potter BK, O'Reilly N, Etchegary H, Howley H, Graham ID, Walker M, Coyle D, Chorny Y, Cappelli M, Boland I. Exploring informed choice in the context of prenatal testing: findings from a qualitative study. Health Expect. 2008;11(4): 355–65.
17. Merkouris A, Yfantopoulos J, Lanara V, Lemonidou C. Developing an instrument to measure patient satisfaction with nursing care in Greece. J Nurs Manag. 1999;7(2):91–100.
18. Nilvér H, Begley C, Berg M. Measuring women's childbirth experiences: a systematic review for identification and analysis of validated instruments. BMC Pregnancy Childbirth. 2017;17(1):203–21.
19. Larkin P, Begley CM, Devane D. Women's experiences of labour and birth: an evolutionary concept analysis. Midwifery. 2009;25(2):e49–59.
20. Shocker AD, Ben-Akiva M, Boccara B, Nedungadi P. Consideration set influences on consumer decision-making and choice: issues, models, and suggestions. Mark Lett. 1991;2(3):181–97.
21. Helkkula A, Kelleher C, Pihlström M. Practices and experiences: challenges and opportunities for value research. J Serv Manage. 2012;23(4):554–70.
22. Helkkula A. Characterising the concept of service experience. J Serv Manage. 2011;22(3):367–89.
23. Helkkula A, Kelleher C. Circularity of customer service experience and customer perceived value. J Cust Behav. 2010;9(1):37–53.
24. Brondino N, Colombini G, Morandotti N, Podavini F, De Vidovich G, Formica M, Arossa A, De Silvestri A, Montanari L, Caverzasi E. Psychological correlates of decision-making during prenatal diagnosis: a prospective study. J Psychosom Obstet Gynaecol. 2013;34(2):68–74.
25. Aune I, Möller A. 'I want a choice, but I don't want to decide': a qualitative study of pregnant women's experiences regarding early ultrasound risk assessment for chromosomal anomalies. Midwifery. 2012;28(1):14–23.
26. Ternby E, Ingvoldstad C, Annerén G, Lindgren P, Axelsson O. Information and knowledge about Down syndrome among women and partners after first trimester combined testing. Acta Obstet Gynecol Scand. 2015; 94(3):329–32.
27. Östlund U, Kidd L, Wengström Y, Rowa-Dewar N. Combining qualitative and quantitative research within mixed method research designs: a methodological review. Int J Nurs Stud. 2011;48(3):369–83.
28. Steckler A, McLeroy KR, Goodman RM, Bird ST, McCormick L. Toward integrating qualitative and quantitative methods: an introduction. Health Educ Q. 1992;19(1):1–8.
29. Foss C, Ellefsen B. The value of combining qualitative and quantitative approaches in nursing research by means of method triangulation. J Adv Nurs. 2002;40(2):242–8.
30. Clarke PN, Yaros PS. Research blenders: commentary and response commentary: transitions to New Methodologies in Nursing Sciences. Nurs Sci Q. 1988;1(4):147–9.
31. Hanson WE, Creswell JW, Clark VLP, Petska KS, Creswell JD. Mixed methods research designs in counseling psychology. J Couns Psychol. 2005;52(2):224–35.
32. Murphy K, Casey D, Devane D, Meskell P, Higgins A, Elliot N, Lalor J, Begley C. Reflections on the added value of using mixed methods in the SCAPE study. Nurse Res. 2014;21(4):13–9.
33. Lalor JG, Casey D, Elliott N, Coyne I, Comiskey C, Higgins A, Murphy K, Devane D, Begley C. Using case study within a sequential explanatory design to evaluate the impact of specialist and advanced practice roles on clinical outcomes: the SCAPE study. BMC Med Res Methodol. 2013;13(1):55–64.
34. Bury M. Illness narratives: fact or fiction? Sociol Health Illn. 2001;**23**(3):263–85.
35. Gill L, Helkkula A, Cobelli N, White L. How do customers and pharmacists experience generic substitution? Int J Pharm Healthc Mark. 2010;4(4):375–95.
36. Pottie K, Haydt S, Farrell B, Dolovich L, Sellors C, Hogg W. Narrative reports to monitor and evaluate the integration of pharmacists into family practice settings. Ann Fam Med. 2008;6(2):161–5.
37. Godin G, Kok G. The theory of planned behavior: a review of its applications to health-related behaviors. Am J Health Promot. 1996;11(2):87–98.
38. Ajzen I. The theory of planned behavior. Organ Behav Hum Decis Process. 1991;50(2):179–211.
39. DeVellis RF. Scale development: theory and applications. 4th ed. Los Angeles: SAGE Publications Inc; 2016.
40. O'Connor AM. User Manual-Decisional Conflict Scale. 1993 [updated 2010]. Ottawa: Ottawa Hospital Research Institute; 2014.
41. O'Connor AM. Validation of a decisional conflict scale. Med Decis Mak. 1995; 15(1):25–30.
42. Marteau TM, Bekker H. The development of a six-item short-form of the state scale of the Spielberger State-Trait Anxiety Inventory (STAI). Br J Clin Psychol. 1992;31(3):301–6.
43. Gourounti K, Zerva C, Gavriil E, Nanou C. Prenatal ultrasound screening for down syndrome and informed choice. Rev Clin Pharmacol Pharmacokinet Int Ed. 2015;29(1):37–41.

44. Porter M, Macintyre S. What is, must be best: a research note on conservative or deferential responses to antenatal care provision. Soc Sci Med. 1984;19(11):1197–200.
45. Carroll JC, Rideout A, Wilson BJ, Allanson J, Blaine S, Esplen MJ, Farrell S, Graham GE, MacKenzie J, Meschino WS. Maternal age-based prenatal screening for chromosomal disorders Attitudes of women and health care providers toward changes. Can Fam Physician. 2013;59(1):e39–47.
46. Légaré F, St-Jacques S, Gagnon S, Njoya M, Brisson M, Frémont P, Rousseau F. Prenatal screening for Down syndrome: a survey of willingness in women and family physicians to engage in shared decision-making. Prenat Diagn. 2011;31(4):319–26.
47. Sharma G, Gold HT, Chervenak FA, McCullough L, Alt AK, Chasen ST. Patient preference regarding first-trimester aneuploidy risk assessment. Am J Obstet Gynecol. 2005;193(4):1429–36.
48. Wong AE, Kuppermann M, Creasman JM, Sepulveda W, Vargas JE. Patient and provider attitudes toward screening for Down syndrome in a Latin American country where abortion is illegal. Int J Gynaecol Obstet. 2011; 115(3):235–9.
49. De Graaf IM, Tijmstra T, Bleker OP, Van Lith JM. Womens' preference in Down syndrome screening. Prenat Diagn. 2002;22(7):624–9.
50. Spencer K, Aitken D. Factors affecting women's preference for type of prenatal screening test for chromosomal anomalies. Ultrasound Obstet Gynecol. 2004;24(7):735–9.
51. Lawson KL, Pierson RA. Maternal decisions regarding prenatal diagnosis: rational choices or sensible decisions? J Obstet Gynaecol Can. 2007; 29(3):240–6.
52. Roberts P, Priest H, Traynor M. Reliability and validity in research. Nurs Stand. 2006;20(44):41–5.
53. Tavakol M, Dennick R. Making sense of cronbach's alpha. Int J Med Educ. 2011;2:53–5.
54. Bagozzi RP, Yi Y, Phillips LW. Assessing construct validity in organizational research. Adm Sci Q. 1991;36(3):421–58.
55. Lewis C, Hill M, Skirton H, Chitty LS. Development and validation of a measure of informed choice for women undergoing non-invasive prenatal testing for aneuploidy. Eur J Hum Genet. 2015;24:809–16.
56. Campbell DT, Fiske DW. Convergent and discriminant validation by the multitrait-multimethod matrix. Psychol Bull. 1959;56(2):81.
57. Witting M, Harala R. The official statistics of finland: Education level of the Finnish population (Finnish title: Suomen virallinen tilasto (SVT): Väestön koulutusrakenne). In: Koulutustilastot 2014. Helsinki: Statistics Finland; 2014.
58. Vuori E, Gissler M. Perinatal statistics: parturients, deliveries and newborns 2015. Helsinki: National Institute for Health and Welfare of Finland (THL); 2016.

5

Adaptation of an evidence-based postpartum depression intervention: feasibility and acceptability of mothers and babies 1-on-1

S. Darius Tandon[1*], Julie A. Leis[2], Erin A. Ward[1], Hannah Snyder[3], Tamar Mendelson[4], Deborah F. Perry[5], Mya Carter[1], Jaime Hamil[1] and Huynh-Nhu Le[3]

Abstract

Background: Mothers and Babies (MB) is a cognitive-behavioral intervention with demonstrated efficacy in reducing depressive symptoms and preventing depressive episodes among perinatal women when delivered in a group format by mental health professionals. Study aims were to describe the adaptation of MB into a 1-on-1 modality (MB 1-on-1) and provide data on the adapted intervention's acceptability and feasibility.

Methods: Seventy-five home visitors trained on MB 1-on-1 delivered the 15-session intervention to 1–2 clients. Client acceptability data assessed intervention enjoyment, comprehension, and usefulness. Home visitor feasibility and acceptability data measured amount of intervention material delivered, client comprehension, and client engagement.

Results: Home visitors were all female with 8.8 years of experience on average. 117 clients completed acceptability surveys. Average client age was 21.9 years and 41% were pregnant. Home visitors completely covered 87.9% of sessions and reported clients totally understood MB material 82.5% of the time across sessions, although variability was found in comprehension across modules. 82.0% of clients found MB 1-on-1 enjoyable and 91.6% said they totally understood sessions, when averaged across sessions. Clients enjoyed content on noticing one's mood and pleasant activities. Implementation challenges were client engagement, facilitating completion of personal projects, and difficulty shifting between didactic and interactive activities.

Conclusions: Clients found MB 1-on-1 to be enjoyable, easily understood, and useful. Home visitors reported excellent implementation fidelity and felt clients understood MB material. A refined 12-session version of MB 1-on-1 should be examined for its effectiveness in reducing depressive symptoms, given encouraging feasibility and acceptability data.

Keywords: Home visiting, Depression, Intervention, Prevention, Implementation

Background

The prevalence of postpartum depression has been estimated at 10–22% and disproportionately affects low-income women of all racial and ethnic groups, with a 20% prevalence rate consistently found among low-income women [1–4]. Postpartum depression is a well-established risk factor for poor parenting practices, with strong and consistent evidence indicating that women experiencing postpartum depression exhibit less maternal responsiveness or sensitivity, less verbal and visual interaction, and more intrusiveness [5–8]. Disparities also exist across socioeconomic lines with respect to prevalence of clinically relevant perinatal depressive symptoms that do not meet DSM criteria for major depression. Studies indicate that rates of clinically elevated perinatal depressive symptoms among low-income women are 30–45% [9, 10] —double the rates of women of higher socio-economic status; these disparities exist irrespective of race, ethnicity, or geography [11–13]. Notably, the presence of subthreshold depressive symptoms are associated with

* Correspondence: dtandon@northwestern.edu
[1]Northwestern University Feinberg School of Medicine, 750 N. Lake Shore Drive, 6th Floor, Chicago, IL 60614, USA
Full list of author information is available at the end of the article

many of the same negative maternal and child health outcomes as major depression [14, 15].

Systematic reviews have highlighted an array of efficacious interventions that reduce the risk of developing postpartum depression [16]. Among interventions that have demonstrated efficacy, the majority use health (e.g., nurses, midwives) or mental health (e.g., psychologists) professionals to deliver individualized or group-based interventions [16]. One exception is the use of peers to deliver support via phone [17], although this study was conducted in Canada with predominately White, upper and middle class women. To our knowledge, there are no interventions led by *non-health or non-mental health professionals* that have demonstrated efficacy in preventing the onset of postpartum depression and reduction of depressive symptoms among low-income women. Interventions delivered by non-health or non-mental health professionals have considerable potential to address the mental health needs of perinatal women, given the stigma associated with seeking mental health services, lack of knowledge about, or limited access to available mental health services [18, 19].

Home visiting programs (HV) are one setting through which perinatal women can receive mental health services via paraprofessionals. Current estimates indicate that more than 750,000 women receive HV services each year, making HV one of the largest avenues through which perinatal women come to the attention of service providers [20]. Home visiting is a service delivery strategy wherein trained paraprofessional or professionals (e.g., social workers, nurses) meet regularly in-home with pregnant women and women with young children. Twenty evidence-based HV models have been identified [20], which—depending on the model—focus on child development and school readiness, positive parenting practices, reduction in child maltreatment, improvement of birth outcomes, and promotion of maternal health. Across different HV models, home visitors tend to see clients weekly or biweekly. Core content of evidence-based HV models typically address: (a) preparation for childbirth and parenting, (b) provision of emotional and tangible support, (c) discussion of infant and child development, (d) linkages to prenatal and pediatric care, and (e) referrals for social and health services.

There is evidence that depression is challenging for HV programs to address and can negatively impact the effects of HV programs on their desired maternal and child health outcomes. Depressed clients in HV require more effort to engage in services [21] and home visitors often feel they do not have appropriate training on how to discuss depression with their clients [22]. Depressive symptoms among HV clients were associated with less parenting self-confidence, higher risk beliefes about parenting and knowledge of child development, and smaller social support networks [23] with other studies indicating that depressed HV clients exhibit more dysfunctional parent-child interactions [24] Recent years have seen increasing calls for and integration of depression screening into HV programs, including through the federal Maternal, Infant, and Early Childhood Home Visiting Program (MIECHV) initiative [25]. Although screening for depression is an important step, research indicates that HV clients who screen positive rarely receive community mental health services [26, 27]. As such, there is a growing need to identify strategies for providing services to HV clients to address this population's mental health needs, which, in turn, may promote greater HV effectiveness in achieving its core outcomes.

To address maternal depression in home visiting, our study team collaborated with HV programs to integrate and evaluate the Mothers and Babies (MB) Course's efficacy in preventing the onset of postpartum depression and worsening of depressive symptoms among HV clients. The MB Course is a manualized cognitive-behavioral intervention that promotes healthy mood management by teaching individuals ways to increase the frequency of thoughts and behaviors that lead to positive mood states. There are three MB modules: (1) behavioral activation to increase enjoyable activities, (2) restructuring harmful cognitions, and (3) increasing social support. MB content is tailored to specific needs and issues related to the perinatal period. A series of randomized controlled trials has demonstrated the association of MB with prevention of major depression onset, reduced depressive symptoms, and improved mood management among perinatal women receiving MB compared to women receiving usual care when MB is delivered in a group format by mental health professionals [28–32]. The most recent of these RCT's have been conducted in HV settings [29, 31, 32].

Despite results showing MB is efficacious in addressing postpartum depression, there are limitations to mental health professionals delivering groups in HV settings: insufficient availability of clinicians, especially in rural areas, untenable costs associated with hiring clinicians, as well as barriers to client attendance such as transportation issues, childcare, and the time commitment to attend group sessions [33]. In response to these challenges, our research team developed and piloted a 1-on-1 adaptation of MB (MB 1-on-1). This article describes the MB 1-on-1 intervention, providing client and home visitor data on the feasibility and acceptability of implementation.

Method

Development of MB 1-on-1

The goal of developing MB 1-on-1 was to adapt intervention content to complement the educational information and supportive communications home visitors provide during visits into 15–20 min segments that could be effectively incorporated during regular home visits. In doing so, care was taken to retain core content of the MB Group curriculum while modifying the intervention to ensure its appropriateness for 1-on-1 delivery. As a starting point, all group activities requiring small or large group conversations were identified; those that required multiple group members were either revised for provider-client interactions or removed. Weekly group relaxation activities were also removed due to the time requirement, while a session teaching relaxation techniques was included in MB 1-on-1. We then removed material that was duplicative across sessions (e.g., multiple discussions of harmful vs. helpful thoughts in the Thoughts module became the focus of a single MB 1-on-1 session). This process resulted in a 15-session version of MB 1-on-1.

Along with modifying the content to be delivered in 15 brief sessions, considerable effort was placed on revising the Instructor's Manual to make it user-friendly for home visitors accessing the Manual in a client's home. Each session consists of two to three topics and a personal project (i.e., homework) for completion between sessions. All topics contain: a) key points for home visitors to communicate to clients as takeaway messages, b) a script to guide home visitors when delivering content, and c) interactive learning activities that help clients practice and understand key concepts.

Setting

In partnership with the Illinois Governor's Office for Early Childhood Development (OECD) an open invitation was offered to HV programs across Illinois to attend one of three regional day and a half-long trainings led by the first author on MB 1-on-1 between February and August 2014. Eighty-one home visitors from 19 HV programs in Illinois attended one of the trainings. Across programs, 14 (74%) used the Healthy Families America model, and 5 (26%) programs employed the Parents as Teachers model. The number of home visitors employed by agency ranged from 1 to 7. Healthy Families America enrolment targets parents facing challenges such as single parenthood, low income, childhood history of abuse and other adverse child experiences, and current or previous issues related to substance abuse, mental health issues, or domestic violence. Individual Healthy Families' sites are given latitude to select specific characteristics of the target population they plan to serve, while enrolling prenatally or within three months of birth [34]. Parents as Teachers provider organizations select the specific characteristics and eligibility criteria of the target population they plan to serve, such as children with special needs, families at risk for child abuse, income-based criteria, teen parents, first-time parents, immigrant families, low literate families, or parents with mental health or substance use issues, enrolling families during pregnancy and the postpartum period [35].

During training, home visitors were provided with an orientation to MB's cognitive-behavioral therapy underpinnings followed by an orientation to implementation guidelines and structure of the Instructor and Participant Manuals. The remainder of the training guided home visitors through each of the 15 sessions. Didactic portions of the training introduced home visitors to key points within each session and potential challenges to communicating material with clients. Training provided ample time for attendees to engage in small and large group activities, including opportunities to practice introducing core MB content, provider-client interactive activities, and personal project presentation, through structured role plays.

OECD was interested in training its HV programs on how to better address maternal depression among its clients and encouraged all HV programs trained to immediately pilot the intervention. Specifically, home visitors attending a training were asked to to implement MB with 1 to 2 clients who were pregnant or had a child < 6 months. In cases where prenatal and recently postpartum clients were not available, home visitors were encouraged to implement MB with clients on their caseload who could benefit from the intervention, with the goal being to practice implementation in close proximity to the training and supervision offered.

Intervention implementation

MB 1-on-1 recommends session delivery every 1–2 weeks, with flexibility to conduct more than one session per week if a home visitor believes the material is particularly salient for a client. Home visitors were trained to deliver a MB session at the beginning or end of a scheduled home visit, with flexibility to conduct a MB session by phone if a client was unable to complete the scheduled home visit. Other individuals were permitted to be present during MB delivery (e.g., father of baby); however, home visitors were encouraged to use professional judgment regarding whether the presence of another individual would compromise MB delivery or client openness. HV clients referred to material in the Participant Manual during sessions. Personal projects for client completion between sessions were described in the Participant Manual. Home visitors were trained to implement MB 1-on-1 chronologically from session 1 through 15.

Each HV program received biweekly phone supervision from the first author upon beginning MB implementation. Supervision was provided for 4–6 months, which corresponded with the length of time it took, on average, for home visitors at a HV program to implement the 15-session curriculum. Supervision calls allowed home visitors to share and receive feedback on both content and implementation process. For example, home visitors posed content-related questions on how to help clients better understand a core MB concept or process-related questions on how to most effectively transition from delivering core HV content to MB material.

Data sources and data collection

The Northwestern University Institutional Review Board reviewed and approved the study protocol and all data collection activities described herein. This protocol was deemed as minimal risk and pursuant to quality assurance activities and was therefore granted a waiver of consent.

Client acceptability

At the end of each of the 15 MB sessions, clients were asked to complete a brief de-identified 5-question survey given to them by their home visitor. Each survey asked the same questions: a) how much did you enjoy today's session (1 = not enjoyable at all, 2 = somewhat enjoyable, 3 = very enjoyable), b) how well did you understand the information in today's session (1 = didn't understand, 2 = somewhat understood, 3 = totally understood), and c) how useful was the information in today's session (1 = not useful at all, 2 = somewhat useful, 3 = very useful). Two open-ended questions were asked: do you have any suggestions on how to make today's session any better, and, was there anything you really enjoyed or thought was really useful in today's session.

Home visitor feasibility & acceptability

Home visitors also completed a survey at the end of each session. Each survey asked the home visitor to indicate for each session topic: a) how much material was covered (not covered, somewhat covered, totally covered), b) how well you think the client understood the topic (did not understand at all, somewhat understood, totally understood), and c) how engaged the client was (not engaged at all, somewhat engaged, very engaged). Home visitors were also given the opportunity to provide open-ended responses indicating if there were challenges when discussing session topics.

Data analysis

Home visitors entered their data directly into a web-based Research Electronic Data Capture (REDCap) survey or emailed or faxed data to the research team who entered the data into REDCap. Client data were collected by home visitors and emailed or faxed to the research team for REDCap data entry. All data were subsequently exported to SPSS 22 for analysis. To analyze client acceptability data, we assessed *enjoyment* by calculating the percentage of women who indicated they found each session very enjoyable, somewhat enjoyable, or not enjoyable at all. We assessed content *comprehension* by calculating the percentage of women who indicated they didn't understand, somewhat understood, or totally understood each session. We assessed perceived usefulness of MB skills by calculating the percentage of women who indicated they found skills not useful at all, somewhat useful, or very useful.

To assess home visitor feasibility and acceptability data, we examined *fidelity of MB implementation* by calculating the percentage of home visitors who reported that they totally covered, somewhat covered, or did not cover each topic within a session. Each session contains between 2 and 4 topics; the percentages for each topic were combined into an average score indicating the extent to which a session was covered. We assessed *client comprehension* by calculating the percentage of home visitors who indicated that a client totally understood, somewhat understood, or did not understand at all the session material for each session. We also estimated *client engagement* by calculating the percentage of home visitors who indicated that a client was totally engaged, somewhat engaged, or not engaged at all for each session.

For each client and home visitor acceptability and feasibility construct, we calculated percentages: a) across all 15 sessions (i.e., the entire intervention) and b) for each MB module [Sessions 1–3 (Overview), Sessions 4–6 (Pleasant Activities); Sessions 7–11 (Thoughts), Sessions 12–15 (Contacts with Others)]. All open-ended client and home visitor responses were exported into Microsoft Excel and coded inductively by a member of the research team; open-ended responses were provided by 95% of clients and 91% of home visitors. The same research team member created two matrices—one for client data and another for home visitor data. Each matrix had a row for each code and a column for each respondent and all open-ended data were placed in one of these matrices. These matrices were then used to guide analysis that identified the most common themes and patterns [36] related to the constructs that the open-ended questions asked about—for example, client enjoyment and home visitors perceptions of intervention fidelity.

Results

Home visitor demographics

Of the 81 home visitors trained, 75 implemented MB 1-on-1. Reasons that home visitors did not implement the intervention included: one HV program decided not to implement MB due to organizational transitions shortly after training ($n = 3$) and staff leaving the agency shortly after training (n = 3). Of the 75 who did implement MB 1-on-1, 68 provided data on implementation. The average age of these 68 female home visitors was 42 years (range 22–66) and the average length of time working as a home visitor was 8.8 years (range < 1 year - 24 years). The majority had at least a 2-year Associate's Degree (72%). The race/ethnicity composition was 36%

African American, 34% White, 25% Latina, 3% Asian-American, and 2% biracial.

Client characteristics

A total of 129 clients received the MB 1-on-1 intervention delivered by the 75 home visitors, of whom 117 (91%) completed client acceptability surveys. Among the 117 study participants, the average age was 21.9 (range 15–36). Forty-five percent of women were African American, 28% White, and 27% Latina. A slight majority of clients (59%) had already delivered their baby when they started receiving MB, with the average number of weeks postpartum being 20 (range 1–96). The remaining 41% of women were pregnant when they received their first MB session, with an average gestational age of 29 weeks (range 10–39). Eighty-eight percent of clients received MB 1-on-1 in English and 12% in Spanish.

Home visitor feasibility and acceptability data

When asked to rate their ability to cover material in a session, home visitors indicated they completely covered 87.9% of the sessions they delivered. Sessions in the Overview module were totally covered most often (92.3%), while the sessions in the other three modules were each totally covered about 85% of the time. Home visitors indicated that clients totally understood MB material 82.5% of the time when averaged across all sessions. There were, however, discrepancies in the extent to which home visitors felt clients understood content in the different modules. Home visitors indicated that clients fully understood the material in the Pleasant Activities module 95.0% of the time, whereas home visitors felt clients totally understood the Contact with Others, Overview and Thoughts Modules less often (Table 1). There was also variability in the extent to which home visitors felt clients were engaged in MB sessions. Similar to home visitors' ratings of client comprehension of MB materials, home visitors felt clients were most often totally engaged with the Pleasant Activities module (79.4%). Each of the other modules was rated as having clients totally engaged between 63.0–69.2% of the time. When asked via open-ended question to indicate challenges with implementing MB, the most commonly reported challenge was the presence of children who were crying or distracting the client from focusing, followed by preoccupation with other household issues. The most commonly reported challenge specific to the MB curriculum was clients not always completing personal projects between sessions. In addition, several home visitors noted that material in the Thoughts module was repetitious. Home visitors also commented that while the script in the Instructor Manual was useful, it felt too long at times and did not clearly indicate when the home visitor should engage in conversation with the client (Table 2).

Client acceptability data

Clients, generally speaking, found MB 1-on-1 sessions to be enjoyable with 82.0% indicating they found sessions very enjoyable when aggregating ratings across all 15 sessions. Pleasant Activities and Contact with Others modules were rated to be slightly more enjoyable than the MB Overview and Thoughts modules (Table 1). Across all MB sessions, clients said they totally understood 91.6% of the sessions. There were minor differences across modules, with clients indicating they understood the pleasant activities module slightly better than the other three modules (Table 1). When asked to indicate perceived usefulness of MB sessions, 85.1% of sessions were rated as very useful when analyzing across all sessions. There was little variation in ratings of usefulness across modules or individual sessions (Table 1). Open-ended comments from client acceptability surveys highlighted several areas that clients particularly enjoyed. In particular, several clients noted they enjoyed using the curriculum's "Quick Mood Scale" as an approach to keep track of their mood during the week. Other clients indicated that they enjoyed developing a list of pleasant activities that they could do by themselves or with others, including their child(ren), and discussing helpful and harmful thoughts (Table 3). Clients also reported on several topics they found useful, including the discussion of how to manage stress (Session 1). Clients consistently highlighted the skills taught in the curriculum as being useful, including generating a list of pleasant activities and strategies to stop harmful thoughts (Table 3).

Discussion

Castro et al. (2004) note that one form of intervention adaptation pertains to modification of program delivery [37]. Accordingly, this study adapted an evidence-based postpartum depression prevention intervention—the Mothers and Babies Course—from a group to an individual modality. In general, clients found MB 1-on-1 to be enjoyable, easily understood, and useful. Home visitors reported excellent fidelity in delivering the intervention and, in general, felt that clients understood the material. However, there appeared to be some discrepancies between home visitor and client ratings of comprehension for specific MB modules. In particular, home visitors felt that clients were less likely to fully understand content in the Thoughts module. Open-ended comments by home visitors also indicated some concern with the repetition of the Thoughts module, as well as a lack of clarity regarding when to engage in conversation with clients instead of doing didactic presentation of material.

In response to these client and home visitor feasibility and acceptability data, we have further modified the MB 1-on-1 curriculum. First, we have shortened the curriculum from 15 to 12 sessions by eliminating two Thoughts sessions and consolidating the Overview sessions into

Table 1 Client Acceptability Data and Home Visitor Acceptability and Feasibility Data

	Client Acceptability Data			Home Visitor Acceptability and Feasibility Data		
	% Rating Very Enjoyable (mean, range)	% Rating Totally Understood (mean, range)	% Rating Very Useful (mean, range)	% Rating Material Totally Covered	% Rating Client Totally Understood Material	% Rating Client as Totally Engaged
Across 15 Sessions	82.0	91.6	85.1	87.9	82.5	71.2
By Module						
MB Overview	81.8 (80.3–82.9)	89.8 (88.0–93.4)	86.1 (84.6–88.1)	92.3	78.7	69.2
Pleasant Activities	84.6 (81.3–87.5)	94.3 (92.5–96.0)	84.7 (80.6–88.0)	85.4	95.0	79.4
Thoughts	79.9 (75.0–81.6)	92.4 (88.1–95.5)	83.6 (80.0–86.8)	84.6	74.5	65.5
Contact with Others	84.4 (76.9–93.3)	92.9 (86.7–100.0)	86.5 (84.6–88.9)	85.7	80.1	63.0

Sessions 1–3 = MB Overview, Sessions 4–6 = Pleasant Activities Module; Sessions 7–11 = Thoughts Module, Sessions 12–15 = Contacts with Others module

Table 2 Challenges Related to Implementing MB: Illustrative Home Visitor Qualitative Responses

MB Implementation Challenge	Quote
Children Distracting Client	"Mother of baby was distracted by the baby's crying. MOB had to try and quiet the baby." "Mom was checking on the baby who was fussy."
Client Preoccupied with other Household Items	"Mom busy with daily chores and is constantly distracted." "Lots of people in the home today. Very noisy."
Client Not Completing Personal Projects	"Client always says that she will try to do personal project but then will say she had too much going on to do it." "Although the client did not complete the pleasant activity personal project, she did verbalize that she engaged in 3 pleasant activities."
Repetition of MB Material	"Some parts of the materials are repetitive but I tried not to repeat too much." "List of harmful thoughts was confusing—it had already been covered last week..."
Instructor Manual Needs to Better Facilitate Conversation	"The script is long. I wonder if open ended questions would engage the client better throughout the session."

two sessions. The Additional file 1 presents the revised 12-session MB curriculum. Second, we modified the Instructor's Manual to indicate in each session where home visitors should engage clients in interactive activities, using call-out boxes within each session. Third, we have added details in the Instructor's Manual on the importance of completing personal projects and strategies to facilitate their completion. The revised version of the MB 1-on-1 curriculum is now being more formally tested via a randomized controlled trial to determine the efficacy of the curriculum in improving maternal mental health outcomes.

Several limitations to this study should be noted. Despite survey instructions to provide honest feedback, some social desirability bias among clients and home visitors may have occurred. In particular, it is possible that home visitors may have overstated client engagement in intervention content in an attempt to portray their intervention delivery in a more favorable light. We were also limited in our measurement of certain constructs. For example, client comprehension of the MB curriculum could have been assessed by asking clients to recall key content after it was delivered to them by their home visitor. Similarly, home visitors' coverage of session material could have been examined using audio and/or video recordings that were rated by members of the research team. We opted to rely on self-report of these constructs at this stage of the research, in large part due to fiscal constraints. We plan more rigorous assessment of client comprehension and observational coding of intervention fidelity in future research.

Conclusions

Given the encouraging findings regarding the feasibility and acceptability of MB 1-on-1, we are currently conducting a randomized controlled trial (RCT) to determine the efficacy of the curriculum in reducing depressive symptoms and preventing new incidence of depressive episodes. In conducting this RCT, we are paying particular attention to potential differences between our MB group and 1-on-1 modalities on promotion of social support, given the potential value of group social support provided via the MB group modality. Given the ubiquity of cell phone users who use text messaging [38], we are also exploring the use of text messaging to reinforce MB skills and encourage completion of personal projects. By virtue of its ability for delivery within home visiting, MB 1-on-1 has the potential to help destigmatize engaging in mental health services and eliminate additional appointments to access mental health services. By using staff already salaried by HV programs to deliver the intervention, we believe MB 1-on-1 has considerable promise to improve maternal mental health on a large scale and in a sustainable manner without increased cost to HV programs.

Table 3 Client Enjoyment and Usefulness of MB Intervention: Illustrative Qualitative Responses

Client Acceptability Domain	Quote
Enjoyment of MB Intervention	"I really enjoyed the mood scale. I liked to learn how to recognize my mood". "I enjoyed making a list of pleasant activities to do" "I enjoyed talking about helpful and harmful thoughts. It's good for me to pay attention to any harmful thoughts or helpful thoughts".
Usefulness of MB Intervention	"I enjoyed the way it explains how to manage stress and how it actually describes my stressors and how to manage. Very helpful". "It made me think about how to make a negative day better and what getting up and doing things can do for you". "It was really helpful because I learned some strategies to stop harmful thoughts".

Additional file

Additional file 1: Detailed Description of MB 1-on-1 Session Content. This file provides a detailed descripton of the key topics found in the 12 sessions of the revised Mothers and Babies (MB) 1-on-1 curriculum.

Abbreviations

HV: home visiting; MB 1-on-1: Mothers and Babies 1-on-1 version; MB: Mothers and Babies; OECD: Illinois Governor's Office for Early Childhood Development; RCT: randomized controlled trial; REDCap: Research Electronic Data Capture

Acknowledgements

The authors would like to thank the home visiting programs part of this study for their participation.

Funding

The authors thank the following funders for their generous support of this project: Friends of Prentice, Illinois Governor's Office for Early Childhood Development. These funders had no role in the design and conduct of the study; collection, management, analysis, and interpretation of the data; preparation, review, or approval of the manuscript; and the decision to submit the manuscript for publication.

Authors' contributions

SDT, EW, HS, JL, TM, DP, and HL were responsible for study concept and design. SDT and EW were responsible for study supervision. SDT, EW, MC, & JH were responsible for acquisition of data. SDT and EW were responsible for statistical analysis and interpretation of data. SDT, JL, EW, TM, DP, and HL were responsible for drafting of the manuscript. All authors read and approved the final manuscript.

Competing interests

The authors declare that they have no competing interests.

Author details

[1]Northwestern University Feinberg School of Medicine, 750 N. Lake Shore Drive, 6th Floor, Chicago, IL 60614, USA. [2]James Bell Associates, 3033 Wilson Blvd, Suite 650, Arlington, VA 22201, USA. [3]Department of Psychology, George Washington University, 2125 G. St. NW, Washington, DC 20052, USA. [4]Department of Mental Health, Johns Hopkins University Bloomberg School of Public Health, 624 N. Broadway, Room 853, Baltimore, MD 21205, USA. [5]Center for Child and Human Development, Georgetown University, 3300 Whitehaven St., Suite 3300, Box 571485, Washington, DC 20057, USA.

References

1. Evans J, Heron J, Francomb H, Oke S, Golding J. Cohort study of depressed mood during pregnancy and after childbirth. BMJ. (Clin Res ed). 2001;323(7307):257–60.
2. Gaynes BN, Gavin N, Meltzer-Brody S, Lohr KN, Swinson T, Gartlehner G, Brody S, Miller WC. Perinatal Depression: Prevalence, Screening Accuracy, and Screening Outcomes. Evidence Report/Technology Assessment No. 119. (Prepared by the RTI-University of North Carolina Evidence-based Practice Center, under Contract No. 290-02-0016.) AHRQ Publication No. 05-E006-2. Rockville, MD: Agency for Healthcare Research and Quality; 2005.
3. Moses-Kolko EL, Roth EK. Antepartum and postpartum depression: healthy mom, healthy baby. Journal of the American Medical Women's Association (1972). 2004;59(3):181–91.
4. Segre LS, O'Hara MW, Arndt S, Stuart S. The prevalence of postpartum depression: the relative significance of three social status indices. Soc Psychiatry Psychiatr Epidemiol. 2007;42(4):316–21.
5. Foster CJ, Garber J, Durlak JA. Current and past maternal depression, maternal interaction behaviors, and children's externalizing and internalizing symptoms. J Abnorm Child Psychol. 2008;36(4):527–37.
6. Horwitz SM, Briggs-Gowan MJ, Storfer-Isser A, Carter AS. Prevalence, correlates, and persistence of maternal depression. Journal of women's health (2002). 2007;16(5):678–91.
7. Lovejoy MC, Graczyk PA, O'Hare E, Neuman G. Maternal depression and parenting behavior: a meta-analytic review. Clin Psychol Rev. 2000; 20(5):561–92.
8. Chronicity of maternal depressive symptoms, maternal sensitivity, and child functioning at 36 months. NICHD Early Child Care Research Network. Dev Psychol 1999, 35(5):1297–1310.
9. Howell EA, Mora PA, Horowitz CR, Leventhal H. Racial and ethnic differences in factors associated with early postpartum depressive symptoms. Obstet Gynecol. 2005;105(6):1442–50.
10. Mora PA, Bennett IM, Elo IT, Mathew L, Coyne JC, Culhane JF. Distinct trajectories of perinatal depressive symptomatology: evidence from growth mixture modeling. Am J Epidemiol. 2009;169(1):24–32.
11. Bennett HA, Einarson A, Taddio A, Koren G, Einarson TR. Prevalence of depression during pregnancy: systematic review. Obstet Gynecol. 2004;103(4):698–709.
12. Dolbier CL, Rush TE, Sahadeo LS, Shaffer ML, Thorp J. Relationships of race and socioeconomic status to postpartum depressive symptoms in rural African American and non-Hispanic white women. Matern Child Health J. 2013;17(7):1277–87.
13. Holzman C, Eyster J, Tiedje LB, Roman LA, Seagull E, Rahbar MH. A life course perspective on depressive symptoms in mid-pregnancy. Matern Child Health J. 2006;10(2):127–38.
14. Cuijpers P, de Graaf R, van Dorsselaer S. Minor depression: risk profiles, functional disability, health care use and risk of developing major depression. J Affect Disord. 2004;79(1–3):71.
15. Wagner HR, Burns BJ, Broadhead WE, Yarnall KS, Sigmon A, Gaynes BN. Minor depression in family practice: functional morbidity, co-morbidity, service utilization and outcomes. Psychol Med. 2000;30(6):1377–90.
16. Dennis CL, Dowswell T. Psychosocial and psychological interventions for preventing postpartum depression. Cochrane Database Syst Rev. 2013;28(2):Cd001134.
17. Dennis CL, Hodnett E, Kenton L, Weston J, Zupancic J, Stewart DE, Kiss A. Effect of peer support on prevention of postnatal depression among high risk women: multisite randomised controlled trial. BMJ (Clinical research ed). 2009;338:a3064.
18. Leis JA, Mendelson T, Perry DF, Tandon SD. Perceptions of mental health services among low-income, perinatal African-American women. Women's health issues : official publication of the Jacobs Institute of Women's Health. 2011;21(4):314–9.
19. Nadeem E, Lange JM, Edge D, Fongwa M, Belin T, Miranda J. Does stigma keep poor young immigrant and U.S.-born black and Latina women from seeking mental health care? Psychiatric services. Washington, DC. 2007;58(12):1547–54.
20. Sama -Miller E, Akers L, Mraz-Esposito A, Zukiewicz M, Avellar S, Paulsell D, Del Grosso P. Home visiting evidence of effectiveness review: executive summary. Office of Planning, research and evaluation, Administration for Children and Families, U.S. Washington, DC: Department of health and human services; 2017.
21. Stevens J, Ammerman RT, Putnam FW, Van Ginkel JB. Depression and trauma history in first-time mothers receiving home visitation. Journal of Community Psychology. 2002;30:551–64.
22. Tandon SD, Mercer C, Saylor E, Duggan AK. Paraprofessional home visitors' perceptions of addressing poor mental health, substance abuse, and domestic violence: a qualitative study. Early Childhood Research Quarterly. 2008;23:419–28.
23. Jacobs S, Easterbrooks MA. Healthy Familes Massachusetts final evaluation report. 2005. [Retrieved January 1, 2009]. from http://ase.tufts.edu/tier/documents/Phase1-FinalReport.pdf.
24. Administration on Children Youth and Families. Making a difference in the lives of children and families: The impacts of early head start programs on infants and toddlers and their families. Washington, DC: U.S: Department of Health and Human Services; 2002.

25. Health Resources and Services Administration. 2018. The Maternal, Infant, and Early Childhood Home Visiting Program. Program Brief. https://mchb.hrsa.gov/sites/default/files/mchb/MaternalChildHealthInitiatives/HomeVisiting/pdf/programbrief.pdf. Accessed 1 Feb 2018.
26. Ammerman RT, Putnam FW, Bosse NR, Teeters AR, Van Ginkel JB. Maternal depression in home visitation: a systematic review. Aggress Violent Behav. 2010;15(3):191–200.
27. Tandon SD, Parillo KM, Jenkins CJ, Duggan AK. Home visitors' recognition of and response to malleable risk factors among low-income pregnant and parenting women. Matern Child Health J. 2005;18:873–81.
28. Le HN, Perry DF, Stuart EA. Randomized controlled trial of a preventive intervention for perinatal depression in high-risk Latinas. J Consult Clin Psychol. 2011;79(2):135–41.
29. McFarlane E, Burrell L, Duggan A, Tandon D. Outcomes of a randomized trial of a cognitive behavioral enhancement to address maternal distress in home visited mothers. Matern Child Health J. 2016;21(3):475–84.
30. Muñoz RF, Le H-N, Ippen CG, Diaz MA, Urizar GG, Soto J, Mendelson T, Delucchi K, Lieberman AF. Prevention of postpartum depression in low-income women: development of the Mamás y Bebés/mothers and babies course. Cogn Behav Pract. 2007;14(1):70–83.
31. Tandon SD, Perry DF, Mendelson T, Kemp K, Leis JA. Preventing perinatal depression in low-income home visiting clients: a randomized controlled trial. J Consult Clin Psychol. 2011;79(5):707–12.
32. Tandon SD, Leis JA, Mendelson T, Perry DF, Kemp K. Six-month outcomes from a randomized controlled trial to prevent perinatal depression in low-income home visiting clients. Matern Child Health J. 2014;18(4):873–81.
33. Bieling PJ, McCabe RE, Antony MM. Cognitive-behavioral therapy in groups: Guilford publications; 2013.
34. Healthy Families America National Office, (2018). Prevent Child Abuse America. Program description Retrieved from: http://www.healthyfamiliesamerica.org
35. Parents as Teachers National Center. (2018). Retrieved from: http://www.parentsasteachers.org.
36. Boyatzis RE: Transforming qualitative information: thematic analysis and code development: SAGE publications; 1998.
37. Castro FG, Barrera M Jr, Martinez CR Jr. The cultural adaptation of prevention interventions: resolving tensions between fidelity and fit. Prevention science : the official journal of the Society for Prevention Research. 2004;5(1):41–5.
38. Hall AK, Cole-Lewis H, Bernhardt JM. Mobile text messaging for health: a systematic review of reviews. Annu Rev Public Health. 2015;36:393–415.

Urinary iodine concentration and thyroid volume of pregnant women attending antenatal care in two selected hospitals in Ashanti Region, Ghana

Daniel Gyamfi[1*], Yaw Amo Wiafe[2], Kwabena Owusu Danquah[1], Ernest Adankwah[1], Gertrude Akua Amissah[1] and Angela Odame[2]

Abstract

Background: Iodine deficiency is a major public health problem affecting people worldwide, particularly pregnant women. Iodine requirements increase substantially during pregnancy making pregnant women vulnerable to iodine deficiency and its disorders such as abortions, stillbirths and pregnancy goitre as well as congenital abnormalities, cretinism and mental retardation in their children. The primary aim of this study was to evaluate the prevalence of iodine deficiency and goitre among pregnant women attending antenatal sessions at two selected hospitals in Ashanti region, Ghana.

Methods: A cross-sectional study was carried out in 239 pregnant women who attended the antenatal clinic at Kwame Nkrumah University of Science and Technology (KNUST) Hospital or Ejura District Hospital, both in Ashanti Region, Ghana. Socio-demographic data and information related to iodine were captured using a questionnaire. Urinary iodine concentration (UIC) was determined on spot urine samples using the Sandell-Kolthoff reaction with ammonium persulfate as digesting agent. Each woman's thyroid volume was also measured by ultrasonography.

Results: The overall median UIC was 155.9 μg/L, indicating adequate iodine intake in the study population. However, goitre prevalence in the pregnant women was 11.3%, denoting mild iodine deficiency. The median UIC for pregnant women who attended KNUST Hospital was higher (163.8 μg/L) than that of Ejura District Hospital (149.0 μg/L). The proportion of women who did not consume iodised salt was significantly higher ($p < 0.001$) in Ejura District Hospital (71.2%) than KNUST Hospital (28.0%). In total, 47.3% of the pregnant women studied had a UIC < 150 μg/L. Only 16.3% knew about the increase in iodine requirement during pregnancy and 21.3% of them had knowledge of the effects of iodine deficiency during pregnancy with most (81.8%) knowing of pregnancy goitre.

Conclusion: There is generally adequate iodine intake among the pregnant women, however, iodine deficiency and goitre still exist among some pregnant women. Thus, assessment and continuous monitoring of iodine nutritional status in pregnant women in the country are warranted. Also, intensification of effective public health campaigns (through radio and television) with regard to iodine utilization and its benefits in pregnancy are still recommended among Ghanaian pregnant women.

Keywords: Iodine deficiency, Excessive iodine intake, Pregnant women, Thyroid volume, Goitre

* Correspondence: danigya2@gmail.com; dgyamfi.chs@knust.edu.gh
[1]Department of Medical Laboratory Technology, Faculty of Allied Health Sciences, Kwame Nkrumah University of Science and Technology, Kumasi, Ghana
Full list of author information is available at the end of the article

Background

Iodine is an important component of the thyroid hormones which regulate the body's metabolic rate and are essential for brain development [1], especially during the gestational period and early childhood [2]. Iodine deficiency during pregnancy results in several problems such as abortions, stillbirths, congenital abnormalities, cretinism, goitre, mental retardation, squinting and mutism [3, 4].

Pregnant women are vulnerable to iodine deficiency since iodine requirements increase substantially during pregnancy [5]. This increase is due to many factors such as an increased demand for thyroxine (T4) in the mother so as to sustain normal metabolism, transport of T4 as well as iodide from the mother to the foetus [2], and an enhanced renal clearance of iodide [6], thus putting pregnant women and their unborn children at high risk of developing a series of functional and developmental abnormalities commonly known as iodine deficiency disorders (IDD) [7]. Based on this increase, the iodine requirement recommended by World Health Organization (WHO) for pregnant women (250 μg/day) is higher than that for adults (150 μg/day) [8].

A prolonged low intake of iodine may cause the thyroid gland of pregnant women to attempt to be more active in order to maintain required levels of thyroid hormones in the blood [9]. This makes the thyroid gland increases in size in order to trap iodine, a condition commonly referred to as pregnancy goitre [10]. The effects of in utero iodine deficiency on the developing foetus may have life-long effects on the offspring [11]. Buxton and Baguune [12] reported that due to iodine deficiency, 120,000 children born each year in Ghana stand a risk of developing intellectual impairment. They also realised that nearly 15,600 (13%) of these children are severely impaired and unable to develop normally, resulting in annual productivity loss of about 22 million dollars [12].

The Declaration for the Survival, Protection and Development of Children, which occurred after the World Summit for Children organized by the United Nations in 1989, stated that every mother is entitled to sufficient iodine nutrition to guarantee the normal brain development of her new-born child [13]. Fortification of salt with iodine - Universal Salt Iodization (USI) - is the most widespread, long-term and effective preventive strategy against IDDs introduced by WHO since 1920 [14]. The USI programme was launched in Ghana in 1995 to improve the consumption of iodised salt [4]. Salt iodization programmes are able in most cases to supply adequate iodine to meet the needs of adults but may not provide enough to meet the needs of pregnant women [15]. It is, therefore, imperative to do a regular check on the pregnant women's iodine status in a population [15]. In order to do this, the WHO and the International Council for the Control of Iodine Deficiency Disorders (ICCIDD) recommended the determination of urinary iodine concentration as a suitable marker for monitoring iodine status in a population as well as measurement of thyroid size by ultrasonography [16]. Urinary iodine concentration is a marker of very recent iodine intake, whereas thyroid volume reflects long-term status rather than current intake [16].

Therefore, it is against this background that this study was organized to evaluate the iodine status in pregnant women who attended antenatal care at Kwame Nkrumah University of Science and Technology (KNUST) Hospital or Ejura District Hospital using urinary iodine concentration and thyroid volume, and to assess the possible sources of iodine consumption, sources of information on iodine utilisation, and knowledge of the increased iodine requirement or the effects of iodine insufficiency during pregnancy.

Methods

Design

This is a cross sectional study to assess urinary iodine concentration and thyroid volume in pregnant women in various trimesters who attended antenatal clinic at KNUST Hospital or Ejura District Hospital from January to April 2016. Prior to the study, a sample size of 222 was determined based on a previous prevalence of iodine deficiency of 42.5% found in pregnant women in the central part of Ghana [17]. The estimate generated was based on a two-sided alpha level of 5%, a marginal error of 6.5% and a confidence interval of 95%. Ethical clearance was sought from and approved by the Committee on Human Research, Publications and Ethics (CHRPE), KNUST, School of Medical Sciences and Komfo Anokye Teaching Hospital. The ethical approval reference number is CHRPE/RC/058/16. Permission to undertake the study at the hospitals was also sought from the hospital management. Written informed consent was obtained from all participants recruited into the study.

Setting

The study was carried out in two randomly selected hospitals in Ashanti Region, Ghana. These hospitals are KNUST and Ejura District Hospitals. The KNUST Hospital is located in Kumasi – the regional capital and the second largest city in Ghana. The KNUST Hospital is the medical arm of the university. The hospital caters for a population of over 200,000 including students, staff and dependants and about 150,000 people from over 30 surrounding communities, including Ayigya, Bomso, Ayeduase, Kotei, Boadi, Deduako, Oforikrom and Anloga. There is a turnover of about 75–100 antenatal cases each week.

The Ejura District Hospital is situated in Ejura, the capital of Ejura-Sekyedumase Municipal Assembly in the Ashanti Region. Ejura is about 96 km from the regional capital, Kumasi. Ejura District Hospital caters for a settlement population of about 39,121 including antenatal cases from surrounding towns such as Miminaso, Anyinasu, Babaso and Sekyedumase.

Participants

Recruitment of participants was done on each clinic day. On each day, every potential participant was approached and those who consented were recruited. Participants were recruited consecutively without specific preference to the trimester of pregnancy. Pregnant women with a history of thyroid disease, on thyroid medication and those who have had thyroidectomy in addition to pregnant women who had a history of smoking [18] were to be excluded, but none of the women approached warranted exclusion. In total, two hundred and thirty–nine (239) women in different trimesters of pregnancy were recruited for the study; 93 from KNUST Hospital and 146 from Ejura District Hospital.

Administration of questionnaire

A questionnaire were designed to obtain information on socio-demographics, medical history, the use of tobacco, sources of iodine utilisation and knowledge of iodine utilisation, knowledge of effects of iodine deficiency or increased iodine requirement during pregnancy (see Additional file 1). The questionnaire was pilot-tested at KNUST Hospital, one of the study sites, by 50 participants and questions were modified based on feedback received. The study questionnaire was administered to participants from both hospitals via face to face interview conducted by trained research staff. The first section of the questionnaire asked about socio-demographic data, in which the women provided descriptive background information, while the second section of the questionnaire was related to consumption of iodised salt at home, intake of marine fish and iodine supplements, and sources of information on iodine utilisation. The third section asked about knowledge of the increase in iodine requirement and the effects of iodine deficiency during pregnancy, as well as medical history and the use of tobacco.

Urinary iodine determination

Spot morning urine samples were collected from the women into clean, sterile, leak-proof plastic urine sample containers. Samples were kept in an ice chest in the antenatal clinics and transported on the same day to the Micronutrient Research Laboratory at Cancer and Infection Research Facility, KNUST. The samples were stored at − 20 °C until analysis. The Micronutrient Research Laboratory is an active participant of Ensuring the Quality of Urinary Iodine Procedures (EQUIP) of the US Centres for Disease Control and Prevention implemented to ensure good laboratory practice and the production of reliable urinary iodine results worldwide [19]. Urinary iodine concentration (UIC) (μg/L) was determined spectrophotometrically using the Sandell-Kolthoff reaction with ammonium persulfate as the digesting agent, one of the three most common methods used by participants of EQUIP programme [20]. This method is based on the principle that iodide released after digestion of urine with ammonium persulfate catalyses the reduction of ceric ammonium sulphate (yellow) to its cerous form (colourless) in the presence of arsenious acid which is detected by the rate of disappearance of the colour [16]. Following the protocol described by EQUIP [20], the participants' urine samples were run in addition to iodine standards (0, 20, 40, 80, 120, 200, and 300 μg/L of iodine prepared from potassium iodate), internal quality control (IQC) samples (low and high concentrations) obtained from pooled urine samples, and external quality control samples from EQUIP.

Briefly, 1 mL of ammonium persulfate was added to 250 μL of urine samples, standards and quality control samples in separate test tubes, vortexed and heated in JB Aqua 18 plus water bath (Grant, UK) at 91-95 °C for 1 h to digest the sample. After cooling to room temperature, arsenious acid (3.5 mL) was added to each tube and incubated for 15 min at room temperature. Ceric ammonium sulphate (400 μL) was then added, vortexed and incubated at room temperature. At exactly 30 min after the addition of the ceric ammonium sulphate, the absorbance was read using LI-722 Visible Spectrophotometer (Lasany, India) at 420 nm. Using the developed iodine standard curve, the urinary iodine concentrations in the samples were obtained and WHO/ICCIDD reference medians for urinary iodine concentration were used to classify iodine intake as deficient (< 150 μg/L), adequate (150–249 μg/L), more than adequate (250–499 μg/L) or excess (≥500 μg/L) [21]. The coefficients of variation of inter-assay of the IQC samples were 8.0 and 9.2% at concentrations of 120 μg/L and 256 μg/L, respectively.

Assessment of thyroid volume

In both centres, thyroid ultrasound was performed for all participants by the same sonographer who had 4 years scanning experience using the same portable machine. All scans were performed with a portable Siemens-Acuson P300 (Siemens Company, USA) equipped with a 7.5–12 MHz linear array transducer. Briefly, the pregnant women were asked to lie in the supine position with hyperextension of the neck. An ultrasound scan of the thyroid gland was then performed. Each lobe of the thyroid gland was assessed separately by measuring the three dimensions (height x width x length). The total volume calculated is the sum of the volumes of the right and left lobes without the inclusion of the isthmus. A normal thyroid gland was classified as the detection of a homogenous thyroid gland which was less than or equal to the 18 mL upper limit for women [22]. A goitre was categorized as a diffuse enlargement of the thyroid gland of more than 18 mL [22]. Texture of the thyroid gland was classified as normal, nodular or diffuse [23].

Data analysis

Data were entered into Microsoft Excel, version 2010 (Microsoft Corporation, USA) and statistical analysis was performed using SPSS Statistics for Windows, version 21 (Armonk, NY: IBM Corp). Simple descriptive statistics such as frequencies and percentages and inferences based on chi-square test were performed on categorical variables such as age categories, stage of trimester, level of education, iodine use, and categories of iodine concentration. Ages of pregnant women were put into 6 categories with a class interval of 5. Kolmogorov-Smirnov test was used to determine the normality of the distribution of numeric data values. Consequently, non-parametric test (Mann-Whitney U test) was utilized to find the association between urinary iodine concentration and categories of thyroid volumes (≤18 mL and > 18 mL). Also, the correlation between two continuous variables (urinary iodine concentration and thyroid volume) was performed using Spearman rank correlation. The iodine status of the study population was calculated as median (interquartile range [IQR]) for UIC and thyroid volume. A two-tailed p value of less than 0.05 was considered as statistically significant.

Results

Socio-demographic and pregnancy-related characteristics of the participants

Of the total number of participants (239), 146 of the pregnant women attended antenatal clinic at Ejura District Hospital and 93 pregnant women at the KNUST Hospital (Table 1). The mean age of the study population was 27.6 ± 6.19 years. Out of the 6 age-categories, most of the women were in the 20–25 (33.5%) and 26–30 (35.6%) age ranges. Majority of the pregnant women were in their third trimester (46.9%) with most of them having no level of formal education (31.8%). The proportion of women with no level of formal education was higher ($p < 0.001$) at Ejura District Hospital (45.9%) than KNUST Hospital (9.7%).

Table 1 Socio-demographic and pregnancy-related characteristics of the pregnant women

	KNUST Hospital n (%)	EJURA Hospital n (%)	Total n (%)	P value*
Age (Years)				0.072
< 20	4 (4.3)	13 (8.9)	17 (7.1)	
20–25	25 (26.9)	55 (37.7)	80 (33.5)	
26–30	33 (35.5)	52 (35.6)	85 (35.6)	
31–35	17 (18.3)	15 (10.3)	32 (13.4)	
36–40	12 (12.9)	6 (4.1)	18 (7.5)	
≥ 40	2 (2.1)	5 (3.4)	7 (2.9)	
Total	93 (100)	146 (100)	239 (100)	
Mean age (years)	28.9	26.7	27.6	0.063
Trimester				0.025
First	29 (31.2)	24 (16.4)	53 (22.2)	
Second	27 (29.0)	47 (32.2)	74 (31.0)	
Third	37 (39.8)	75 (51.4)	112 (46.9)	
Total	93 (100)	146 (100)	239 (100)	
Level of Education				< 0.001
None	9 (9.7)	67 (45.9)	76 (31.8)	
Primary	2 (2.2)	29 (19.7)	31 (13.0)	
JHS	28 (30.1)	32 (21.9)	60 (25.1)	
SHS	35 (37.6)	10 (6.9)	45 (18.8)	
Tertiary	19 (20.4)	8 (5.5)	27 (11.3)	
Total	93 (100)	146 (100)	239 (100)	

JHS: Junior High School; SHS: Senior High School
*p values are based on chi-square test

Urinary iodine concentration and thyroid volume in the study population

The overall median urinary iodine concentration (UIC) of the pregnant women was 155.9 μg/L (109.4–235.3), showing an adequate iodine intake. However, the median UIC was higher in pregnant women who attended the antenatal clinic at KNUST Hospital [163.8 μg/L (107.3–258.4)] [adequate iodine intake] than those who attended the Ejura District Hospital [149.0 μg/L (108.9–224.4)], though the difference was not statistically significant. In total, 47.3% of the pregnant women studied had a UIC < 150 μg/L. Only 30.5% of the pregnant women had a UIC of 150–249 μg/L with 21.3 and 0.8% recording UIC of 250–499 μg/L and ≥ 500 μg/L, respectively. The proportion of pregnant women with UIC < 150 μg/L was higher in Ejura District Hospital (50.7%) than KNUST Hospital (41.9%), however, the difference was not

Table 2 Comparison of iodine status and sources of iodine utilisation of pregnant women who attended KNUST Hospital and Ejura District Hospital

	KNUST Hospital *n* (%)	EJURA Hospital *n* (%)	Total *n* (%)	*P* value*
Urinary Iodine Concentration (μg/L) (*n* = 239)				0.221
< 150	39 (41.9)	74 (50.7)	113 (47.3)	
150–249	29 (31.2)	44 (30.1)	73 (30.5)	
250–499	25 (26.9)	26 (17.8)	51 (21.3)	
≥ 500	0 (0.0)	2 (1.4)	2 (0.8)	
Use of Iodised Salt (n = 239)				< 0.001
Yes	67 (72.0)	42 (28.8)	109 (45.6)	
No	26 (28.0)	104 (71.2)	130 (54.4)	
Marine Fish Consumption (n = 239)				0.295
Yes	91 (97.8)	139 (95.2)	230 (96.2)	
No	2 (2.2)	7 (4.8)	9 (3.8)	
Usage of iodine supplement (n = 239)				0.777
Yes	2 (2.2)	4 (2.7)	6 (2.5)	
No	91 (97.8)	142 (97.3)	233 (97.5)	

*p values are based on chi-square test

statistically significant (Table 2). Also, the proportion of women who did not use iodised salt was significantly higher ($p < 0.001$) in Ejura District Hospital (71.2%) than KNUST Hospital (28.0%).

The median thyroid volume of the study population was 8.4 mL (6.5–10.9). Prevalence of goitre among the pregnant women was 11.3%. About 2.9% had diffuse goitre whilst 8.4% had nodular goitre. In the goitrous population, the prevalence of diffuse goitre was higher among pregnant women who attended Ejura District Hospital (38.5%) as compared to pregnant women who attended KNUST Hospital (14.3%). There was slightly larger proportion of women with thyroid volume > 18 mL in the second and third trimesters (4.1 and 2.7%, respectively) than the first trimester (1.9%). A greater number of women (4.6%) who did not use iodised salt had thyroid volume of > 18 mL, compared to those (0.9%) who used iodised salt (Table 3). However, all these differences were not statistically significant.

Table 3 Thyroid volume and its relationship with trimester and use of iodised salt

	Thyroid volume ≤ 18 mL *n* (%)	Thyroid volume > 18 mL *n* (%)
Trimester		
First (*n* = 53)	52 (98.1)	1(1.9)
Second (*n* = 74)	71 (96.0)	3 (4.1)
Third (*n* = 112)	109 (97.3)	3 (2.7)
Use of Iodised Salt		
Yes (*n* = 109)	108 (99.1)	1 (0.9)
No (*n* = 130)	124 (95.4)	6 (4.6)

Relationship between urinary iodine concentration and other parameters studied

The study observed a clinically significant negative weak correlation between urinary iodine concentration and thyroid volume ($r = -0.142$; $p = 0.028$). A greater proportion of pregnant women with lower UIC (< 150 μg/L) had thyroid volume > 18 mL (71.4%) whereas 46.6% of pregnant women with lower UIC had thyroid volume ≤ 18 mL (Table 4). Pregnant women who had a UIC of 150–249 μg/L with thyroid volume ≤ 18 mL were 31.0% as against 14.3% pregnant women who had thyroid volume > 18 mL. The median UIC was 132.5 μg/L (44.6–221.0) and 156.9 μg/L (110.8–236.8) in pregnant women who had thyroid volume > 18 mL and ≤ 18 mL, respectively. However, the difference was not statistically significant.

The age of the pregnant women, gestational age, level of education, gravidity and the use of iodised salt did not associate significantly with UIC (Table 4). However, the number of pregnant women with a UIC of 150–249 μg/L was higher in the first trimester (22/52) compared with the second (19/74) and third (32/112) trimesters. In addition, pregnant women who had no level of education recorded the highest number of women with a UIC < 150 μg/L (41/113). Similarly, a high number of pregnant women who did not use iodised salt had a UIC < 150 μg/L (67/113).

Table 4 Relationship of urinary iodine concentration with various parameters

	Urinary Iodine Concentration [*n* (%)]					*P* value
	< 150(μg/L)	150–249(μg/L)	250–499(μg/L)	≥500(μg/L)	TOTAL	
Age group (years)						0.801
< 20	7 (41.2%)	9 (52.9%)	1 (5.9%)	0 (0.0%)	17 (100%)	
20–25	44 (55.0%)	20 (25.0%)	15 (18.8%)	1 (1.3%)	80 (100%)	
26–30	36 (42.4%)	30 (35.3%)	19 (22.4%)	0 (0.0%)	85 (100%)	
31–35	15 (46.9%)	9 (28.1%)	8 (25.0%)	0 (0.0%)	32 (100%)	
36–40	9 (45.0%)	3 (15.0%)	8 (40.0%)	0 (0.0%)	20 (100%)	
> 40	2 (40.0%)	2 (40.0%)	0 (0.0%)	1 (20.0%)	5 (100%)	
Trimester						0.755
First	23 (43.4%)	22 (41.5%)	8 (15.1%)	0 (0.0%)	53 (100%)	
Second	33 (44.6%)	19 (25.7%)	22 (29.7%)	0 (0.0%)	74 (100%)	
Third	57 (50.9%)	32 (28.6%)	21 (18.8%)	2 (1.8%)	112 (100%)	
Education						0.445
None	41 (54.0%)	21 (27.6%)	13 (17.1%)	1 (1.3%)	76 (100%)	
Primary	17 (54.8%)	8 (25.8%)	5 (16.1%)	1 (3.2%)	31 (100%)	
JHS	24 (40.0%)	25 (41.7%)	11 (18.3%)	0 (0.0%)	60 (100%)	
SHS	19 (42.2)	13 (28.9%)	13 (28.9%)	0 (0.0%)	45 (100%)	
Tertiary	12 (44.4%)	6 (22.2%)	9 (33.3%)	0 (0.0%)	27 (100%)	
Gravidity						0.562
< 3	62 (48.1%)	37 (28.7%)	29 (22.5%)	1 (0.8%)	129 (100%)	
3–5	43 (47.8%)	26 (28.9%)	20 (22.2%)	1 (1.1%)	90 (100%)	
> 5	8 (40.0%)	10 (50.0%)	2 (10.0%)	0 (0.0%)	20 (100%)	
Use Of Iodised Salt						0.115
Yes	46 (42.2%)	34 (31.2%)	28 (25.7%)	1 (0.9%)	109 (100%)	
No	67 (51.5%)	39 (30.0%)	23 (17.7%)	1 (0.8%)	130 (100%)	
Thyroid volume (ml)						0.028
≤ 18	108 (46.6%)	72 (31.0%)	50 (21.6%)	2 (0.9%)	232 (100%)	
> 18	5 (71.4%)	1 (14.3%)	1 (14.3%)	0 (0.0%)	7 (100%)	

P values are based on chi-square test

Knowledge of increased iodine requirement or effects of iodine insufficiency and sources of information on iodine intake during pregnancy

Most of the participants (83.7%) had no knowledge of the increased iodine requirements during pregnancy (Table 5). Only 21.3% pregnant women out of the total study population had knowledge of the benefits of iodine consumption during pregnancy. It was observed that most of the women had no knowledge (86.2%) of the effects of iodine insufficiency in the mother or child. Out of those who had knowledge (13.8%), a greater proportion knew about pregnancy goitre (81.8%), followed by mental retardation (48.5%), cretinism (21.2%) and squinting (3.0%), but none had knowledge of both mutism and stillbirth (data not shown). Radio and television constituted the major sources of information on iodine and its benefits among the participants (91.6%). Only a few of the women (6.0%) had received information on iodine through health workers in their various hospitals and no pregnant woman had learnt about iodine from fliers or posters (Table 5).

Discussion

Iodine is required for the synthesis of thyroid hormones, which are crucial regulators of early brain development. Iodine requirement increases during pregnancy and insufficiency during pregnancy can cause maternal hypothyroidism leading to pregnancy goitre and foetal hypothyroidism, which causes impaired neurological development of the foetus [1]. The study mainly sought to determine the urinary iodine concentration and thyroid volume in pregnant women who attended antenatal clinics at two selected hospitals - KNUST Hospital and Ejura District Hospital, all in Ashanti Region, Ghana.

Table 5 Knowledge of iodine requirement and iodine insufficiency effects and sources of information on iodine utilisation

	KNUST Hospital	EJURA Hospital	Total
	n (%)	*n* (%)	*n* (%)
Knowledge of increased iodine requirement			
Yes	17 (18.3)	22 (15.1)	39 (16.3)
No	76(81.7)	124 (84.9)	200(83.7)
Knowledge of effects of iodine insufficiency during pregnancy			
No	77 (82.8)	129 (88.4)	206 (86.2)
Yes	16 (17.2)	17 (11.6)	33 (13.8)
Sources of information			
Radio and television	76(81.7)	143(98.0)	219(91.6)
School	12(12.9)	2(1.4)	14(5.9)
Health Workers	5(5.4)	1(0.7)	6(2.5)
Fliers	0(0.00)	0(0.0)	0(0.0)
Posters	0(0.00)	0(0.0)	0(0.0)

Generally, the median UIC obtained in the study population (155.9 μg/L) indicates adequate iodine intake according to WHO criteria [20]. However, of the 239 pregnant women recruited, 113 (47.3%) had a UIC < 150 μg/L as judged by urinary iodine concentration. A similar finding was obtained in a recent study carried out among pregnant women by Simpong et al. [17] at Kissi Health Centre in the Central Region of Ghana where 42.5% of pregnant women were iodine deficient by the same method. However, Simpong et al. [17] did not assess the thyroid volume in their study. Our study showed goitre prevalence of 11.3%, indicating mild iodine deficiency among the pregnant women [24]. These results suggest that some Ghanaian pregnant women are still not meeting the higher iodine requirements during pregnancy; this may lead to a negative effect on foetal brain development [25–27] and thus a general survey of iodine nutritional status in pregnancy is recommended.

In this study, it was found that the iodine status of pregnant women who attended antenatal care at Ejura District Hospital (located far from the regional capital) was just below the cut-off for sufficiency as recommended by WHO, with median UIC of 149 μg/L (generally adequate) whereas pregnant women who attended antenatal care at the KNUST Hospital (found in the regional capital) had median UIC of 164 μg/L (adequacy). Additionally, thyroid volume was found to be increased in 38.5%(7) of pregnant women who attended antenatal at Ejura District Hospital as compared to 14.3% of pregnant women attending KNUST Hospital. The difference in the median UIC and thyroid volume in these areas can be attributed to iodised salt intake since consumption of table salt is the main factor that influences iodine intake in countries which have implemented the universal salt iodization programme [28]. This study found that iodised salt intake in pregnant women at Ejura District Hospital was 28.8% as compared to 72.0% seen in pregnant women at KNUST Hospital. A similar trend was reported by Habimana et al. [29] who also obtained median UIC to be lower in a suburban area than urban area in Republic of Congo. Sultanalieva et al. [30] and Simpong et al. [17] also concluded that the iodine nutritional status was highly responsive to the use of iodised salt. This means that there should be continuous monitoring and education among pregnant women on the need to use iodised salt.

It was observed in this study that the association between urinary iodine concentration and thyroid volume was clinically significant ($p = 0.028$). Median UIC was 138.2 μg/L in pregnant women who had thyroid volume > 18 mL and 155.9 μg/L in those who had ≤18 mL. Research conducted in various countries to assess maternal urinary iodine concentration and thyroid volume indicated that in iodine deficient pregnant women, thyroid volume increased significantly [31–35]. During pregnancy, the thyroid becomes more active leading to the production of about 50% more thyroid hormones than usual [36]. Giusti et al. [10] stated that a reduced intake of iodine for a long period of time may stimulate the thyroid gland of pregnant women to be more active to maintain the correct level of thyroid hormones in the blood. This means that the thyroid increases in size in order to trap more iodine, which leads to pregnancy goitre (thyroid volume > 18 mL). This could account for the increased thyroid volume seen in pregnant women with UIC < 150 μg/L in this study.

The finding of slightly higher thyroid volume values during the second and third trimesters of pregnancy than the first trimester is consistent with previous reports from other researchers [29, 31, 37]. This could be explained by the increase in oestrogen concentration during pregnancy which peaks during the third trimester to enable the uterus and placenta to improve vascularization [38]. Oestrogen induces increased synthesis of thyroid hormone binding proteins and since greater than 99% of thyroid hormones in the blood are attached to these proteins, the total thyroid hormone concentration in the blood consequently increases [39]. This implies that more iodine is needed for the increased thyroid hormone synthesis across the first trimester to the third [5]. A relatively low iodine intake during pregnancy with time, leads to thyroidal stress, with increases in thyroid size [40]. This thus calls for education and monitoring of iodine status in pregnant women during early stage of the pregnancy and thereafter.

Only fifty-one (21.3%) of the pregnant women had knowledge of the effect of iodine deficiency during pregnancy with knowledge of pregnancy goitre being the highest (81.8%). A similar study performed at Kaneshie Polyclinic in the Greater Accra Region of Ghana revealed that 79.4% of pregnant women knew about pregnancy goitre more than the other effects [41]. Most participants reported getting knowledge of iodine intake from radio and television (91.6%). A few obtained the knowledge from school (5.9%) and health workers at their hospitals (2.5%). However, a study in Australian pregnant women showed that most pregnant women obtained knowledge of iodine and its effects from their healthcare professionals (49.0%) at various health centres, with 35.2% of them not having any knowledge of iodine [42]. This indicates that public health campaign strategic on the importance of iodine consumption involving radio and television needs to be utilised more in Ghana besides encouraging health workers in our antenatal care centres to intensify the education on iodine and its importance during pregnancy.

Conclusion

These findings suggest that after more than two decades of the implementation of the universal salt iodisation programme in Ghana, iodine intake in our study population is adequate, however, iodine deficiency still exists in some pregnant women and these women are at risk of iodine deficiency disorders. Also, utilization of iodised salt as well as knowledge of increased requirement of iodine during pregnancy is generally low among the women especially those in areas far from the regional capital. Efforts need to be intensified through better educational programmes on the benefits and increased use of iodised salt during pregnancy in such areas. Further research is recommended to look at the possible barriers to the use of iodised salt especially in areas far from the regional capitals. Also, longitudinal study can be conducted to find the changes in iodine status over the course of pregnancy in the women in our setting.

Abbreviations

CHRPE: Committee on Human Research, Publications and Ethics; EQUIP: Ensuring the Quality of Urinary Iodine Procedures; ICCIDD: International Council for the Control of Iodine Deficiency Disorders; IDD: Iodine deficiency disorders; IQC: Internal quality control; IQR: Interquartile range; KNUST: Kwame Nkrumah University of Science and Technology; T4: Thyroxine; UIC: Urinary iodine concentration; WHO: World Health Organization

Acknowledgments

We are grateful to the authorities of KNUST and Ejura District Hospitals for allowing us to carry out this study on the pregnant women attending antenatal care in their facilities.

Authors' contributions

DG and YAW contributed substantially to the conception and design, acquisition of data, analysis and interpretation of data, and writing of the manuscript. KOD and EA made substantial contributions to the conception and design, analysis and interpretation of data, and writing of the manuscript. GAA and AO made substantial contributions to the acquisition of data, analysis and interpretation of data, and writing of the manuscript. All authors read and approved the final manuscript.

Competing interests

The authors declare that they have no competing interests.

Author details

[1]Department of Medical Laboratory Technology, Faculty of Allied Health Sciences, Kwame Nkrumah University of Science and Technology, Kumasi, Ghana. [2]Department of Sonography, Faculty of Allied Health Sciences, Kwame Nkrumah University of Science and Technology, Kumasi, Ghana.

References

1. Mobasseri M, Roshanravan N, Mesri Alamdari N, Ostadrahimi A, Asghari Jafarabadi M, Anari F, et al. Urinary and milk iodine status in neonates and their mothers during congenital hypothyroidism screening program in eastern Azerbaijan: a pilot study. Iran J Public Health. 2014;43(10):1380–4.
2. Bath SC, Rayman MP. Iodine deficiency in the U.K.: an overlooked cause of impaired neurodevelopment? Proc Nutr Soc. 2013;72:226–35.
3. Nair S, Joshi K. Effect of double fortified salt supplementation on iodine and hemoglobin status of school children of rural Vadodara, India. Int J Appl Biol Pharm Technol. 2014;5(2):8–13.
4. Kissi PO. Utilization of iodised salt among households in the Danfa community [internet]. University of Ghana Digital Collections. University of Ghana; 2012. Available from: http://ugspace.ug.edu.gh/handle/123456789/5883. Accessed 19 Jan 2016.
5. Delange F. Iodine requirements during pregnancy, lactation and the neonatal period and indicators of optimal iodine nutrition. Public Health Nutr. 2007;10(12A):1571–80.
6. Lazarus JH. Thyroid function in pregnancy. Br Med Bull. 2011;97:137–48.
7. Kapil U. Health consequences of iodine deficiency. Sultan Qaboos Univ Med J. 2007;7(3):267–72.
8. Andersson M, de Benoist B, Delange F, Zupan J. Prevention and control of iodine defi ciency in pregnant and lactating women and in children less than 2-years-old: conclusions and recommendations of the technical consultation. WHO Secretariat Public Health Nutr. 2007;10:1606–11.
9. Berghout A, Wiersinga W. Thyroid size and thyroid function during pregnancy: an analysis. Eur J Endocrinol. 1998;138:536–42.
10. Giusti M, Orlandi D, Melle G, Massa B, Silvestri E, Minuto F, et al. Is there a real diagnostic impact of elastosonography and contrast-enhanced ultrasonography in the management of thyroid nodules? J Zhejiang Univ Sci B. 2013;14(3):195–206.
11. Untoro J, Mangasaryan N, de Benoist B, Darnton-Hill I. Reaching optimal iodine nutrition in pregnant and lactating women and young children: programmatic recommendations. Public Health Nutr. 2007;10:1527–9.
12. Buxton C, Baguune B. Knowledge and practices of people in Bia District, Ghana, with regard to iodine deficiency disorders and intake of iodised salt. Arch Public Heal. 2012;70(1):5.
13. United Nations. World summit for children. World declaration and plan of action for implementing the world declaration on the survival, protection and development of children in the 1990s. New York: United Nations; 1990.
14. Chirawurah D, Apanga S, Addah J. Assessing iodised salt use in rural northern Ghana : a mixed method approach. Food Public Heal. 2015; 5(3):70–6.
15. Bath SC, Walter A, Taylor A, Wright J, Rayman MP. Iodine deficiency in pregnant women living in the south east of the UK: the influence of diet and nutritional supplements on iodine status. Br J Nutr. 2014;111(9):1622–31.

16. WHO. Assessment of iodine deficiency disorders and monitoring their elimination: a guide for programme managers. Geneva: WHO; 2007.
17. Simpong DL, Adu P, Bashiru R, Morna MT, Yeboah FA, Akakpo K, et al. Assessment of iodine status among pregnant women in a rural community in Ghana - a cross sectional study. Arch Public Heal. 2016;74(8):1–5.
18. Steinmaus C, Miller MD, Howd R. Impact of smoking and thiocyanate on perchlorate and thyroid hormone associations in the 2001–2002 National Health and nutrition examination survey. Environ Health Perspect. 2007; 115(9):1333–8.
19. Caldwell KL, Jones RL, Hollowell JG. EQUIP: a worldwide program to ensure the quality of urinary iodine procedures. Accred Qual Assur. 2005;10:356–61.
20. Makhdmudov AA, Caldwell KL. The challenge of iodine deficiency disorder: a decade of CDC's ensuring the quality of urinary iodine procedures program. [Internet]. 2011. Available from: http://www.cdc.gov/labstandards/pdf/equip/EQUIP_Booklet.pdf. Date accessed 15 Jan 2016.
21. WHO. Urinary iodine concentrations for determining iodine status deficiency in populations [Internet]. Vitamin and Mineral Nutrition Information System. 2013. Available from: http://www.who.int/nutrition/vmnis/indicators/urinaryiodine. Date accessed 16 Jan 2016.
22. Report of a joint WHO/UNICEF/ICCIDD consultation, 3–5 November 1992. Geneva: World Health Organization; 1993. [19 June 2014]. Indicators for assessing iodine deficiency disorders and their control programmes. Review version September 1993. WHO/NUT 93.1; http://www.who.int/iris/handle/10665/62614. Date accessed 15 Aug 2017.
23. Menon VU, Chellan G, Sundaram KR, Murthy S, Kumar H, Unnikrishnan AG, et al. Iodine status and its correlations with age, blood pressure, and thyroid volume in south Indian women above 35 years of age (amrita thyroid survey). Indian J Endocrinol Metab. 2011;15(4):309–15.
24. WHO. Goitre as a determinant of the prevalence and severity of iodine deficiency disorders in populations. Geneva: WHO; 2014.
25. de Escobar GM, Obregón MJ, del Rey FE. Iodine deficiency and brain development in the first half of pregnancy. Public Health Nutr. 2007;10: 1554–70.
26. Vitti P, Delange F, Pinchera A, Zimmermann M, Dunn JT. Europe is iodine deficient. Lancet. 2003;361:1226.
27. Zimmermann MB. The effects of iodine deficiency in pregnancy and infancy. Paediatr Perinat Epidemiol. 2012;26:108–17.
28. Andersen SL. Iodine status in pregnant & breastfeeding women A Danish regional investigation. Dan Med J. 2015;62(5):B5974.
29. Habimana L, Twite KE, Wallemacq P, De Nayer P, Daumerie C, Donnen P, et al. Iodine and iron status of pregnant women in Lubumbashi, Democratic Republic of Congo. Public Health Nutr. 2013;16(8):1362–70.
30. Sultanalieva RB, Mamutova S, van der Haar F. The current salt iodization strategy in Kyrgyzstan ensures sufficient iodine nutrition among school-age children but not pregnant women. Public Health Nutr. 2010;13(5):623–30.
31. Costeira MJ, Oliveira P, Ares S, de Escobar GM, Palha JA. Iodine status of pregnant women and their progeny in the Minho region of Portugal. Thyroid. 2009;19(2):157–63.
32. Castañeda R, Lechuga D, Ramos RI, Magos C, Orozco M, Martínez H. Endemic goiter in pregnant women: utility of the simplified classification of thyroid size by palpation and urinary iodine as screening tests. BJOG. 2002; 109:1366–72.
33. Glinoer D. The importance of iodine nutrition during pregnancy. Public Health Nutr. 2007;10:1542–6.
34. Pedersen KM, Laurberg P, Iversen E, Knudsen PR, Gregersen HE, Rasmussen OS, et al. Amelioration of some pregnancy-associated variations in thyroid function by iodine supplementation. J Clin Endocrinol Metab. 1993;77(4): 1078–83.
35. Rasmussen LB, Ovesen L, Knudsen N, Laurberg P, Perrild H. Relations between various measures of iodine intake and thyroid volume, thyroid nodularity and serum thyroglobulin. Am J Clin Nutr. 2002;76:1069–76.
36. Zimmermann MB. Iodine deficiency in pregnancy and the effects of maternal iodine supplementation on the offspring: a review. Am J Clin Nutr. 2009;89(suppl):668S–72S.
37. Novosel S, Roncevic S, Lukinac L, Nothig-Hus D, Herman R, Kusic Z. Ultrasonographic analysis of the thyroid gland during pregnancy. Acta Clin Croat. 2000;39:71–5.
38. Brucker-Davis F, Ferrari P, Gal J, Berthier F, Fenichel P, Hieronimus S. Iodine status has no impact on thyroid function in early healthy pregnancy. J Thyroid Res. 2012;2012:1–6.
39. Hansen D, Bennedbaek FN, Hansen LK, Hoier-Madsen M, Jacobsen BB, Hegedus L. Thyroid function, morphology and autoimmunity in young patients with insulin-dependent diabetes mellitus. Eur J Endocrinol. 1999; 140:512–8.
40. Meng F, Zhao R, Liu P, Liu L, Liu S. Assessment of iodine status in children, adults, pregnant women and lactating women in iodine-replete areas of China. PLoS One. 2013;8(11):1–7.
41. Tweneboa, M. Determinants of the use of iodised salt among pregnant women attending ante-natal clinic at the Kaneshie Polyclinic. [Internet]. University of Ghana Digital Collections. University of Ghana; 2015. Available from: http://ugspace.ug.edu.gh/handle/123456789/9001. Accessed 19 Jan 2017.
42. Charlton K, Yeatman H, Lucas C, Gemming L. Poor knowledge and practices related to iodine nutrition during pregnancy and lactation in Australian women: pre-and post-iodine fortification. Nutrients. 2012;4(9):1317–27.

7

Pregnant women's experiences with an integrated diagnostic and decision support device for antenatal care in Ghana

Ibukun-Oluwa Omolade Abejirinde[1,2,3*], Renate Douwes[4], Azucena Bardají[3], Rudolf Abugnaba-Abanga[5], Marjolein Zweekhorst[1], Jos van Roosmalen[1,6] and Vincent De Brouwere[2]

Abstract

Background: Quality antenatal care (ANC) is recognised as an opportunity for screening and early identification of pregnancy-related complications. In rural Ghana, challenges with access to diagnostic services demotivate women from ANC attendance and referral compliance, leading to absent or late identification and management of high-risk women. In 2016, an integrated diagnostic and clinical decision support system tagged 'Bliss4Midwives' (B4M), was piloted in Northern Ghana. The device facilitated non-invasive screening of pre-eclampsia, gestational diabetes and anaemia at the point-of-care. This study aimed to explore the experiences of pregnant women with B4M, and its influence on service utilisation ("pull effect") and woman-provider relationships ("woman engagement").

Methods: Through an embedded study design, qualitative methods including individual semi-structured interviews and non-participant observation were employed. Interviews were conducted with 20 pregnant women and 10 health workers, supplemented by ANC observations in intervention facilities. Secondary data on ANC registrations over a one-year period were extracted from health facility records to support findings on the perceived influence of B4M on service utilisation.

Results: Women's first impressions of the device were mostly emotive (excitement, fear), but sometimes neutral. Although it is inconclusive whether B4M increased ANC registration, pregnant women generally valued the availability of diagnostic services at the point-of-care. Additionally, by fostering some level of engagement, the intervention made women feel listened to and cared for. Process outcomes of the B4M encounter also showed that it was perceived as improving the skills and knowledge of the health worker, which facilitated trust in diagnostic recommendations and was therefore believed to motivate referral compliance.

Conclusions: This study suggests that mHealth diagnostic and decision support devices enhance woman engagement and trust in health workers skills. There is need for further inquiry into how these interventions influence maternal health service utilization and women's expectations of pregnancy care.

Keywords: mHealth, Antenatal, Woman-provider interaction, Prenatal screening, Ghana, Clinical decision support

* Correspondence: i.o.abejirinde@vu.nl
[1]Athena Institute, Faculty of Science, Vrije Universiteit, Amsterdam, The Netherlands
[2]Department of Public Health, Institute of Tropical Medicine, Maternal and Reproductive Health Unit, Antwerp, Belgium
Full list of author information is available at the end of the article

Background

Worldwide, significant progress has been made to reduce maternal mortality and morbidity. However, many low and middle-income countries (LMICs) remain significantly burdened by preventable maternal deaths and pregnancy-related morbidities [1, 2]. Substantive efforts to improve maternal health globally is therefore a key agenda under the Sustainable Development Goals [3, 4]. Furthermore, there is an observed shift from higher proportions of maternal deaths due to direct causes such as haemorrhage and sepsis, to increasing mortality related to indirect causes such as heart disease and anaemia, i.e. the obstetric transition [5, 6].

Quality antenatal care (ANC) is widely recognised as an important opportunity for screening and early identification of pregnancy-related complications such as pre-eclampsia, anaemia, and gestational diabetes [7, 8]. In cases of late or failure to diagnose, these conditions may cause severe morbidity and mortality. It is estimated that haemorrhage, often in combination with anaemia, as well as preeclampsia, account for about 27 and 14% of all maternal deaths worldwide [9, 10]. Specifically, in Ghana, the Maternal Mortality Ratio (MMR) in 2015 was reported at 319 per 100,000 live births with a large range of uncertainty (from 216 to 458) [11]. Haemorrhage (39%), hypertensive disorders (35%) and unsafe abortions (7%) were the main direct causes, while indirect causes (26%) include severe anaemia, diabetes and malaria [12].

In rural and remote areas of Ghana, comprehensive ANC is often hampered by staff shortages, lack of diagnostic equipment and supplies or weak referral linkages [13, 14]. Pregnant women are therefore often referred to distant health facilities, laboratories or private facilities for routine diagnostics. The resultant loss of time and money required to visit these facilities, demotivate women from ANC attendance and referral compliance, and may result in late identification and management of pregnancy-related complications.

Mobile Health (mHealth) solutions, defined as "the provision of health services and information via mobile technologies" [15] have been reported as beneficial for improving ANC services in LMICs [16–18]. There is a growing body of literature stating that mHealth solutions can potentially reduce gaps and inefficiencies in health service delivery including point-of-care screening, integration of records and streamlining care processes [19–22]. However, there is sparse evidence on the influence of such interventions on service utilisation and woman engagement. Using a mHealth intervention in rural Ghana as a case study, this paper aims to address this gap.

In 2016, a one-year proof-of-concept study tagged Bliss4Midwives (B4M) was launched in two regions of Northern Ghana- Upper East and Northern regions, with a goal to improve ANC services. The B4M device is an integrated diagnostic and Clinical Decision Support System (CDSS) that enables non-invasive point-of-care screening for pre-eclampsia, gestational diabetes and anaemia. B4M components include a non-invasive device for measuring haemoglobin via infrared sensors mounted on a finger clip; a self-inflating blood pressure cuff; and an automated reader for urinary protein and glucose through dipsticks. Data from all diagnostic devices are automatically or manually linked to an android tablet equipped with decision support algorithms. Additionally, a traffic light system (red, orange and yellow colours) visually indicates risk category or referral urgency for pre-eclampsia, gestational diabetes and anaemia, while prompting the health worker on counselling and treatment. Before commencing the pilot project, users (midwives and community health nurses) were trained on the technical and operational functions of the device. Training also included modules on the principles of quality ANC and management of pregnancy complications.

The project hypothesised that through this mHealth-health worker interface, the interpersonal process of care- a component of quality ANC- would improve. It was also expected that coupled with treatment or referral advice, the traffic light signalling would increase women's engagement with the midwife, and women's compliance. Additionally, by being responsive to the needs of pregnant women for screening tests, the project anticipated that use of B4M would increase demand and utilisation of ANC services. Summarily, the pilot project offered the opportunity to assess the influence of mHealth on ANC demand or service utilization ("pull effect"), and on the interpersonal process of care ("woman engagement").

This paper therefore explores the experiences of women exposed to the B4M device, to answer the research questions: i) How did women experience the use of Bliss4Midwives during their routine antenatal care consultations? ii) What influence did Bliss4Midwives have on woman-provider relationships and on ANC service utilization?

Due to inactive use of B4M devices in the Northern region at the time of data collection, only findings in the Upper East region are reported.

Methods

Design

Qualitative methods including individual semi-structured interviews and non-participant observation were employed. Data collection was embedded into a broader realist evaluation of midwives' adoption and utilization of the B4M device.

Setting

The Upper East region (UER) is one of the 10 administrative regions in Ghana and is further sub-divided into districts and municipalities. The B4M project was piloted in Bawku municipal (one health facility- identified as Facility A) and Binduri district (three health facilities- identified as B, C and D) in the UER. Both Bawku municipal and Binduri district are predominantly rural and about half of their population is illiterate [23, 24]. Three B4M devices were placed in health facilities on a fixed (permanently stationed in facilities A and D) or rotational basis (one device shared by facilities B and C) and used to screen women attending ANC.

Data collection

Exit interviews following ANC screening were conducted using a semi-structured interview guide. Questions explored women's initial reactions to the device, its perceived benefits, their views on its (potential) effect on ANC uptake behaviour (i.e. pull effect), quality of service delivery and their desire for continued use of the device.

Interview guides for pregnant women were developed in English language and translated to the local language-Kusaal (see Additional file 1). These were discussed with local program managers before piloting and subsequent modification (ambiguous words identified and refined, exclusion of questions perceived to be culturally inappropriate). The first author and a trained female Research Assistant (RA) who is fluent in both English and Kusaal conducted 20 interviews with pregnant women in June 2017. Sixteen exit interviews were conducted in the four health facilities immediately after ANC visits with B4M use. Using disaggregated data from the project database and with the help of health facility staff, additional women who had been exposed to the device during past ANC visits were traced at community level and invited to the health facility for retrospective interviews ($n = 4$). Respondents were selected by convenience sampling based on their attending ANC at the health facility during data collection, or based on previous ANC screening with the device and availability for interview. Women were interviewed irrespective of gestation and type of ANC visit (i.e. first or follow-up). Interviews were conducted in locations close to health facilities, but not in the immediate vicinity of ANC consultations. Based on the level of education and preference of the respondent, interviews with pregnant women were conducted in English or Kusaal. Depending on the nature and unique circumstances related to timing and respondents' convenience, the RA was sometimes the main interviewer while the principal researcher observed or functioned as the main interviewer, with the RA translating.

In addition, 10 semi-structured interviews in English were conducted with health workers (midwives and community health nurses) who operated the B4M device in intervention facilities and thereby were engaged in the B4M-ANC care process (see Additional file 2). This was done to understand the experience of use and nature of the mHealth-mediated consultation from different actors. Health workers were asked to share their perceptions of the influence of B4M on women's behaviour, compliance to referral or clinical recommendations, and on women's attitudes to the use of mHealth for ANC. As part of the realist evaluation in which this study was embedded, workers were asked to respond to a colour-guided Likert five-point scale (ranging from 'strongly disagree' to 'strongly agree') in response to specific questions about B4M use. The questionnaire section of the interview explored perceptions of how women responded to the device. Specifically: *"I think more pregnant women are coming for ANC now that we use B4M in the Health Facility"* and *"I think that pregnant women follow my advice more now that I use B4M for consultation."* Responses to these questions were therefore included in the analysis for this paper. We aimed to interview all health workers who had been trained in B4M use, had used the device at least once post-training and were available at the time of data collection. Due to staff rotations, not all midwives who were initially trained were available to be interviewed and not all health workers in each facility were trained on the use of B4M. A summary of the number and category of interviews is presented in Table 1.

All interviews were audio recorded and later transcribed and translated where necessary to English language. Two independent individuals transcribed a random number of interviews done in Kusaal to assure the quality of transcription and translation. Duration of interviews with pregnant women was between 11 and 34 min (median 21.36 min). Because interviews with health workers were part of a broader evaluation objective, these lasted longer- from 35 to 91 min (median 52.29 min).

In order to triangulate and validate findings from interviews, one researcher using a semi-structured checklist and observation guide conducted non-participant

Table 1 Categories of respondents per health facility

	Health Workers	Pregnant Women	
		Exit interviews	Retrospective interviews
Health Facility[a]			
Facility A	3	6	0
Facility B	2	7	0
Facility C	3	0	1
Facility D	2	3	3
TOTAL	10	16	4

[a]Facility A is a district hospital in Bawku Municipality and is the first level referral point for facilities B, C and D which are health centers in Binduri district

observations of ANC consultations in three intervention sites (facilities A, B and D). These were documented using handwritten notes. Non-participant observation is stated here to mean that the researcher is not an active participant in the facility, but interacts occasionally with the people in a non-intrusive way through questions and active listening, if the opportunity presents itself [25].

Secondary data on first ANC visits (i.e. registrations) over a one-year period- from December 2015 to December 2016 (i.e. 6 months before and 6 months after the pilot commenced in June 2016) were extracted from health facility records to supplement findings on the perceived pull effect of B4M.

Data analysis

All transcripts were read and a preliminary codebook was developed guided by the main themes explored in the interviews. Two researchers developed codes inductively. One researcher coded all transcripts while another coded a random number of six transcripts to test consistency of codes and support data analysis. Codes were clustered into themes based on similar or recurring patterns. Qualitative data analysis was supported using NVivo qualitative data analysis Software; QSR International Pty Ltd. Version 11, 2014.

Ethical considerations

Approval for this study was granted by the Navrongo Health Research Centre Institutional Review Board (Approval ID: NHRCIRB18) and the EMGO+ Scientific Committee of the Amsterdam Public Health Institute (Reference Number: WC2017–026). Verbal and or written consent was secured from all respondents. Consent was secured prior to all interviews, and respondents signed or appended their thumbprints to an informed consent form. Respondents for exit interviews received transport reimbursement (equivalent value of USD$1 - $2). Health workers were not reimbursed since interviews were conducted at their work place.

Results

Between June 2016 and April 2017, 950 ANC screenings (including follow-up visits) were conducted with the B4M device in the UER; 284 screenings from health

Table 2 Socio-demographic characteristics of respondents

Characteristic	Pregnant women ($n = 20$)	Health workers ($n = 10$)
Age		
< 18	1	0
18–24	8	1
25–29	3	2
30–34	1	5
35–39	2	1
40+	1	1
Missing data	4	0
Number of Births		
0–1	12	
2–3	4	
4–5	2	
Missing data	2	
ANC Observations Conducted		
Yes	14	
No	6	
Cadre		
Midwife		8
Enrolled Nurse [a]		1
Community Health nurse		1
Years of Experience		
0–4		4
5–9		5
> 10		1

[a]An auxiliary cadre similar to health assistants

facility A, 69 in health facility B, 129 in C and 468 in D. Socio-demographic characteristics of interviewees are presented in Table 2.

Women's first impressions of B4M

Pregnant women's first impressions of the Bliss4Midwives device ranged from fear and happiness to curiosity or a neutral disposition (Table 3). The non-invasive Haemoglobin clip required women to insert an index finger into the peg-like clip and was a main reason for fear. This was because some beneficiaries did not know what to anticipate on insertion. Two women specifically reported a feeling of discomfort during the screening.

Happiness was related to technological novelty or appreciation for easier and additional diagnostic services. As noted during ANC observations, some attendees were neutral- rarely questioning or initiating conversations with the health worker, and were passive actors in the consultation process. Notably, the few women who demonstrated curiosity were formally educated (completed basic primary education). Health workers also corroborated reports of happiness and fear.

The ability of providers to clearly explain the device function and help women understand its benefits facilitated a positive disposition to B4M. Attempts by health workers to incorporate use of B4M while handling a high volume of work in understaffed settings, sometimes resulted in situations where not all women attending ANC were screened with B4M. An unintended consequence of this adaptation strategy was that while some women felt special for being selected, others felt otherwise excluded or came up with plausible explanations of why they were not screened with the device.

Perceived benefits of B4M

ANC respondents felt satisfied about the services offered at the facilities. When asked to rate the quality of their just concluded ANC visit on a scale of 1–10, most respondents gave scores between 6 and 10 points with specific credit given to counselling and staff attitude (e.g. health workers are friendly and not shouting). However, these ratings could not be directly attributed to the B4M device, although a few respondents specifically stated that their satisfaction of the visit was because of the otherwise absent diagnostic service provided by B4M. Analysis showed that pregnant women appreciated the device for detecting their health problems and saving time and money that would have been otherwise expended on diagnostic referrals. Some women also believed the device improved the knowledge of health workers and made them pay closer attention to specific aspects of the woman's health (Table 4).

Prior to the intervention, diagnostic screening was not frequently conducted at the point of care and now constituted an additional task in the ANC workflow, necessitating more time. For this reason, a drawback on the perceived benefits of B4M use was that the ANC process took longer time, which made women impatient. Health workers interpreted this impatience to mean that women were not accepting the device. Reports on time estimates and perceived delays with B4M use ranged from 10 to 30 min extra as compared to the standard workflow. Technical difficulties (software freezes, slow response time), and procedural issues (low user dexterity with operating the device) were two main factors that contributed to delays. While there were reports of rare occasions where one or two respondents voiced their displeasure about time delays, midwives more commonly observed signs of displeasure through body language. One midwife mentioned an extreme case where the turnaround time was too long, and a woman got restless and left the facility.

Interestingly, while ANC attendees in the district hospital (facility A) were particularly grateful to B4M for saving time, their peers in the health centres did not make this association. Contrarily, up to two women from health centres B, C and D associated the use of B4M with a time delay. Observations revealed that the reported time saving benefits of B4M from respondents in facility A was connected to women otherwise having to spend up to 2 hours at the hospital laboratory to

Table 3 Initial reactions of ANC attendees to B4M device

Reaction	Supporting Quote
Fear	*"It was because I had never seen it and that was my very first time of seeing it, so I was afraid"* -Pregnant woman 1, Facility D
Happiness	*"I was excited because I was hopeful that if I have any sickness in my system, the machine will let me know."* -Pregnant woman 3, Facility A *"I would say for us here, when you hear that you have a device that is going to help you do something, they get excited.... some (women) get excited, but others.... it is the explanation that you have given them of what (the box) can do so that they can accept it."* -HCW 3, Facility A
Neutral	*"I wasn't happy and wasn't afraid as well, I just knew it was part of the care they were providing"* -Pregnant woman 6, Facility B *"I thought using the box is only when it becomes necessary. So whether or not she uses it, it is the same... They are the professionals and know the best for me. As for me, I cannot tell."* -Pregnant woman 1, Facility A
Curiosity	*"That, because after she said she was going to use it for this particular thing, when she was doing it, I was eager and ready to see whether I belong to any of the diseases she has mentioned or I'm free, so I was just waiting to see what the machine will tell me"* -Pregnant woman 2, Facility B

Table 4 Pregnant women's Perceptions of B4M

Factor	Supporting Quote
Service Provision	*"(I like) every part of the machine. I like it because the machine will tell you the right BP.... and then it will tell you the types of disease or the problems you are finding in your system."* -Pregnant woman 2, Facility B
Improved Knowledge	*"(I think the midwife has more knowledge). Because it is through those things that she used to get the information about my condition. If not, (the results I got from) outside, she could have recorded it and give me the card to go away, but because of the machine she has took her time to also take me through this procedure to know whether it is really true that I have this disease and ...she is sure that what they brought outside is comparing to her machine."* - Pregnant woman 2, Facility B
Efficiency	*"It has helped to make her efficient. It is because the things we could have gone to the lab to do that requires so much time, this one is faster and easier."* -Pregnant woman 3, Facility A
Time delays	*"I: So in your opinion which particular place do you spend a lot of time?* *R: At the machine* *I: So where do you think when worked on, will help reduce the time spent? At the records, the machine, the palpation area, the dispensary?* *R: No, just at the machine* *I: ....so the machine is what causes the delay* *R: Yes"* -Pregnant woman, Facility D

process routine tests. Except where other laboratory tests had to be conducted, B4M therefore became a welcome time-efficient alternative in the larger facility.

ANC workflow is usually structured in stations such that women have to move from one point to another for specific tests or different aspects of the consultation (palpation, updating records, weight, height and blood pressure check, collection of routine drugs). In this context, workers felt the integrated function of B4M made ANC routine easier and more comfortable. However, one minor but crucial deviation from the perception that B4M facilitated focused antenatal care was noted in observation visits showing that workflow was still broken when women needed to provide their urine samples. This usually necessitated going to an outhouse, which prolonged consultation time and was sometimes frowned upon by other workers within the facility who saw this as an interruption of the general workflow.

In health facilities where workers helped women (re)-negotiate their ANC experience and workflow, women better understood the value and benefits of the box and this improved acceptability while diminishing complaints about time delays. As one health worker put it *"they develop some love in it and every time they come, even if it is wasting time, they will still wait"*- an indication that women may have also adjusted their expectations and factored in the extra time needed for use of the device.

Women's engagement with B4M

Prior to using B4M for the first time, the project required that health workers informed women about the device using a structured information sheet. Following this, the woman was required to confirm consent by appending a thumbprint or signature. This mandatory step served as an opening for interactive communication, but was not always carried out. Observations showed that not all women received a full explanation about the device, its functions and the procedures for the screening. On the other hand, the structured format of B4M compelled prolonged woman-provider interaction leading to improved counselling that was otherwise previously rushed or absent.

Observations and follow-up questions to workers revealed that most women were indifferent about the details of care and did not necessarily want to be involved. Women were reportedly more keen to receive assurances about their health status without spending much time at the facility. In two of the three facilities where B4M use was observed, the physical positioning of the device relative to the woman and B4M user prohibited (in the case of opposite seating) or was suboptimal for (e.g. screen not within field of vision) visual engagement by the woman.

With a few exceptions, midwives would usually explain the summary of the B4M encounter to the woman after screening and use the tests results as an opportunity to educate them on diet, birth preparedness and pregnancy care prior to scheduling the follow-up appointment. Although this partly explained why the B4M encounter took longer, pregnant women also felt listened to and more included in the care process.

> *"Because I saw that everything, everything was ok. But that place (i.e. another health facility) I can't see. But here, everything is plain and I will know that... I can see it. I see what are the problems, what they are advising me on and other things."* -Pregnant woman 6, Facility D.

Trust and compliance with B4M

Prior to project implementation, it was found that apart from challenges in the health system with referral linkages, women would often not comply with referral recommendations. Reasons for this included doubt in the severity of their problem, concerns about cost and time implications, and fear of being unattended or getting lost in an unfamiliar large health facility.

One of the B4M intervention hypotheses was that the traffic-light module of the system (which should be visible to the woman during ANC consultations) would facilitate women's engagement and motivate referral compliance. Interviews explored the confidence of women in the diagnostic decisions from B4M and the possibility that women were more assured about the validity and necessity of referral instructions if it came from a digital third party. Analysis showed that most women were confident with the screening results and a couple of respondents noted that they would not have believed a referral recommendation if it had not come from the device.

> *"Using the box makes me actually believe that it is indeed true, because with the box she is telling me what she has seen"* -Pregnant woman 7, Facility B.

However, there were a few reports of women who while acknowledging benefits of the device, did not necessarily trust its decisions or recommendations. In negotiating this digital trust, educated respondents were found most likely to critically reflect on results and recommendations from B4M.

All health workers agreed to varying extents (eight strongly agreed and two slightly agreed) to the question *"I think pregnant women follow my advice more now that I used the box for consultation"*. Reasons included the perception that women's respect for workers increased- an extension of additional skills acquired through B4M. Many health workers felt that women's compliance to referral and counselling recommendations happened because the machine, which was seen as a more knowledgeable or accurate medium, was 'demanding' it.

Some health workers were also of the opinion that the device mediated woman-provider relationship by enhancing trust.

> *"Even here the moment you work with them and they have trust with you, that is all. They believe and they trust whatever you tell them.... And with the box, it has even enhanced our work. They believe and they trust that if we tell them something, it is true because the box has actually said it."* -HCW 2, Facility D.

Interestingly, some women personified the device, reporting that the box "advised them" while others described what "the machine said". Just as the receipt of routine drugs (iron and folate) at the end of a visit was considered proof that ANC had been effectively carried out, two pregnant women said interaction with the box was proof that ANC was properly completed.

> *"You know when I come and they don't use it to attend to me and I just get back home like that, it doesn't actually feel like you came"* -Pregnant woman 3, Facility B.

Pull effect

An anticipated effect of B4M use in health facilities was that its innovativeness and the provision of diagnostic options for women would encourage more first time (registrants) and follow-up ANC visits (attendants). Interviews revealed that all, except two health workers, felt that the use of B4M in their health facility created a demand for ANC services. In some cases, it was believed that B4M attracted women from other health centres to theirs. In response to the Likert-scale question *"I think that more pregnant women are coming for ANC now that we have this device in our health facility"*, two health workers neither agreed nor disagreed, three slightly agreed and five were strongly in agreement. A minority, however, felt that more women were now registering for ANC, but that this was unrelated to B4M.

Health workers attributed this perception of a positive pull effect to women spreading news about the device within their communities, especially following a testimony of improved wellbeing after adhering to the B4M advice.

> *"When they saw it the first time and those (I screened) and told them their problem, they were telling their colleagues- 'Oh I went to the hospital, they are now having a machine'. So everybody wants to come and see the machine."* -HCW 2, Facility B.

However, no pregnant woman reported discussing the availability of the device with any of their peers or learning about its presence in the facilities from a third party.

Although we did not have enough data points to determine the extent to which number of ANC visits was associated with the presence of B4M in health facilities, we compared descriptive data on ANC registrations (1st visits) in UER intervention facilities 6 months prior to B4M (December 2015–May 2016) and 6 months following commencement of the pilot (July 2016–December 2016). Interestingly, results did not show a dramatic increase in total visit numbers. In some instances, we noticed a decline over time (Table 5).

When women were asked to comment on their disposition to return for ANC even in the absence of the box, all noted that it would not influence their attendance of follow-up visits, although they may be curious or

Table 5 Number of ANC registrants 6-months pre- and 6-months post- B4M initiation[a]

	Facility A[b]	Facility B	Facility C	Facility D
Dec 2015- May 2016	792	199	79	171
July 2016- Dec 2016	647	205	88	135
Difference	– 145	+ 6	+ 9	–36

[a]Data from June 2016 was not included in this analysis because the intervention commenced in the middle of the month
[b]Facility A is a district hospital in Bawku Municipality and is the first level referral point for facilities B, C and D which are health centers in Binduri district

slightly disappointed if it was absent. This may have been due to the lack of alternatives as pointed out by one respondent:

> *"Of course I will (keep visiting this health facility). Where else will I go? I was even coming here when the box was not here"* - Client 1, Facility B.

Although most women felt their future ANC behaviour would not be motivated by the presence of the device, their expectation for future use was affirmative.

Discussion

This paper aimed to explore the experiences of pregnant women screened with B4M device and its influence on ANC service utilization and woman-provider relationships. There has been significant focus on the feasibility and acceptability of mHealth from the lens of the technology user. However, less attention has been paid to the views and perceptions of the end beneficiary- perspectives which are equally important in the outcome and long-term use of mHealth devices [26].

The reported enthusiasm of women to B4M can be linked to the novelty effect of mHealth and are similar to reactions of health worker users in other studies [21, 27]. While there are mHealth innovations where the user is the direct beneficiary of the functions offered [16, 28], the nature and function of B4M necessitated a triad relationship between the device, the health worker user and the direct beneficiary i.e. pregnant women. Findings that some women were initially fearful of the device shed light on the importance of incorporating both technology users and beneficiaries in the mHealth-assimilation process. Specifically, reactions of fear in the B4M study were directly related to device components, which can be overcome with careful explanation and guidance from health workers. The potential risk of skipping this process of careful negotiation is the spread of myths and misconceptions, which could hamper eventual integration of mHealth into routine care.

The neutral disposition of some pregnant women to B4M may have been related to low literacy levels and feelings of inadequacy about questioning the competence of a trained professional. Given the intervention context- predominantly rural with high illiteracy levels, it was not surprising that only a couple of B4M beneficiaries who are also educated, were engaged actively in the care process [29]. Future interventions of a similar nature should go beyond technical training; additional training in communication and negotiation skills is necessary to facilitate acceptability and to actively involve women in the care process.

This study found that although pregnant women could not fully engage with the B4M-mediated process, they were still satisfied with the care received. The design of B4M compelled health workers to follow structured guidelines and procedures, such that they had to directly communicate with women. In so doing, the device served as a platform for improved woman-provider interaction. This made women feel heard and listened to, although an indirect consequence of this was longer consultation time. Missed opportunities for improved engagement occurred when workers did not take the entry point offered by the intervention to explain its function to end-beneficiaries. By virtue of providing diagnostic services, which would otherwise take a longer time or incur additional time and financial commitments of pregnant women, B4M served to overcome gaps in unnecessary diagnostic referral while influencing the likelihood that women would comply with referral recommendations. A note of warning, however, is that if women become only compliant to clinical recommendations when delivered by technology, there is risk of a dilemma should woman-mHealth trust rank above woman-provider trust.

While technology has shown promise in improving access and efficiency of some health care processes, it is generally agreed that it is not yet a substitute for real-time face-to-face interaction and interpersonal relationship [30]. There are mixed reports on how mHealth may facilitate or hinder woman-provider interaction [30–32]. A study on the perceptions of community health workers in Brazil to the use of a data collection and transmission tool, reported social barriers to utilizing the cell phone intervention despite its reported advantages [31]. Such barriers included the negative impact of the tool on social interaction (i.e. interpersonal connection) with pregnant women. Interrupted eye contact and passive involvement especially with illiterate and older women impeded trust building and effective engagement. On the other hand, assessment of the *mobile santé Nouna* intervention in rural Burkina Faso showed expectations of improved relationships between the health facility and the community with mHealth as an intermediary [33].

The meanings of expertise that women attached to the B4M device while personifying it were notable. This made B4M seem like an active expert-participant in the consultation. A review of studies found that when beneficiaries of care attribute a status of specialised or "higher up" knowledge to CDSS, it enhances their trust in results and recommendations [21]. Woman-provider trust has been shown to play a role in the continuity of maternal care and in women's preferences for facility delivery [34, 35] and ANC visits have been earmarked as an entryway to establish such trust [7]. Although some health workers believed that the B4M device mediated the woman-provider relationship by enhancing trust, we could not ascertain the pattern of interactions regarding the trust effect. Were ANC attendees trusting health workers more because they used the device, or did it only enhance existing trust? Especially with B4M where screening results required voluntary compliance from women to seek further care, their trust in test results and the midwife's recommendations was crucial. Screening, which is only one of many steps in the chain of care is therefore only relevant when followed by prompt and proper management of the conditions detected. Unfortunately, broader health system deficiencies such as lack of resources and fragmented referral systems limit the capability for a full chain of service delivery, which is beyond the scope of what mHealth can do.

Interestingly, perceptions of time efficiency differed between types of health facility. The mixed reports about the time efficiency of B4M use in health centres (facilities B, C, D) and the hospital (facility A) appeared to be linked to the workload associated with the latter. B4M allowed women bypass burdensome bottlenecks of the care process in the bigger health facility. Studies have shown that service delivery advantages of mHealth vary depending on characteristics of the facility in which it is placed and aspect of care it is used for. Reports from a multi-country study show greater time efficiency when CDSS was used in the delivery room than for ANC [36]. This may explain why B4M was considered more time efficient at the district hospital than at lower levels where women had more direct contact with all points of the ANC workflow without too many interruptions in the care process. Overall, our findings show that B4M saves time compared to the standard where women from health centres have to delay screening and travel a distance for tests. In this standard scenario, ANC consultation becomes interrupted till a later date, after test results have been acquired. These are time inefficient processes that may not be immediately appreciated by pregnant women and overall influence the timeliness of treatment and continuity of care.

In the last decade, the effect of community focused information, education and communication campaigns about the value of ANC seems to have paid off. Even in rural areas of Northern Ghana, studies have reported impressive rates (up to 90%) of ANC attendance and utilization of skilled delivery [37]. While this study could not prove increased ANC registrations due to B4M use, health workers had a strong perception of a pull effect. The counter-intuitive results from B4M facilities with continuous use versus rotating use, where registrations marginally decreased in the former group compared to the latter, further caution against hasty conclusions regarding a pull effect and hint at other factors at play to explain these differences. However, some studies in similar settings have reported improvements in health service utilization, specifically ANC attendance, due to mHealth [28, 38, 39]. In addition to a small data set, the absence of agreement between workers' perceptions and routine data from the B4M sites may be due to incomplete records, pre-existing trends of high ANC coverage in study regions, or minimal options at competing health facilities from which clients could be pulled. In light of updated guidelines recommending eight ANC contacts during pregnancy [7], and the continued expansion of mHealth use in LMICs, it is beneficial to identify the contexts and mechanisms by which mHealth positively influences demand and service utilization.

Study limitations

The B4M intervention was a short-term proof of concept and as such its use was confined to a limited number of health facilities in study regions. Retrospective interviewing of some pregnant women as well as B4M users who had not used the device for up to 2 months before the interview, introduced a risk of recall bias. We attempted to counter this by using visual cues of the device and prompting respondents with specific events associated with device use. In addition we used multiple data sources for triangulation. By conducting women's exit interviews in locations removed from the immediate service delivery environment, other biases (e.g. social desirability and confirmation) were minimized. A researcher who was not familiar with the local language conducted observations. This limited the ability to fully capture verbal elements of what was observed. However, when possible, information gaps were filled by follow-up questions to health workers. Research bias due to the researchers' presence during the initial sets of observations was inevitable. To counter the observer effect, multiple observation visits were conducted over a number of days, with the expectation that those being observed will resume their natural behaviour over time [40]. Not all respondents declared their age and health record booklets were not readily accessible, leading to information gaps on socio-demographic characteristics.

Conclusions

Pregnant women's experiences and perceptions of mHealth-supported service delivery can influence how the implementation process translates to desired care outcomes. The B4M proof-of-concept showed that mHealth influences the trust ANC attendees have in health workers and in referral recommendations, which may positively impact compliance of women to treatment. Additionally, by fostering some level of engagement, the intervention made women feel listened to and cared for. There is, however, a need for further inquiry into how mHealth shapes women's expectations of maternal care and the perceived pull effect. Future studies should also focus on how beneficiaries, in addition to mHealth users, directly or indirectly influence mHealth adoption, utilization and health outcomes.

Abbreviations

ANC: Antenatal care; B4M: Bliss4Midwives; CDSS: Clinical decision support system; LMICs: Low and middle-income countries; mHealth: Mobile health; RA: Research assistant; UER: Upper East Region

Acknowledgements

The authors would like to thank the Bliss4Midwives implementing organizations (Stichting Cordaid; Relitech B.V.; Ned. Org. voor Toegepast Natuurwetenschappelijk Ond. TNO; Stichting Simavi; Stichting Enviu Nederland; Association of Church-based Development NGOs, Ghana; and Presbyterian Health Services-North, Ghana) for their support in carrying out this study and in facilitating evaluation activities. We would also like to thank the local research assistants, translators and transcribers, study participants, and the district administrators and health facility personnel involved. The first author appreciates the additional financial support of Professor Vincent De Brouwere towards the stakeholders' dissemination meeting organized at the end of the study.

Funding

The Bliss4Midwives proof-of-concept was funded by the Life Sciences and Health for Development (LS&H4D) grant: Number- LSH14GH16, from the Dutch Ministry of Foreign Affairs (RVO). The LS&H4D grant, as well as the Erasmus Mundus Joint Doctorate Fellowship Specific Grant Agreement 2015–1595, which IOA is a beneficiary of, financed data collection activities. Funding agencies had no role in study design, analysis, or preparation of the manuscript.

Authors' contributions

IOA led study design, data collection, analysis, interpretation and writing; RD contributed to design, analysis, interpretation and writing; RAA contributed to data collection and writing; AB, MZ, JvR and VDB supervised the study and contributed to design, interpretation and writing. All authors have read and approved the final manuscript.

Competing interests

RD and RAA work for organizations involved in the implementation of the Bliss4Midwives proof-of-concept and were actively involved in the project. JvR is a member of the editorial board (section editor) of BMC Pregnancy and Childbirth. Other authors declare no competing interests.

Author details

[1]Athena Institute, Faculty of Science, Vrije Universiteit, Amsterdam, The Netherlands. [2]Department of Public Health, Institute of Tropical Medicine, Maternal and Reproductive Health Unit, Antwerp, Belgium. [3]ISGlobal, Hospital Clínic- Universitat de Barcelona, Barcelona, Spain. [4]Simavi, Amsterdam, The Netherlands. [5]Presbyterian Health Services-North, BolgatangaUpper East RegionGhana. [6]Department of Obstetrics, Leiden University Medical Centre, Leiden, The Netherlands.

References

1. WHO. Trends in Maternal Mortality: 1990 To 2015: estimates by WHO, UNICEF, UNFPA. Geneva: World Bank Group and the United Nations Population Division; 2015.
2. Filippi V, Chou D, Ronsmans C, Graham W, Say L. Levels and Causes of Maternal Mortality and Morbidity. In: Black RE, Laxminarayan R, Temmerman M, Walker N, editors. Reproductive, Maternal, Newborn, and Child Health. Third Edit ed. Washington (DC): The International Bank for Reconstruction and Development / The World Bank; 2016.
3. Requejo JH, Bhutta ZA. The post-2015 agenda: staying the course in maternal and child survival. Arch Dis Child. 2015;100:76–81.
4. Scott H, Isabella D. Accountability for improving maternal and newborn health. Best Pract Res Clin Obstet Gynaecol. 2016;36:45–56.
5. Graham W, Susannah W, Peter B, Filippi V, Giorgia G, Sandra V, et al. Diversity and divergence: the dynamic burden of poor maternal health. Lancet. 2016;388:2164–75. https://doi.org/10.1016/S0140-6736(16)31533-1.
6. Souza JP, Tunçalp Ö, Vogel JP, Bohren M, Widmer M, Oladapo OT, et al. Obstetric transition: the pathway towards ending preventable maternal deaths. BJOG. 2014;121(Supplement 1):1–4.
7. World Health Organisation. WHO Recommendations on Antenatal Care for a Positive Pregnancy Experience. Geneva: WHO Press; 2016. http://apps.who.int/iris/bitstream/10665/250796/1/9789241549912-eng.pdf .
8. Requejo JH, Bryce J, Barros AJD, Berman P, Bhutta Z, Chopra M, et al. Countdown to 2015 and beyond: fulfilling the health agenda for women and children. Lancet. 2015;385:466–76. https://doi.org/10.1016/S0140-6736(14)60925-9.
9. Say L, Chou D, Gemmill A, Tunçalp Ö, Moller A-B, Daniels J, et al. Global causes of maternal death: a WHO systematic analysis. Lancet Glob Health. 2014;2:e323–33. https://doi.org/10.1016/S2214-109X(14)70227-X.
10. Menéndez C, Romagosa C, Ismail MR, Carrilho C, Saute F, Osman N, et al. An autopsy study of maternal mortality in Mozambique: the contribution of infectious diseases. PLoS Med. 2008;5:e44. https://doi.org/10.1371/journal.pmed.0050044.
11. WHO, UNICEF, UNFPA, World Bank Group, United Nations population division. Trends in Maternal Mortality: 1990 to 2015: estimates by WHO, UNICEF, UNFPA, World Bank Group and the United Nations Population Division. Geneva, Switzerland: WHO Press; 2015. http://www.afro.who.int/sites/default/files/2017-05/trends-in-maternal-mortality-1990-to-2015.pdf
12. Ghana Health Service. Family Health Division Annual Report for 2015. 2015. http://www.ghanahealthservice.org/downloads/2015_FAMILY_HEALTH_DIVISION_ANNUAL_REPORT.pdf.
13. Ayanore MA, Pavlova M, Groot W. Focused maternity care in Ghana: results of a cluster analysis. BMC Health Serv Res. 2016;16:395. https://doi.org/10.1186/s12913-016-1654-5.
14. Amoakoh-Coleman M, Agyepong IA, Kayode GA, Grobbee DE, Klipstein-Grobusch K, Ansah EK. Public health facility resource availability and provider adherence to first antenatal guidelines in a low resource setting in Accra, Ghana. BMC Health Serv Res. 2016;16:505. https://doi.org/10.1186/s12913-016-1747-1.
15. Hagan D, Uggowitzer S. Information and communication Technologies for Women's and Children's health- a planning workbook. Geneva: WHO Press; 2014. http://www.who.int/pmnch/knowledge/publications/ict_mhealth.pdf.
16. Oliveira-Ciabati L, Vieira CS, Franzon ACA, Alves D, Zaratini FS, Braga GC, et al. PRENACEL – a mHealth messaging system to complement antenatal care: a cluster randomized trial. Reprod Health. 2017;14:146. https://doi.org/10.1186/s12978-017-0407-1.
17. Feroz A, Perveen S, Aftab W. Role of mHealth applications for improving antenatal and postnatal care in low and middle income countries: a systematic review. BMC Health Serv Res. 2017;17:704. https://doi.org/10.1186/s12913-017-2664-7

18. Amoakoh-Coleman M, Borgstein AB-J, Sondaal SFV, Grobbee DE, Miltenburg AS, Verwijs M, et al. Effectiveness of mHealth interventions targeting health care workers to improve pregnancy outcomes in low- and middle-income countries: a systematic review. J Med Internet Res. 2016;18:e226. https://doi.org/10.2196/jmir.5533.
19. Hall CS, Fottrell E, Wilkinson S, Byass P. Assessing the impact of mHealth interventions in low- and middle-income countries – what has been shown to work? Glob Health Action 2014;7:10.3402/gha.v7.25606. doi:https://doi.org/10.3402/gha.v7.25606.
20. Aranda-Jan CB, Mohutsiwa-Dibe N, Loukanova S. Systematic review on what works, what does not work and why of implementation of mobile health (mHealth) projects in Africa. BMC Public Health. 2014;14:188. https://doi.org/10.1186/1471-2458-14-188.
21. Adepoju I-OO, Albersen BJA, De Brouwere V, van Roosmalen J, Zweekhorst M. mHealth for clinical decision-making in sub-Saharan Africa: a scoping review. JMIR mHealth uHealth. 2017;5:e38. https://doi.org/10.2196/mhealth.7185.
22. Gbadamosi OS, Eze C, Olawepo OJ, Iwelunmor J, Sarpong FD, Ogidi GA, et al. A Patient-Held Smartcard With a Unique Identifier and an mHealth Platform to Improve the Availability of Prenatal Test Results in Rural Nigeria: Demonstration Study. J Med Internet Res. 20:e18. https://doi.org/10.2196/jmir.8716.
23. Ghana Statistical Service. 2010 Population and Housing Census, Regional Analytical Report, Upper East Region. 2013. http://www.statsghana.gov.gh/docfiles/2010phc/2010_PHC_Regional_Analytical_Reports_Upper_East Region.pdf.
24. Ghana Statistical Service. 2010 Population and Housing Census, District Analytical Report, Binduri District. 2014. http://www.statsghana.gov.gh/docfiles/2010_District_Report/Upper East/BINDURI.pdf.
25. Feng L, Maitlis S. Non-Participant Observation. In: Mills AJ, Durepos G, Wiebe E, editors. Sage Encyclopedia of case study research. Los Angeles: Sage Publications Ltd; 2010.
26. Latulippe K, Hamel C, Giroux D. Social health inequalities and eHealth: a literature review with qualitative synthesis of theoretical and empirical studies. J Med Internet Res. 2017;19:e136. https://doi.org/10.2196/jmir.6731.
27. Agarwal S, Perry HB, Long L-A, Labrique AB. Evidence on feasibility and effective use of mHealth strategies by frontline health workers in developing countries: systematic review. Trop Med Int Heal. 2015;20:1003–14. https://doi.org/10.1111/tmi.12525.
28. Lund S, Nielsen BB, Hemed M, Boas IM, Said A, Said K, et al. Mobile phones improve antenatal care attendance in Zanzibar: a cluster randomized controlled trial. BMC Pregnancy Childbirth. 2014;14:29. https://doi.org/10.1186/1471-2393-14-29.
29. Sen A. Health: perception versus observation : self reported morbidity has severe limitations and can be extremely misleading. BMJ Br Med J. 2002; 324:860–1. http://www.ncbi.nlm.nih.gov/pmc/articles/PMC1122815/
30. Håland E, Melby L. Negotiating technology-mediated interaction in health care. Soc Theory Heal. 2015;13:78–98. https://doi.org/10.1057/sth.2014.18.
31. Schoen J, Mallett JW, Grossman-Kahn R, Brentani A, Kaselitz E, Heisler M. Perspectives and experiences of community health workers in Brazilian primary care centers using m-health tools in home visits with community members. Hum Resour Health. 2017;15:71. https://doi.org/10.1186/s12960-017-0245-9.
32. Vedanthan R, Blank E, Tuikong N, Kamano J, Misoi L, Tulienge D, et al. Usability and feasibility of a tablet-based decision-support and integrated record-keeping (DESIRE) tool in the nurse Management of Hypertension in rural western Kenya. Int J Med Inform. 2015;84:207–19. https://doi.org/10.1016/j.ijmedinf.2014.12.005.
33. Duclos V, Yé M, Moubassira K, Sanou H, Sawadogo NH, Bibeau G, et al. Situating mobile health: a qualitative study of mHealth expectations in the rural health district of Nouna, Burkina Faso. Heal Res Policy Syst. 2017; 15(Suppl 1):47. https://doi.org/10.1186/s12961-017-0211-y.
34. Jack SM, DiCenso A, Lohfeld L. A theory of maternal engagement with public health nurses and family visitors. J Adv Nurs. 2005;49:182–90. https://doi.org/10.1111/j.1365-2648.2004.03278.x.
35. Sheppard VB, Zambrana RE, O'Malley AS. Providing health care to low-income women: a matter of trust. Fam Pract. 2004;21:484–91. https://doi.org/10.1093/fampra/cmh503
36. Mensah N, Sukums F, Awine T, Meid A, Williams J, Akweongo P, et al. Impact of an electronic clinical decision support system on workflow in antenatal care: the QUALMAT eCDSS in rural health care facilities in Ghana and Tanzania. Glob Health Action. 2015;8 https://doi.org/10.3402/gha.v8.25756.
37. Gudu W, Addo B. Factors associated with utilization of skilled service delivery among women in rural northern Ghana: a cross sectional study. BMC Pregnancy Childbirth. 2017;17:159. https://doi.org/10.1186/s12884-017-1344-2.
38. Atnafu A, Otto K, Herbst CH. The role of mHealth intervention on maternal and child health service delivery: findings from a randomized controlled field trial in rural Ethiopia. mHealth; Sept 2017. 2017. http://mhealth.amegroups.com/article/view/16495.
39. Shiferaw S, Spigt M, Tekie M, Abdullah M, Fantahun M, Dinant G-J. The effects of a locally developed mHealth intervention on delivery and postnatal care utilization; a prospective controlled evaluation among health Centres in Ethiopia. PLoS One. 2016;11:e0158600. https://doi.org/10.1371/journal.pone.0158600.
40. Liu F, Maitlis S, Observation N. In: Mills AJ, Durepos G, Wiebe E, editors. Encyclopedia of case study research. London: SAGE; 2010. p. 610–2. https://doi.org/10.4135/9781412957397.n229.

8

Spatial distribution of antenatal care utilization and associated factors in Ethiopia: evidence from Ethiopian demographic health surveys

Abraham Yeneneh[1], Kassahun Alemu[2], Abel Fekadu Dadi[2*] and Atinkut Alamirrew[1]

Abstract

Background: Antenatal care (ANC) is one of the components of care to be provided to pregnant women. In Ethiopia, characterizing the spatial distribution of antenatal care utilization is essential to prioritize risk areas where ANC is needed and facilitate interventions. Therefore, this spatial analysis was performed to assess the spatial distribution of ANC utilization between 2000 and 2011 and to identify factors associated with ANC utilization in Ethiopia.

Methods: A total of 23,179 women who had a live birth in the five years preceding the surveys were included in the study. The spatial data were created in ArcGIS10.1 for each study clusters. The Bernoulli model was used by applying Kulldorff methods using the SaTScan™ software to analyze the purely spatial clusters of ANC utilization. Multiple logistic regression analysis was used to identify predictors affecting ANC utilization.

Results: ANC utilization had spatial variations across the country. Spatial scan statistics identified 49 high performing clusters (LLR = 111.92, $P < 0.001$) in 2000, 51 (LLR = 114.49, $P < 0.001$) in 2005 and, 86 (LLR = 121.53, $P < 0.001$) in 2011. ANC utilization was higher among mothers; with richest wealth quintiles, lowest number of birth order, who are living in urban areas, younger and educated.

Conclusion: These results provide further insight into differences in ANC utilization in the country and highlight high and modest performing clusters. This could enable efficient and timely spatial targeting to improve ANC service up take in Ethiopia.

Keywords: Antenatal care utilization, Spatial distribution, Ethiopia

Background

Antenatal care refers to the regular medical and nursing care recommended for women during pregnancy to prevent, detect and treat complications [1]. Timely initiation of antenatal care is an opportunity to prevent the direct causes of maternal deaths and reduce fetal and neonatal deaths related to obstetric complications [2].

* Correspondence: Fekten@yahoo.com
[2]College of Medicine and Health Sciences, Institute of Public Health, Department of Health Informatics, Department of Epidemiology and Biostatistics, University of Gondar, Gondar, Ethiopia
Full list of author information is available at the end of the article

Globally, about 300,000 women die each year as a result of pregnancy related complications [3], 2.6 million babies are estimated to be stillborn [4], and 4 million newborns die in the neonatal period. In sub-Saharan Africa and other resource-poor settings, maternal mortality remains a major public health problem [3, 5]. Such deaths could be prevented if pregnancy and birth-related complications are managed properly through the expansion and uptake improvement of basic antenatal care service [6].

In Ethiopia, the levels of maternal and infant morbidity and mortality are among the highest in the world [7]. These major problems could be addressed

Table 1 Socio-demographic characteristics of women participated on EDHS (2000, 2005, 2011), Ethiopia

	Year					
	2011		2005		2000	
Variables	Frequency ($n = 7909$)	Percent	Frequency ($n = 7304$)	Percent	Frequency ($n = 7967$)	Percent
Place of residence						
Urban	1189	15	633	8.7	906	11.4
Rural	6720	85	6671	91.3	7061	88.6
Age at birth						
15–19	402	5.1	440	6.0	472	5.9
20–24	1608	20.3	1473	20.2	1727	21.6
25–29	2383	30.1	1960	26.8	2021	25.6
30–34	1489	18.8	1427	19.5	1493	18.6
35–39	1239	15.7	1138	15.6	1219	15.3
40–44	572	7.2	578	7.9	706	8.9
45–49	216	2.7	288	4.0	329	4.1
Birth order						
1	1399	17.7	1190	16.3	1362	17.1
2–4	3465	43.8	3024	41.4	3259	40.9
> =5	3045	38.5	3090	42.3	3346	42.0
Level of education						
No education	2506	31.7	5734	78.5	6539	82.1
Primary	3483	44.1	1205	16.5	1003	12.6
Secondary	1068	14.5	325	4.5	400	5.0
Higher	852	10.7	40	0.5	25	0.3
Wealth quintile						
Poorest	1739	22.0	1520	20.8		
Poorer	1696	21.5	1553	21.26		
Middle	1628	20.6	1585	21.71		
Richer	1494	18.8	1451	19.86		
Richest	1352	17.1	1195	16.37		
Region						
Tigray	530	6.7	480	6.6	536	6.7
Affar	78	0.9	68	0.9	85	1.1
Amhara	1991	25.2	1856	25.4	2222	27.8
Oromia	3116	39.4	2723	37.3	3057	38.4
Somali	198	2.5	288	3.9	84	1.1
Benishangul-gum	92	1.2	68	0.9	81	1.0
SNNP	1634	20.7	1631	22.3	1689	21.2
Gambela	31	0.4	23	0.3	22	0.3
Harari	19	0.2	15	0.3	16	0.2
Addis Ababa	193	2.4	128	1.8	148	1.9
Dire Dawa	27	0.4	24	0.3	27	0.3

by proper utilization of ANC, skilled delivery and postnatal care services [8]. Geographic accessibility of the services is one of the most important factors associated with utilization of maternity care [9]. Rural populations are particularly disadvantaged as they often lack reliable means of transport [10]. Women who have a higher density of clinics nearby have a lower risk of starting antenatal care late [11].

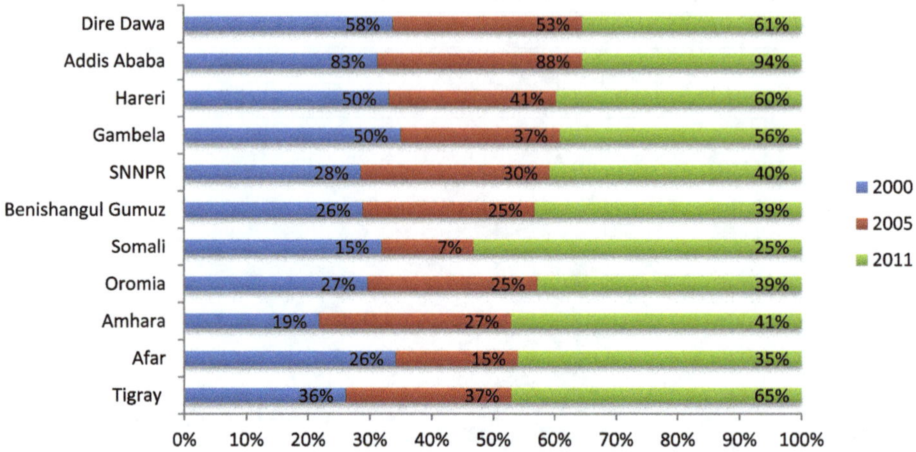

Fig. 1 Trends in ANC utilization overtime by regions, in 2000, 2005 and 2011, Ethiopia

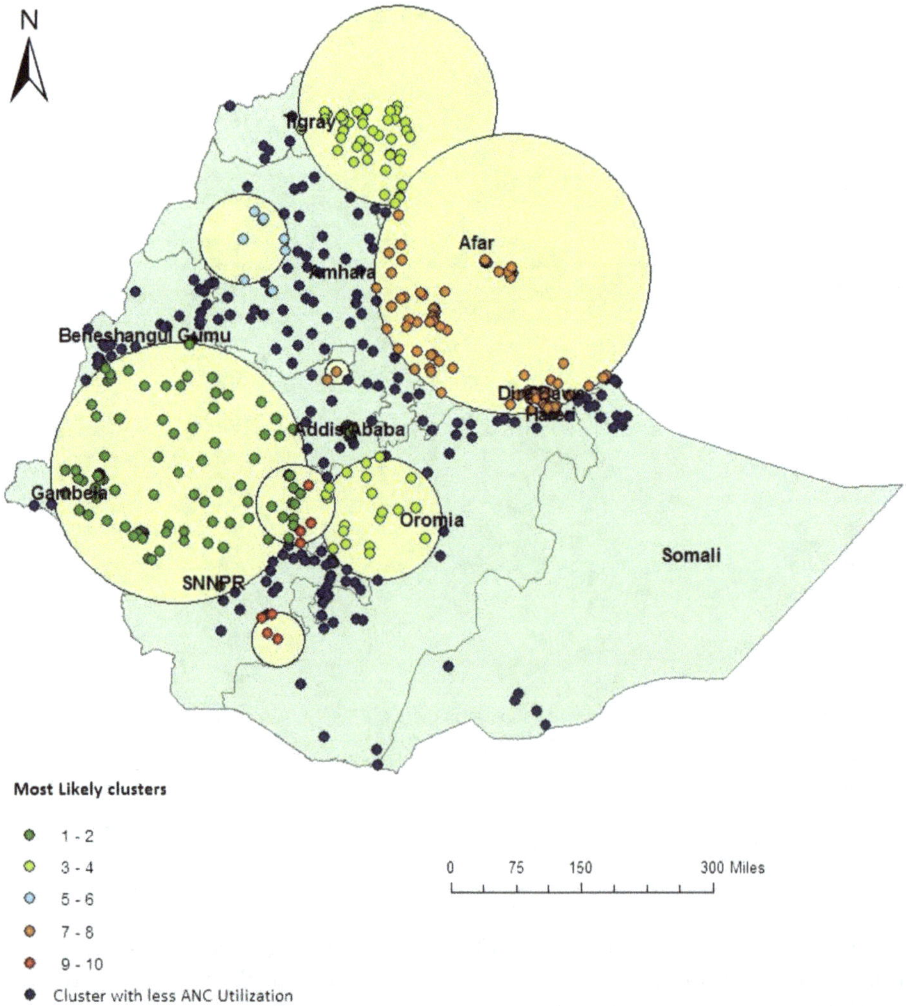

Fig. 2 Spatial distribution of ANC utilization in 2000 EDHS

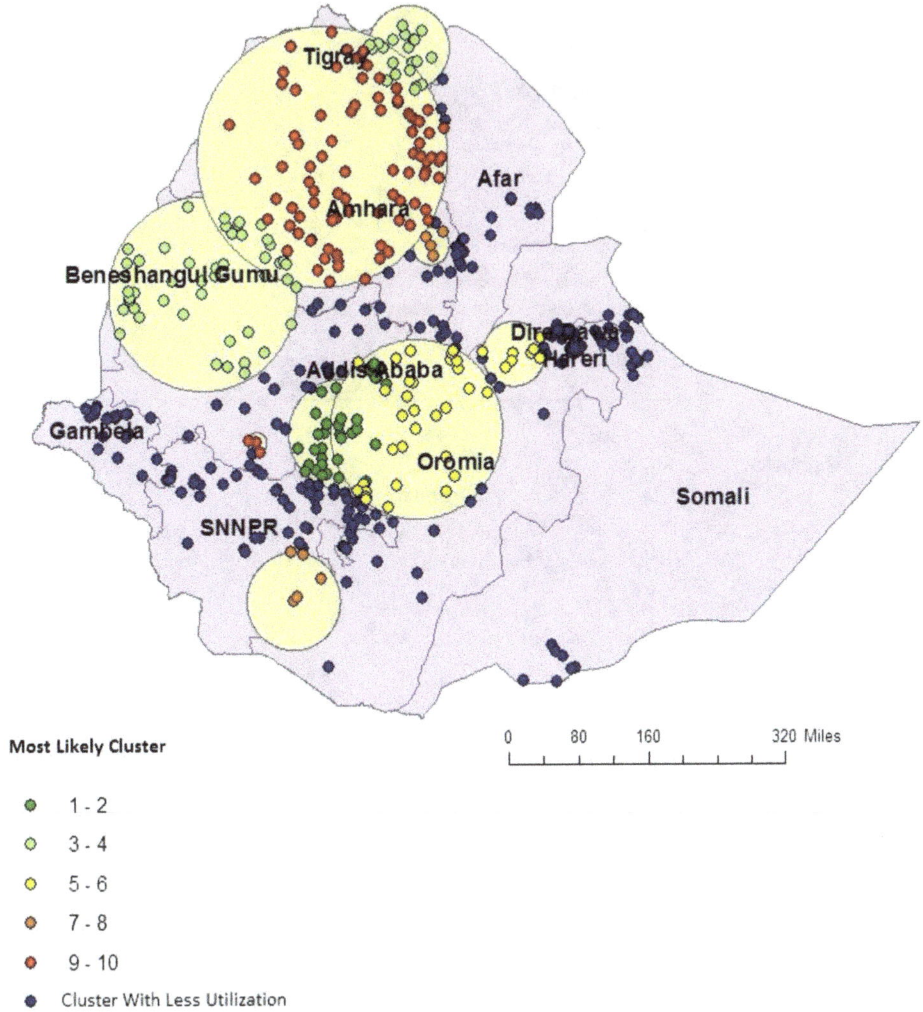

Fig. 3 Spatial distribution of ANC utilization in 2005 EDHS

Understanding the levels and geographical variations of ANC utilization would help policymakers, planners, programmers and partners in the health sector to formulate appropriate strategies and interventions and provide quality reproductive health services. The aim of this study was to assess the spatial distribution and identify factors associated with ANC utilization using evidence from the Ethiopian Health and Demographic Surveys between 2000 and 2011.

Methods

Study design and study settings

A repeated cross sectional study design was employed using the Ethiopian Demography and Health Surveys (EDHS) in 2000, 2005, and 2011 to assess spatial pattern of ANC utilization. Ethiopia is located in the horn of Africa. It has a total area of 1,100,000 km^2 and lies between latitudes 3° and 15°N, and longitudes 33° and 48°E. Ethiopia has been divided into nine ethnic based and politically autonomous regional states and two cities (Addis Ababa and Dire Dawa). The Regions are subdivided into sixty-eight zones, and then further into 817 districts which are further divided into around 16,253 Kebeles (the lowest local administrative units).

Study population

The source population was all women of childbearing age (15–49 years) in Ethiopia. The study population was all women who had a live birth in the five years preceding the survey just to minimize the recall bias arising from the time relapse. The most recent birth was considered for women with two or more live births during the five-year period. All records related to ANC utilization, which had complete records in all EDHS (EDHS-2000, 2005 and 2011) documents were included in the study.

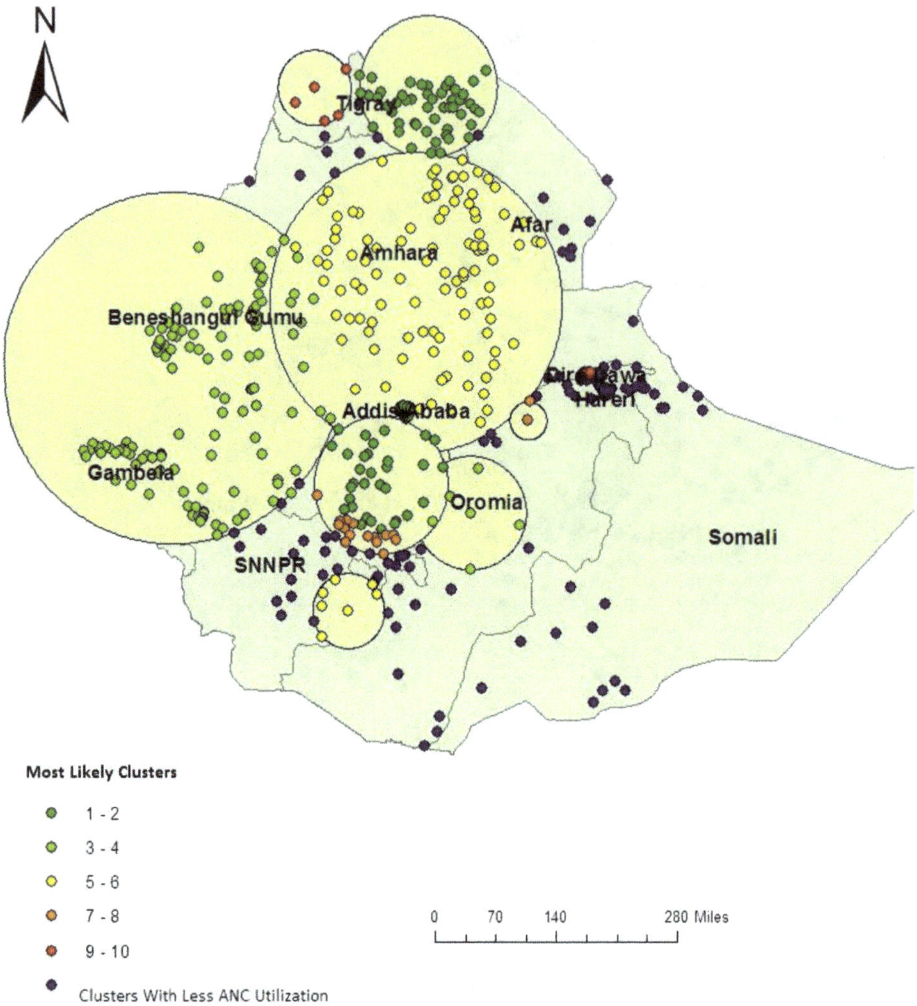

Fig. 4 Spatial distribution of ANC utilization in 2011 EDHS

Sample size and sampling procedure

A total of 23,179 women (7967 women in 2000, 7304 women in 2005 and, 7909 women in 2011) were included in the study. Weighted values were used because weights restore the representativeness of sampled data. Sample weights were calculated and included in each EDHS recoded file. Data were extracted using STATA version 12.0 and SPSS version 20 software.

A Multi-stage stratified sampling technique was used for all three EDHS. In 2000 and 2005, sampling was based on the Census Enumeration Areas (CEAs) of the 1994 Population and Housing Census of Ethiopia [12]. In 2011, sampling was based on the 2007 National Population and Housing Census of Ethiopia [13].

In 2000 and 2005, a total of 540 (139 urban and 401 rural) CEAs were selected using systematic sampling from all regional states in the country. Then, in 2000, 27 households per CEA and in 2005, 24 to 32 households per CEA were selected systematically. In 2011, a total of 624 CEAs (187 urban and 437 rural) were selected using systematic sampling technique.

Data collection tools and procedures

ANC data were obtained from central statistics agency (CSA) using www.dhsprogram.com. The web provided the data only for authorized users. Data also comprised the location data (latitude and longitude coordinates).

Statistical analysis

Descriptive and multivariable logistic regression analyses were carried out using STATA 12. Independent variables were age, birth order, region, education, wealth index, and ANC accessibility (e.g. residence, transport and distance). Both bi and multivariable binary logistic regression models were used to identify factors that affect ANC utilization. Those variables with P-value < 0.2 in bi-variable logistic regression model were entered in the multivariable logistic

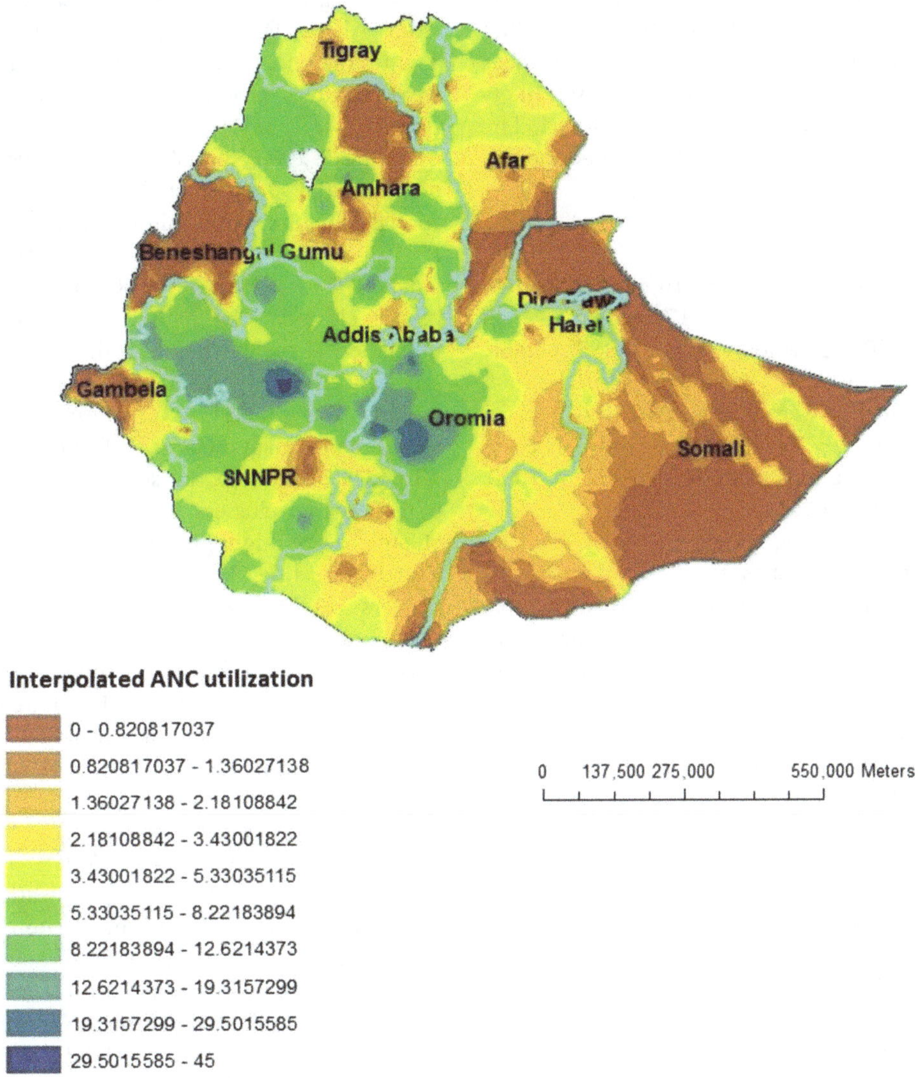

Fig. 5 Interpolated special distribution of ANC utilization in 2000, EDHS

regression model to measure the effect of each variable after adjusting for the effect of other variables using Backward Logistic Regression. Variables with p-value < 0.05 were considered as statistically significant.

A Bernoulli-based model was used in which events at particular places were analyzed if women use ANC or not represented by a 0/1 variable. The scan statistics developed by Kulldorff and SaTScan™ software version 9.4 [8] were used to identify the presence of purely spatial low ANC utilization clusters. Scan statistics did scanning gradually across the space to identify the number of observed and expected observations inside the window at each location. The scanning window with the maximum likelihood was the most likely high performing clusters, and a p-value was assigned to this cluster. The window centered on each of the several possible grid points positioned throughout the study areas. For each grid point, the radius of the window differed continuously in size from zero to a specified maximum value. ANC utilization clusters centered on one of the grid squares used as spatial units of observation.

Spatial interpolation technique was applied to predict the unsampled/unmeasured value from sampled measurements. In the DHS survey ANC utilization is known for all census enumeration areas, but ANC utilization for other unselected locations in Ethiopia is also of interest. The one with the maximum likelihood comprised the highest performing cluster. The p-value was obtained through the Monte Carlo hypothesis testing by comparing the rank of the maximum likelihood from the real datasets with the maximum likelihoods from the random datasets. The number of replications were 999. Secondary clusters were identified in the datasets in addition to the most likely cluster and we ordered them according to their likelihood ratio test statistic. The inferences of secondary clusters were adjusted for more likely clusters in the data using an iterative manner. The maximum cluster size was set at 50% of the population at risk.

Results

There are 14,642 households and 15,716 eligible women in 2000, 14,645 households and 14,717 eligible women in 2005, and 18,720 households and 17,385 eligible women in 2011. From this, a response rates for the first, second, and third surveys were 97.8% ($n = 15{,}370$), 95.6% ($n = 14{,}069$), and 95% ($n = 16{,}515$), respectively. The actual women included in this study were 7967 in 2000, 7304 in 2005, and 7909 in 2011.

Socio-demographic characteristics

Of the total respondents, in 2000, 7061 (88.6%), in 2005, 6673 (91.3%), and in 2011, 6720 (85%) were rural residents. The majority of women ages during birth were between 25 to 29 years old. Women who had 2 to 4 birth order were 3259 (43.8%) in 2000, 3026 (41.4%) in 2005, and 3464 (40.9%) in 2011. In 2000, 6539 (82.0%), in 2005, 5734 (78.5%), and in 2011, 5270 (66.6%) women were uneducated. Of the total women in 2005, 1520 (20.8%) and in 2011 1739 (22.0%) were in the lowest wealth quintile (Table 1). Despite the low coverage of ANC utilization, all regions registered an increasing trend from 2000 to 2011 (Fig. 1).

Spatial distribution of ANC utilization

Spatial variation was found in ANC utilization at regional levels. Of a total of 7909 women interviewed, 3361 (42.5%) women utilized ANC by skilled health care providers. The highest utilization of ANC was spatially clustered in Addis Ababa. On the other hand, Somali Region was the lowest in ANC utilization (Table 1). Of a total of 7304 women interviewed in 2005, 2016 (27.6%) utilized ANC. Of a total of 7967 women interviewed in 2011, 2127 (26.7%) utilized ANC. Out of these, the highest ANC utilization was in Addis Ababa, Dire Dawa, Hareri and Gambela sequentially, while Amhara and Somali Region showed the lowest ANC utilization (Table 1).

Spatial pattern of ANC utilization

In EDHS 2000, spatial scan statistics identified a total of 145 high and modest performing spatial clusters of ANC utilization. Of these, 49 clusters were high performing clusters) (LLR = 111.92, $P < 0.001$) accounting for 33.7% and 96 clusters were modest performing clusters (LLR = 71.15, $P < 0.001$) accounting for 66.3%. The highest performing clusters of ANC utilization were detected in Addis Ababa, Dire Dawa, Harari, Oromia, Gambela and Tigray regions. The modest ANC utilization clusters were located around Somali and Amhara Regions (Fig. 2).

In EDHS 2005, spatial scan statistics identified a total of 78 spatial clusters of ANC utilization. Of these, 51 spatial clusters were high performing (LLR = 114.49, $P < 0.001$) and 27 clusters were modest performing clusters (LLR = 99.04, $P < 0.001$) and accounted 53.9% of the clusters. The high performing clusters of ANC utilization were detected in Addis Ababa, Dire Dawa, Harari, some part of SNNP, Benishangul Gumuz and Tigray regions. The modest ANC utilization clusters were detected in Somali and Gambela Regions (Fig. 3).

In EDHS-2011, spatial scan statistics identified a total of 136 spatial clusters of ANC utilization. Of these, 86 clusters were high performing clusters (LLR = 121.53, $P < 0.001$) while 50 clusters were modest perfuming clusters (LLR = 61.87, $P < 0.001$). The high performing spatial clusters of ANC utilization were detected in Addis Ababa, Dire Dawa, Harari, Gambela, Benishangul Gumuz and Tigray regions. The modest antenatal care service utilization clusters were mostly located around Somali and some part of Afar Regions (Fig. 4).

Interpolation using GIS mapping

Based on EDHS-2000 sampled data, geostatistical analysis predict that highest ANC utilization rates were detected in South-West Oromia region, some Northern part of Oromia and some parts of southern SNNPR. In contrast, relatively low ANC utilization areas were predicted in Beneshangul Gumuz, Western part of Gambela, Northern part of Affar and most part of Somali. Based on EDHS-2005 Geostatistical analysis, high ANC utilization was detected in Southwest part of Amhara, Northeast Oromia and Southeast part of SNNPR. In contrast to this, low ANC utilization places were in the Eastern part of Somali, most part of Affar and Gambela and Western part of Beneshangul Gumuz. From the third EDHS sampled data in 2011, geostatistical analysis predicted that most part of Oromia, Northern Amhara and some part of Western SNNPR contained the highest ANC utilization areas, while most parts of Afar, Somali, Beneshangul Gumuz and Gambela contained modest ANC utilization areas (Figs. 5, 6 and 7).

Factors associated with ANC utilization for EDHS-2011

After adjusting for different confounding variables, place of residence, age at birth, level of education, region, birth order and wealth status were significantly associated with ANC utilization (Table 2).

Women who lived in urban areas were 1.55 times more likely to utilize ANC than women living in rural

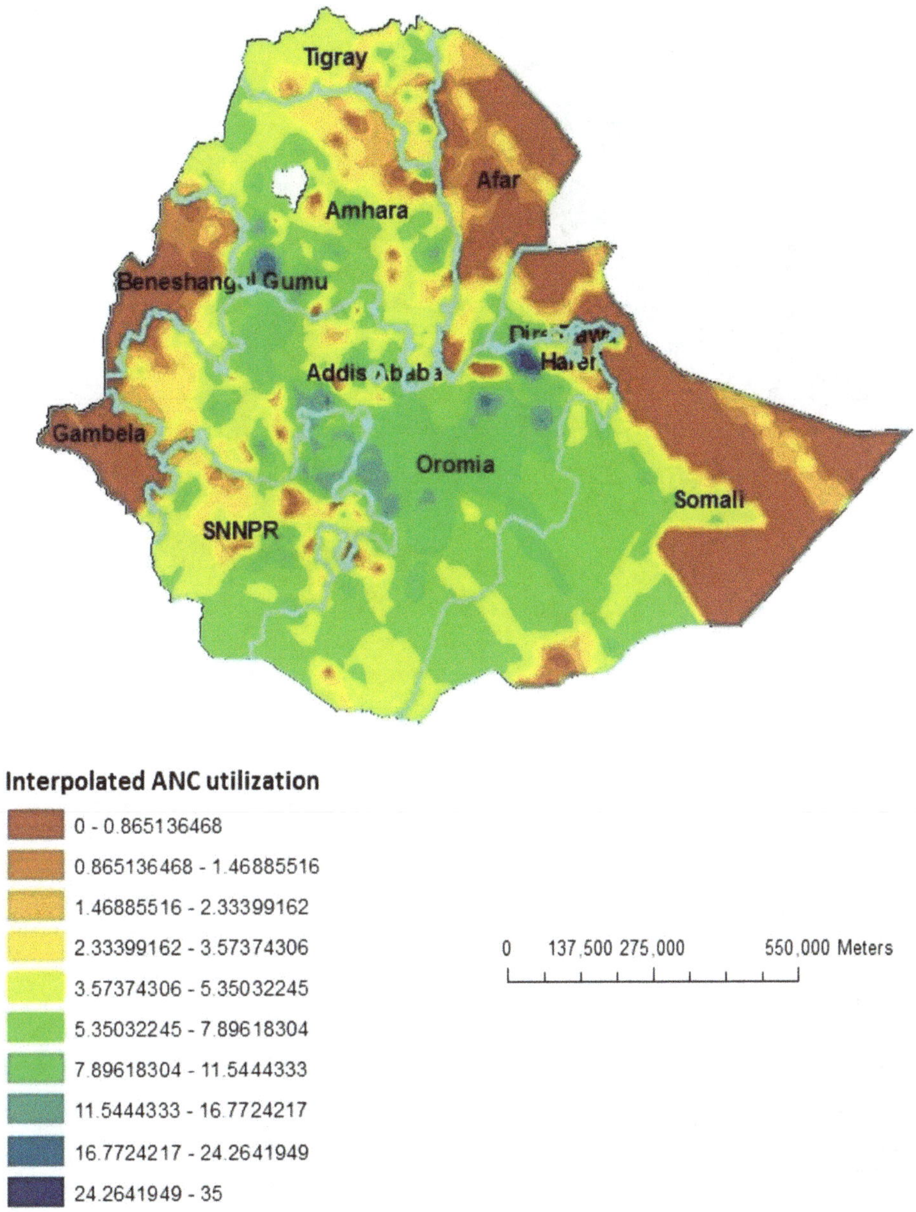

Fig. 6 Interpolated special distribution of ANC utilization in 2005, EDHS

areas [AOR = 1.55; 95% CI; 1.22–1.97]. As the wealth of the women increases the odds of utilizing ANC also increases. The odds of ANC utilization was 0.31 [AOR = 0.31; 95%CI; 0.23–0.56] times lower among non-educated group, 4.67 [AOR = 4.67; 95%CI; 4.02–6.65] times higher among mothers with secondary education and 7.44 [AOR = 7.44; 95%CI; 6.98–9.01] times higher among mothers with higher education as compared to mothers with primary level of education. Women's in age group of 30–34 and 45–49 were 20% [AOR = 0.80; 95%CI; 0.68–0.95] and 41% [AOR = 0.59; 95%CI; 0.41–0.85] less likely to utilize ANC as compared to women in the age group of 25–29. Mothers whose their pregnancy is for the first time were 1.34 times more likely to utilize ANC [AOR = 1.34; 95%CI; 1.13–1.59]. Compared to women living in Oromia region, those living in Tigray [AOR = 2.85; 95%CI; 2.28–3.57] and Addis Ababa [AOR = 4.00, 95%CI; 2.14–7.48) were more likely to utilize ANC (Table 2).

Discussion

SaTScan and GIS-based spatial statistical techniques provide an opportunity to clarify and identify antenatal care utilization within a country and help future investigations into factors responsible for increased antenatal care utilization. Geographic visualization of

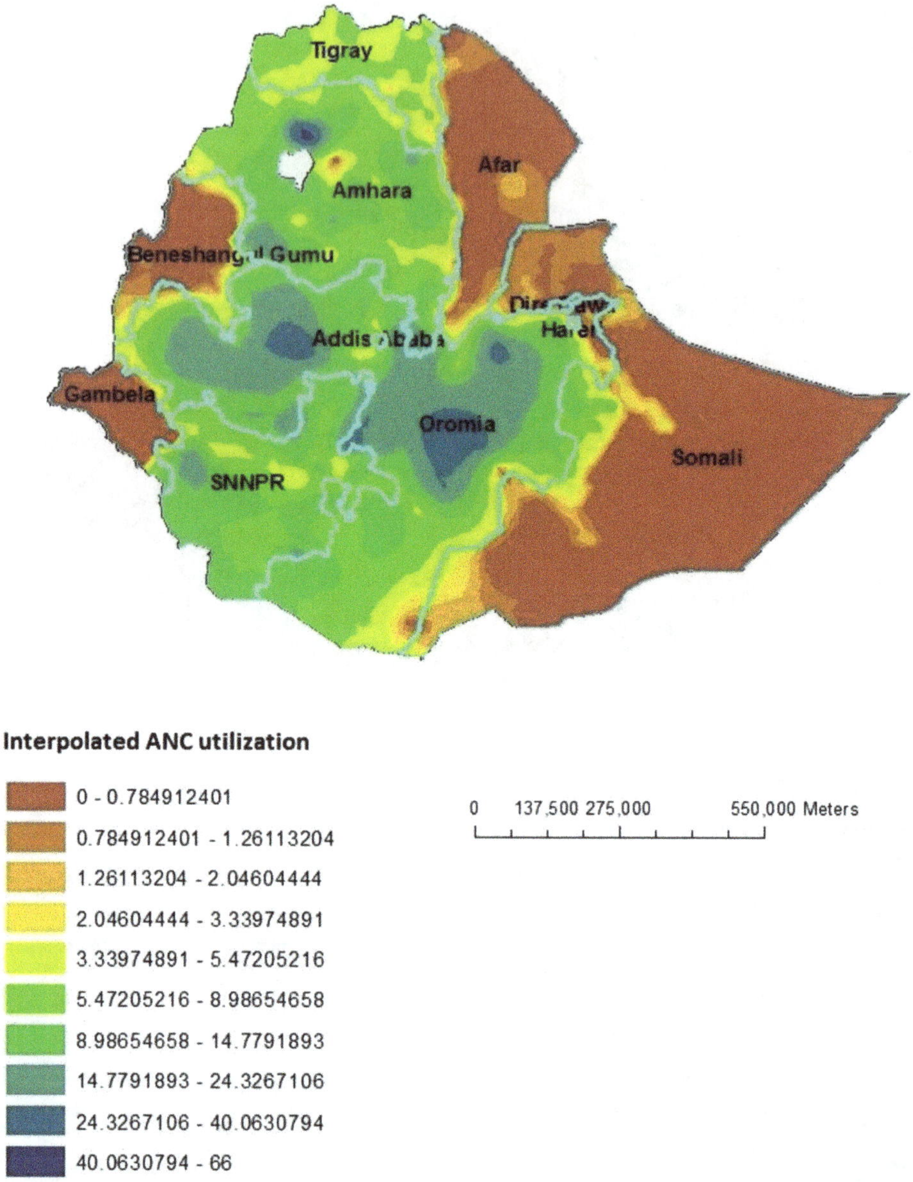

Fig. 7 Interpolated special distribution of ANC utilization in 2011, EDHS

ANC utilization using these tools was instrumental to understand highest and modest utilization level and target interventions in high-risk areas. This study has provided a visually powerful analysis of spatial variation in antenatal care utilization among women in Ethiopia.

ANC utilization rate has substantially increased from 26.7% in 2000 to 27.6% in 2005 and 42.5% in 2011 in Ethiopia. High variations, however, are observed between rural and urban areas. This variation may be because of proximity of the health facility in the village and the geographical distribution of ANC clinics. These reasons are consistent with findings of another study in Brooklyn, US [11]. In all surveys, women from urban areas had less numbers than women from rural areas (11.4% versus 88.6%, in 2000, 8.7% versus 91.3% in 2005, and 15% versus 85% in 2011, respectively. There is also variation in antenatal care utilization across the country's regions. Highest antenatal care utilization rates were reported in Addis Ababa, Dire Dawa, Harari, whereas comparatively modest utilization was reported in Somali regions and Affar. These regions are relatively urban in which health facilities are more accessible and women are more aware of maternal health services. The multivariable model also revealed consistent finding in which Tigray and Addis Ababa were the places where the highest ANC utilization is recorded and Somali is found to be the place where small number of mothers

Table 2 Women's socio-demographic characteristics and its association with utilization of antenatal care service 2011, Ethiopia

Variable	Received ANC		Crude odds ratio (95% CI)	Adjusted odds ratio (95% CI)
	Yes	No		
Place of residence				
Urban	893	297	5.21 (4.52–5.99)	1.55 (1.22–1.97)
Rural	2471	4248	1	1
Age at birth				
15–19	160	242	0.82 (0.66–1.02)	0.80 (0.61–1.06)
20–24	787	822	1.19 (1.05–1.36)	1.18 (1.00–1.38)
25–29	1059	1324	1	1
30–34	577	912	0.79 (0.69–0.90)	0.80 (0.68–0.95)
35–39	512	727	0.88 (0.77–1.01)	0.94 (0.78–1.13)
40–44	207	364	0.71 (0.59–1.86)	0.83 (0.65–1.06)
45 49	63	153	0.52 (0.38–0.70)	0.59 (0.41–0.85)
Birth order				
1	753	646	1.53 (1.35–1.74)	1.34 (1.13–1.59)
2-4	1495	1969	1	1
>=5	1117	1929	0.76 (0.69–0.84)	1.01 (0.87–1.18)
Mothers Education				
No education	888	1618	0.45 (0.40–0.49)	0.31 (0.23–0.56)
Primary	1916	1567	1	1
Secondary	943	125	6.17 (5.06–7.52)	4.67 (4.02–6.65)
Higher	796	56	11.62 (8.79–15.36)	7.44 (6.98–9.01)
Wealth quintile				
Poorest	436	1303	1	1
Poorer	593	1103	1.607 (1.39–1.86)	1.54 (1.31–1.81)
Middle	616	1012	1.82 (1.57–2.11)	1.86 (1.58–2.19)
Richer	704	790	2.66 (2.30–3.09)	3.01 (2.54–3.56)
Richest	1016	336	9.07 (7.69–10.68)	5.79 (4.52–7.40)
Region				
Tigray	328	202	2.76 (2.28–3.34)	2.85 (2.28–3.57)
Affar	27	51	0.82 (0.51–1.31)	0.86 (0.49–1.51)
Amhara	794	1197	1.01 (0.90–1.14)	1.02 (0.89–1.17)
Oromia	1232	1884	1	1
Somali	50	148	0.52 (0.37–0.72)	0.37 (0.25–0.55)
Benishangul	37	55	1.03 (0.67–1.56)	1.02 (0.63–1.65)
SNNP	660	974	1.04 (0.92–1.17)	1.13 (0.98–1.31)
Gambela	18	13	2.03 (0.99–4.15)	2.03 (0.86–4.75)
Harari	11	8	2.22 (0.89–5.52)	1.02 (0.35–2.97)
Addis Ababa	180	13	21.54 (12.16–38.16)	4.00 (2.14–7.48)
Dire Dawa	16	11	2.29 (1.05–5.03)	1.14 (0.44–2.94)

got ANC as compared to the biggest region (Oromia). These reasons are consistent with the findings of another study in Ethiopia [14].

Another factor that affected ANC utilization was the income of the mother, the odds of ANC utilization being higher among women in the richest wealth quintile. Even though, ANC is currently under exempted service in health facilities in Ethiopia, it was not like this before and women should pay to get the service. In addition, income would also affect health seeking behavior of the mother in which poor mothers had low health seeking behavior [15, 16].

Age of the mother and birth order are the other predictor variables reported to have an association with ANC utilization. Relatively younger women and whose pregnancy is for their first time were more likely to attend ANC service as compared to older and multiparous women. Similar studies have also reported an indirect relationship between parity and maternal services; women's of high parity tend to use ANC less [17, 18]. This could be explained by low to no experience about the current pregnancy will make the new mother to have some sort of fear of risks associated with her pregnancy that make her more curios to have frequent ANC visits. The perception that they had better knowledge about pregnancy complications would be another factor that explains low ANC uptake by mothers who had more number of children as compared to new mothers [19].

Like previous studies [17–19], in the current analysis, educated women were more likely to utilize ANC as compared to those relatively educated. It is true that education enhances the health seeking behavior of the mother, it also make the mother to actively involved in different knowledge enhancement activities like reading materials, service promotions, and peer discussions. It is also believed that more educated mothers would tend to give better care and concern for their health and their fetus and they are also more likely to strive to know benefits of the service and associated pregnancy complications.

Conclusion

This study identified spatial clusters of ANC utilization in Somalia Region with low utilization rates and Addis Ababa with the highest utilization rate. Richest wealth quintiles, lowest number of birth order, educated, living in urban areas and being younger increased the likelihood of utilizing ANC. These results provide further insights into identifying the true picture of ANC utilization clusters in the country and enable efficient and timely spatial targeting factors triggering low utilization of antenatal care.

Abbreviations

ANC: Antenatal care; AOR: Adjusted Odds ratio; CSA: Central statistics agency; EDHS: Ethiopian demographic and health survey; IRB: Institutional Review Board; SNNPR: Southern Nations and Nationality and peoples region; SPSS: Statistical package for social sciences

Acknowledgements

The authors gratefully acknowledge support received from University of Gondar for providing fund. We also thank the Ethiopian Central Statistics Agency for providing us with the data and shape files for the study area.

Authors' contributions

Conception and design of the work, acquisition of data, analysis and interpretation of data was done by AY, KA, and AA. Drafting the article, revising it critically for intellectual content, and final approval of the version to be published was done by AY, KA, AF and AA. All authors read and approved the final manuscript.

Competing interests

The authors declare that they have no competing interests.

Author details

[1]College of Medicine and Health Sciences Institute of Public Health, Department of Health Informatics, University of Gondar, Gondar, Ethiopia. [2]College of Medicine and Health Sciences, Institute of Public Health, Department of Health Informatics, Department of Epidemiology and Biostatistics, University of Gondar, Gondar, Ethiopia.

References

1. Organization WH. Making pregnancy safer: a health sector strategy for reducing maternal and perinatal morbidity and mortality. Geneva: World Health Organization; 2005.
2. Reynolds HW, Wong EL, Tucker H. Adolescents' use of maternal and child health services in developing countries. Int Fam Plan Perspect. 2006;32(1)
3. Lozano R, Wang H, Foreman KJ, Rajaratnam JK, Naghavi M, Marcus JR, et al. Progress towards millennium development goals 4 and 5 on maternal and child mortality: an updated systematic analysis. Lancet. 2011;378
4. Mondal D, Galloway TS, Bailey TC, Mathews F. Elevated risk of stillbirth in males: systematic review and meta-analysis of more than 30 million births. BMC Med. 2014;12(220)
5. Hogan MC, Foreman KJ, Naghavi M, Ahn SY, Wang M, Makela SM, et al. Maternal mortality for 181 countries, 1980–2008: a systematic analysis of progress towards millennium development goal 5. Lancet. 2010;
6. Kinney MV, Kerber KJ, Black RE, Cohen B, Nkrumah F, Coovadia H, et al. Sub-Saharan Africa's mothers, newborns, and children: where and why do they die? PLoS Med. 2010;7(6)
7. CSA. Ethiopia Demographic and Health Survey 201, 1Central Statistical Agency Addis Ababa, Ethiopia ICF International Calverton. Maryland, USA: CSA; 2011.
8. Kulldorffand M. Spatial disease clusters: detection and inference. Stat Med. 1995;14(8)
9. Ronsmans C, Graham WJ. Maternal mortality: who, when, where, and why. Lancet. 2006;368:1189–200.
10. Ibnouf AH, van den Borne HW, Maarse JA. Utilization of antenatal care services by sudaneses women in their reproductive age. Saudi Med. 2007;28(5)
11. McLafferty S, Grady S. Prenatal care need and access: a GIS analysis. McLafferty and Grady. 2004;
12. Central Stastical Agency of Ethiopia; The 2007 population and house census of Ethiopia; results at country level.
13. [Ethiopia] CSA. The 2007 Population and Housing Census of Ethiopia. Statistical Summary Report at National Level. Addis Ababa, Ethiopia; 2008.
14. Tewodros B, G/Mariam A, Dibaba Y. Factors affecting antenatal care utilization in yem special woreda, Southwestern Ethiopia Ethiop J Health Sci 2009;Vol. 19(01).
15. Goland E, Hoa DT, Malqvist M. Inequalities in maternal health care utilization in Veitnam. Int J Equity Health. 2012;11:24. https://doi.org/10.1186/1475-9276-11-24.
16. Rahman M, Haque SE, Mostofa G, Tarivonda L, Shuaib M. Wealth inequality and utilization of reproductive health services in the Republic of Vanuatu: insights from the multiple indicator cluster survey, 2007. Int J Equity Health. 2011;10:58.
17. Simkhada B, Teijlingen ER v, Porter M, Simkhada P. Factors affecting the utilization of antenatal care in developing countries: systematic review of the literature. J Adv Nurs. 2008;61:244–60. https://doi.org/10.1111/j.1365-2648.2007.04532.x.
18. Fekede B, G/Mariam A. Antenatal care services utilization and factors associated in Jimma Town (South West Ethiopia). Ethiop Med J. 2007; 45(2):123–33.

The role of timely initiation of antenatal care on protective dose tetanus toxoid immunization: the case of northern Ethiopia post natal mothers

Muhabaw Shumye Mihret[*†], Miteku Andualem Limenih[†] and Temesgen Worku Gudayu[*]

Abstract

Background: Globally, tetanus toxoid protective dose immunization of the mothers is one of the strategies of maternal and neonatal tetanus prevention. Ethiopia has planned the national tetanus protection at birth coverage to reach 86% by the year 2015. However, there is still low coverage with less identified associated factors. Therefore; the purpose of this study was to assess tetanus toxoid protective dose immunization at last birth and associated factors among mothers who gave birth within one year prior to the study in Debretabor town, Northwest Ethiopia, 2016.

Methods: A community based cross sectional study was conducted from May 1 to June 10 / 2016. A total of 511 mothers were included in the study. Structured questionnaire and checklists were used to collect the data. Face to face interview with cross checking documented record were employed. A systematic random sampling technique was used. The data were entered in to Epinfo version 7.0 and then exported to SPSS version 20.0 for analysis. Both bivariate and multivariable logistic regression model were fitted and crude and Adjusted Odds ratio with 95% confidence interval were computed. Finally, statistically significant association of variables was determined based on Adjusted Odds ratio with its 95% confidence interval and p-value ≤0.05.

Result: The proportion of tetanus toxoid protective dose immunization among mothers was 56.2% (95% CI: 52–60%). In the multivariable analysis; formal education (AOR = 2.09; 95%CI: 1.12, 3.90), planned last pregnancy (AOR = 6.63; 95%CI: 2.36, 18.63), four or more antenatal care visits (AOR = 5.16; 95%CI: 2.93, 11.14), timely antenatal care visit (AOR = 4.29; 95%CI: 1.94, 9.49), and perceived good quality of service (AOR = 2.20; 95% CI: 1.26, 3.84) were positively associated with tetanus toxoid protective dose immunization.

Conclusion: In this study, protective dose tetanus toxoid immunization is lower than the national target. Strengthening information education communication regarding tetanus and its prevention and encouraging timely initiation of and complete attendance of antenatal care is recommended.

Keywords: Debretabor, Immunization, Protective dose, Tetanus toxoid

* Correspondence: muhabawshumye@gmail.com; teme.worku@gmail.com
[†]Muhabaw Shumye Mihret and Miteku Andualem Limenih contributed equally to this work.
Department of Midwifery, College of Medicine and Health Sciences, University of Gondar, Po. Box 196, Gondar, Ethiopia

Background

Protected at birth (PAB) against tetanus is the proportion of births protected from tetanus infection at birth by tetanus toxoid protective dose immunization (TTPDI) of the mothers before birth [1, 2]. World Health Organization (WHO) recommends 5 consecutive doses of tetanus toxoid (TT) vaccination for child bearing age women (CBAW) per schedule to protect the birth against tetanus [3]. Tetanus is a highly fatal, non-communicable, toxin-mediated disease caused by Clostridium tetani bacteria [3, 4]. Women and their newborns are at high risk of acquiring tetanus related to the birthing process [5]. Globally, tetanus toxoid (TT) immunization of the mothers is one of the preventive strategies of maternal and neonatal tetanus (MNT) at birth [5–7].

Maternal and neonatal tetanus (MNT) is a public concern mainly accreditable to low maternal TT vaccination [8]. Fortunately, almost all developed countries have achieved maternal and neonatal tetanus (MNT) elimination prior to 1999 either by full coverage of TT immunization or by hygienic birth practice [9]. However, it has been a big deal in developing regions. Between 1999 and 2014, still about 33 million child bearing age women (CBAW) didn't receive two or more doses of TT vaccination [9]. Worldwide, about 36% of mothers were not immunized with TT protective dose at birth against tetanus [10]. Consequently; about 49,000 neonates and a significant numbers of mothers died of tetanus [11]. This problem is much higher in South East Asian (SEA) and Sub-Saharan African (SSA) countries where 90% of maternal and neonatal tetanus (MNT) appeared and almost all cases ended with death [11]. In Ethiopia, about 51% of pregnant women were not received valid TT vaccination [12]. The problem magnified in Amhara regional state where 56% infants were not protected at birth(PAB) against tetanus [13].

To alleviate this problem, TT vaccination of pregnant women was included in World Health Organization's (WHO) Expanded Program on Immunization (EPI) [14, 15]. World Health Organization (WHO) and its partners jointly have been working for global elimination of MNT basically through maternal TT vaccination. Accordingly, they had planned a targeted date for this goal, a reduction of neonatal tetanus incidence to below one case per 1000 live births per year in every district of the globe, to be at 1995. However, it was postponed many times due to inability to achieve the goal [14, 15]. In Ethiopia context, the Federal Ministry of Health (FMOH), in collaboration with Expanded Program of Immunization (EPI) partners, started implementing TT supplemental immunization since 1999 with the aim of MNT elimination. Moreover, the country introduced the protection at birth(PAB) method for tetanus toxoid (TT) immunization monitoring in 2009 [1]. By August 2015, 21 countries have still not reached the MNT elimination status including Somali region of Ethiopia [11].

Despite impressive efforts, coverage of PAB against tetanus is still low [9, 13–20]. Though, Ethiopia planned the national tetanus PAB coverage to reach 86% by the year 2015, it is still only 49% as of EDHS 2016 [12, 21]. Even, this magnitude is based mostly on health institutional data. Thus, this secondary data often may not depict the actual condition since the situation tends to happen in a communities with restricted access and/ or use of health facilities [22].

Therefore; with the current universal push of ending preventable deaths of newborns and children under 5 years of age, a reliable community based study on preventive strategies like TTPDI and associated factors to have representative data, is required. Having this point of view, this community based study was conducted to assess TTPDI and associated factors at last birth among mothers delivered within one year prior to the study in Debretabor town, North West Ethiopia, 2016.

Methods

A community based cross sectional study was conducted at DebreTabor town which is the largest town in South Gondar zone Amhara regional state, Northwest Ethiopia. The town is located at 665 km from Addis Ababa (the capital city of Ethiopia) in Northwest direction.

Based on the 2007 National Census conducted by Central Statistical Agency of Ethiopia (CSAE), the projected total population in the town is about 55,596 of whom 27, 644 (49.7%) are men and 27,952 (50.3%) are women. Orthodox Christians' are 96.72% of the population of the town and 2.54% are Muslims [23]. The town is divided in to four small administrative units called kebeles and has one general hospital, 3 health centers and 4 Health posts [23].

In the study area, antenatal health services are not active. In other words, if women did not attend the clinic, health providers don't go to the door to give the care. However, the health extension workers (HEWs) are responsible to go to the community home –to- home to mobilize the pregnant women, their family and the community at large so as to visit the health facilities during pregnancy for antenatal care (ANC) service. In addition, HEWs provide information for the client on the importance of antenatal care follow up by moving door to door. As far as duties for provision of ANC services concerned, midwives are primarily responsible at the health centers as well as at the hospitals. Whereas, health extension workers are responsible at health post (i.e. the smallest unit of health facility). Furthermore, there is a consultancy system between midwives and other health care professionals.

Sample size for the study was determined using an Open-Epi Version 2 software by considering the following assumptions: ratio among married and unmarried women 1:1, OR 1.83, power 80%, CI 95%and the proportion of births PAB against tetanus among married women 77.9% [24]. So, the largest sample size for this study was 460 and by assuming 10% non response rate the final sample size turned to be 511.

All mothers in the town who gave birth within one year before the study period were included in the study. Mothers who came from other places to the town for the first time after delivery and also who resided in the town for less than six months were excluded.

First, total numbers of households (HHs), (13,837), were obtained from DebreTabor town administrative office. The sampling interval was made by dividing the total households (HHs) for total sample sizes by assuming every household (HH) had at least one eligible mother, (that is, 13,837/511 = 27). The first HH was then selected by using lottery method among the first 1–27 HHs. And then, selection was proceeded every 27 HHs interval by employing systematic random sampling technique. Finally, a total of 511 HHs with eligible mothers were selected. In case of no eligible woman in the HH, the interviewer approached to the next closest HH. In the selected HH, adequate explanation offered; presence of eligible mother confirmed; written informed consent requested and obtained; and then the HH identification code placed at questionnaire as well as at the door. Face to face interview was then proceeded by using structured and pretested questionnaire. At times, clients have been categorized as ever or never taking TT based on their verbal history. For those mothers who admitted ever history of receiving TT dose(s), documented evidences (either TT card or EPI registration book) was reviewed. Finally, mothers categorized as whether receiving tetanus toxoid protective dose immunization or not based on the listed criteria.

Tetanus toxoid protective dose immunization (TTPDI) was defined as proportion of mothers who have been received any of the following documented TT doses:

1. Two tetanus toxoid injections during that pregnancy
2. Two or more injections, the last one within 3 years of the birth
3. Three or more injections, the last one within 5 years of the birth
4. Four or more injections, the last one within 10 years of the birth
5. Five or more injections at any time prior to the birth

Socio-demographic, obstetric and health service related variables such as maternal age, mother's educational status, husband's educational status, marital status, religion, mother's occupation, husband's occupation, family monthly income, ethnicity, owing radio /television, parity, planned last pregnancy, having ANC visit during the recent pregnancy, number of ANC visit, time of initiating ANC visit, place of ANC visit, client perceived quality of services, time to cover the distance home to health facility, client perceived confidentiality, client trust on TT service, client perceived behavior of service provider, client perceived providers' respect of clients, purpose of taking the vaccine and reason for not taking the vaccine. In addition, checklists on regarding TT vaccination status in the recent pregnancy as well as in life like ever taking the vaccination, number of doses, timing(interval) among doses, source of information for vaccination status which categorized as history alone, card(document) alone, or both history and card. Finally, TT protective dose immunization status (yes or no) was included.

The questionnaires were first prepared in English [Additional file 1] and translated into Amharic and finally, translated back to English. Six unemployed midwifery professional graduates were recruited for data collection process. These include, four diploma midwives for data collection and two BSc midwives for supervision. A one day training was given for data collectors and supervisors. In addition, data collectors had employed the interview guide during discussion [Additional file 2]. A pretest study was done on 5% of sample size. Data were checked, coded and entered to EPI INFO version 7. Then, it was exported to SPSS version 20 for analysis. Both descriptive and analytical statistical procedures were utilized. Descriptive statistics were carried out and the results were presented using tables and texts. Binary logistic regression was used to identify factors associated with TTPDI at last birth. Then, those variables with P-value < 0.2 from Bivariate analysis, were fitted to multivariable logistic regression with Backward Stepwise Likelihood Ratio. Both COR and AOR with the corresponding 95%CI were computed to show the strength of the association. Finally, statistically significant association of variables was determined based on Adjusted Odds ratio with its 95% confidence interval and p-value ≤ 0.05.

Result

Socio-demographic and economic characteristics

A total of 511 women were interviewed.

The median age of the participants was 27 years with (IQR =7). Majority, (83.8%), of the participants were in age group 20–34 years. More than half, (50.9%), of women were housewife by occupation and 99, (19.4%), women have never attended any formal education. Large segment, (77.5%), of respondents' family earned more than 36.00 US dollar per month [Table 1].

Obstetric and health service related factors

More than half, (52.8%), and 226, (44.2%), of the participants were primipara and grand-multipara, respectively.

Table 1 Socio-demographic and economic characteristics of women, Debre Tabor town, Northwest Ethiopia, 2016 ($n = 511$)

Variables	Frequency	Percentage
Age (years		
18–19	15	2.9
20–34	428	83.8
35–49	68	13.3
Mothers' educational status		
Never attend formal education	99	19.4
Primary school	46	9
Secondary school and above	366	71.6
Mother's occupation		
House wife	260	50.9
Government employee	120	23.5
Merchant	68	13.3
Student	53	10.4
Others[a]	10	2
Marital status		
Married	476	93.2
Divorced	28	5.5
Others[b]	7	1.4
Family monthly income(in US dollar)		
≤ 18	22	4.3
18.01–36.00	93	18.2
≥ 18.01	396	77.5
Religion		
Orthodox	476	93.1
Muslim	33	6.5
Catholic	2	0.4
Radio /Television		
Yes	475	93.0
No	36	7.0
Husbands' occupation		
Governmental employee	320	62.6
Merchant	69	23.5
Student	55	10.8
Farmer	43	8.4
Daily laborer	24	4.7
Husband's education		
Never attend formal education	14	2.7
Primary school	92	18
Secondary school and above	405	79.3

[a]Daily labored and house worker
[b]Windowed and never married

Considerable, (90%), of participants' last pregnancy were planned. Substantial proportion, (95.3%), of the respondents have had ANC visit with the mean ± SD of 2.14 ± 1.01 visits and about 36.6% of them have had 4 or more ANC visits. More than two-third, (74.2%), of women perceived as good quality of health services and 472, (92.4%), thought as the service provider respected the women. Majority, (86.1%), women believed as there was no confidentiality problem while about 480, (93.9%), of them trusted health care providers [Table 2].

Proportion of tetanus toxoid protective dose immunization

Proportion of mothers who have been immunized with TT protective dose immunization were 56.2% (95%CI: 52–60%). Among mothers who did not take TT immunization properly; majority, (53.26%), replied that no one advised them and others reasons were not known (30.43%), no problem faced (11.96%), distance barrier (3.26%) and no service provider (1.09%).

Factors influencing tetanus toxoid protective dose immunization

Bivariate analysis

Finding from bivariate logistic regression analysis showed that mother's age, mother's educational status, marital status, ever having ANC visit, parity, perceived behavior of service providers, place of ANC visit, time of initiating ANC visit, planned last pregnancy, number of ANC visit and perceived quality of service were associated with TTPDI at last birth [Table 4]. Whereas, among socio-demographic variables, only mothers' age and educational status were stasticaly associated with ever taking TT vaccination [Table 3].

Multivariable analysis

In the multivariable logistic regression analysis; mother's educational status, planned pregnancy, perceived quality of service, time of initiation and number of ANC visit remained statistically significantly associated with TTPDI.

Accordingly, mothers with formal education were 2.09 times more likely to have been immunized with protective doses of TT than uneducated mothers (AOR = 2.09; 95 CI: 1.12, 3.90).

Besides, the odds of having TT protective dose immunization were nearly 4 times higher among mothers who have initiated ANC visits with in first trimester compared to their counterparts (AOR = 4.29; 95%CI: 1.94,9.49). Similarly, mothers who had four or more ANC visits during the last pregnancy were 5.16 times more likely to have been immunized with TT protective dose than those who had below four ANC visit (AOR = 5.16; 95%CI: 2.93, 11.14). This study also depicted that mothers with planned last pregnancy were 6.63 times more probably to receive TT protective dose immunization than their counterpart (AOR = 6.63; 95% CI: 2.36, 18.63).

Table 2 Obstetric and health service related factors among mothers in DebreTabor town, Northwest Ethiopia, 2016 ($n = 511$)

Variables	Frequencies	Percentage
Parity		
1	270	52.8
2–4	15	2.9
> 5	226	44.2
ANC visit		
Yes	487	95.3
No	24	4.7
Time of starting ANC visit ($n = 487$)		
< 13 wks	112	23
13–28 wks	256	52.6
> 28wks	119	24.4
Number of ANC visit ($n = 487$)		
One	38	7.8
Two	90	18.5
Three	172	35.3
Four or more	187	38.4
Site of ANC visit ($n = 487$)		
Health post	10	2.1
Health center	223	45.8
Hospital	254	52.2
Client perceived Quality of TT service		
Good	379	74.2
Poor	132	25.8
Client perceived behaviour of service providers		
Good	434	84.9
Poor	77	15.1
Time to cover the distance		
Less than 1 h	350	68.5
Between 1 and 2 h	134	26.2
More than 2 h	27	5.3
Ever received TT		
Yes	477	93.3
No	34	6.7
Number of TT vaccination ($n = 477$)		
One	100	20.96
Two	242	50.73
Three	68	14.26
Four	53	11.11
Five or above	14	2.94
Purpose of taking TT vaccination ($n = 477$)		
For the mother	28	5.9
For the newborn	43	9.0
For both	393	82.4
Not known	13	2.7

Finally, Mothers, having good perceived quality of service were 2.20 times more probably to have been immunized with protective doses of TT than their congruent (AOR = 2.20; 95% CI:1.26, 3.84) [Table 4].

Discussion

This study assessed proportion of tetanus toxoid protective dose immunization and associated factors among mothers who gave birth within one year prior to data collection period. The odds of TT protective dose immunization was higher among mothers who have attended formal education, have initiated early ANC visit, with planned last pregnancy, achieving two or more ANC visit, and with perceived good quality of service.

The study illustrated that the proportion of Tetanus toxoid protective dose immunization among mothers found to be 56.2%. The finding is in line with the Nigeria national coverage (55%) [25]. On the other hand, this magnitude is higher as compared to the study done in Lagos Nigeria (20%) [26], Umuahia Nigeria (50%) [27], Ankara Turk (27.8%) [28] and Ibadan Nigeria (38.1%) [29].

This result was also larger as compared to the Ethiopian national PAB coverage (49%) [12] and other local reports, such as Ambo town,(26.8%) [24], Afar regional (26.7%), [16] and Amhara regional PAB coverage, (43.2%), [16].

This disparity could be explained by variation in tools used to measure the outcome variable: some studies were laboratory based which measured the actual serum antibody level enough to protect against tetanus where as the current study used documented evidence to measure proportion of TT protective dose. So, the tool used in the current study might brought about higher magnitude as compared to that of the actual serum antibody measurement [29]. Besides, the discrepancy could be due to variation in the study setting; some studies have included both urban and rural residents. Studies showed that rural dwellers were less educated as compared to urban women. As the current and other studies showed, TT vaccination utilization predicted by level of mother's education (13). So, the higher magnitude of TT protective dose immunization in the current studies might be attributable to composition of the study participants that is including only urban women. In addition, as studies elucidated, lack of TT vaccination occurred in the communities with limited access to and use of healthcare services, and maternal TT vaccination was predicted by distance from the nearest immunization centre, and level of contact with health worker (35, 38, 45). Thus; those women resided in the rural and remote areas would not easily accessed to health facilities as compared to urban women although the TT service was free of charge [24]. Furthermore, the discrepancy could be variation in time of the study: some studies were done back to 5 years. But, currently trends on educational status and awareness toward the importance

Table 3 Comparisons of socio-demographic variables across TT ever and never vaccinated women in Debretabor town, Northwest Ethiopia, 2016

Socio demographic Variables	Ever taking TT Vaccine?		COR with 95% CI	AOR with 95% CI
	Yes n (%)	No n (%)		
Mothers' age (in years)				
18–29	349 (91.6)	32 (8.4)	1	1
30–49	128 (98.5)	2 (1.5%)	5.87 (1.39,24.84)*	7.27 (1.70,31.15)*
Mothers' religious				
Orthodox Tewahido	445 (93.5)	31 (6.5)	1.35 (0.39,4.64)	1.17 (0.29,4.67)
Others[a]	32 (91.4)	3 (8.6)	1	1
Mothers' educational status				
Never attend formal education	87 (87.9)	12 (12.1)	1	1
Attend formal education	390 (94.7)	22 (5.3)	2.45 (1.17,5.13)*	4.02 (1.69,9.58)*
Mother's occupation				
House wife	244 (93.8)	16 (6.2)	1.18 (0.59,2.37)	2.13 (0.94,4.81)
Others[b]	233 (92.8)	18 (7.2)	1	1
Marital status				
Currently Married	446 (93.7)	30 (6.3)	1.92 (0.64,5.79)	2.15 (0.67,6.98)
Currently not married	31 (88.6)	4 (11.4)	1	1
Family monthly income(in US dollar)				
≤ 36	108 (93.9	7 (6.1)	1	1
> 36	369 (93.2)	27 (6.8	0.89 (0.38,2.09)	0.57 (0.07,5.04)
Have Radio /Television				
Yes	442 (93.1)	33 (6.9)	0.38 (0.05,2.88)	0.28 (0.04,2.21)
No	42 (97.2)	1 (2.8)	1	1
Husbands' occupation				
Governmental employee	300 (93.8)	20 (6.2)	1.19 (0.59,2.41)	1.14 (0.52,2.51)
Others[c]	177 (92.7)	14 (7.3)	1	1
Husband's education				
Never attend formal education	463 (93.2)	34 (6.8)	NA	NA
Attend formal education	14 (100)	0		

*P-value < 0.05
[a]Catholic and protestant
[b] Daily labored, house worker, merchant and student
[c] Student, merchant, farmer and daily labored

of TT changed across a time. These all mentioned explanation possibly could answer why TT protective dose immunization in the current study was higher.

However, the result was considerably lower as compared to findings from national PAB coverage in Ghana (82.6%) [30] and local studies in: Pakistan in 2007-(87%)-[31], Pakistan in 2011-(90.5%)-[32], Ghana (82.6%) [30], Sudan (83%) [33] and Ethiopia (82.3%) [13]. This variation might be due to the method employed to measure the outcome variable; the current study used proofed (documented) evidence for maternal vaccination status whereas most other studies described primarily based on maternal verbal history which was prone to recalled bias and might be resulted in over estimation in the latter studies [30–33].

As this study demonstrated, the odd of TT protective dose immunization was 2.09 times among mothers with formal education than that of uneducated women. This finding is in line with the study done in different settings: in Bangladesh [34], in France [35] and in Ethiopia [24, 36]. This might be due to the fact that education increases awareness of women on the benefits of immunization, a greater decision-making power at home and perhaps escalate capacity to travel outside the home to seek health care (26).

This study also revealed that planned last pregnancy was statistically significantly associated with TT protective dose immunization; women with planned last pregnancy were more than six times more likely to have been

Table 4 Factors influencing tetanus toxoid protective dose immunization among mothers, DebreTabor town, Northwest Ethiopia, 2016 ($n = 511$)

Variables	TT Protective dose		Crude Odds Ratio 95% C1	*P*-Value	Adjusted Odds Ratio 95% C1
	Yes n (%)	No n (%)			
Age					
18–29	203 (53.3)	178 (46.7)	0.63 (0.41,0.94)	0.02	0.59 (0.33,1.08)
30–49	84 (64.6)	46 (35.4)	1		1
Religion					
Orthodox	271 (56.9)	205 (43.1)	1.57 (0.32,1.27)	0.2	NA
Others[a]	16 (45.7)	19 (4.3)	1		
Educational status					
Ever attended	249 (60.4)	163 (39.6)	2.45 (1.56, 3.890	0.000	2.09 (1.12,3.90)*
Never attended	38 (38.4)	61 (61.6)	1		1
Marital status					
In marital relation	277 (58.2)	199 (41.8)	3.48 (1.64,7.41)	0.002	1.58 (0.50,4.98)
No marital relation	10 (28.6)	25 (71.4)	1		1
Husband educational status					
Ever attended	282 (56.7)	215 (43.3)	2.36 (0.78–7.15)	0.16	1.16 (0.19,7.07)
Never attended	5 (35.7)	9 (64.3)	1		1
Mother's occupation					
House wife	145 (55.8)	115 (44.2)	0.97 (0.68,1.37)	0.86	NA
Others[b]	142 (56.6)	109 (43.4)	1		
Husband's occupation					
Governmental employee	182 (56.9)	138 (43.1)	1.08 (0.75,1.55)	0.68	NA
Others[c]	105 (55)	86 (45)	1		
Owing radio/Television					
Yes	263 (55.4)	212 (44.6)	0.62 (0.30,1.27)	0.20	NA
No	24 (66.7)	12 (33.3)	1		
Planned last pregnancy					
Yes	278 (60.4)	182 (39.6)	7.13 (3.39–15.00)	0.000	6.63 (2.36,18.63)*
No	9 (17.6)	42 (82.4)	1		1
Time to cover distance					
< 1 h	179 (51.14)	171 (48.86)	1.03 (0.47,5.38)	0.36	NA
> or = 1 h	81 (50.31)	80 (49.69)	1		
Family monthly income(in US dollar)					
< or = 36	57 (49.6)	58 (50.4)	1		
> 36	230 (58.1)	166 (41.9)	1.41 (0.93,2.14)	0.20	NA
Ever having ANC visit					
Yes	289 (58.7)	201 (41.3)	3.49 (2.28,4.86)	0.000	1.48 (0.70,3.09)
No	7 (29.17)	17 (70.83)	1		1
Place of ANC visit in recent pregnancy(n = 487)					
Hospital	132 (51.97)	122 (48.03)	1.00 (0.36,3.72)	0.53	NA
Health Center/Post	121 (51.93)	112 (48.07)	1		
Timing of initiating ANC visit(n = 487)					
Within 1st trimester	101 (90.2)	11 (9.8)	9.43 (4.9,18.14)	0.000	4.29 (1.94,9.49)**
After 1st trimester	185 (49.3)	190 (50.7)	1		1

Table 4 Factors influencing tetanus toxoid protective dose immunization among mothers, DebreTabor town, Northwest Ethiopia, 2016 ($n = 511$) *(Continued)*

Variables	TT Protective dose		Crude Odds Ratio 95% C1	*P*-Value	Adjusted Odds Ratio 95% C1
	Yes n (%)	No n (%)			
Parity					
Two or more	113 (46.9)	128 (53.1)	0.49 (0.336,0.684)	0.000	0.94 (0.48,1.85)
One	174 (64.4)	96 (35.6)	1		
Number of ANC visit (n = 487)					
Four or above	151 (80.7)1	36 (19.3)	5.13 (3.34,7.87)	0.000	5.16 (2.93,11.14)
Three or below	135 (45)	165 (55)	1		1
Client perceived quality of service					
Good	249 (65.7)	130 (34.2)	4.74 (3.08,7.30)	0.000	2.20 (1.26,3.84)*
Poor	38 (28.8)	94 (71.2)	1		1
Client perceived behavior of service provider					
Good	270 (62.2)	164 (37.8)	5.81 (3.28,10.30)	0.000	1.84 (0.84,4.05)
Poor	17 (22.1)	60 (77.9)	1		1

*P-value < 0.05
[a]Catholic and protestant
[b]Daily labored, house worker, merchant and student
[c]Student, merchant, farmer and daily labored

immunized with TT protective dose than women whose pregnancy was unplanned. This is in accordance with the study done in Bangladesh [37], Kenya [38] and Ambo town,Ethiopia [24]. This might be due to the logic those mothers with planned pregnancy possibly ready themselves to overcome physical barriers like distance, to allocate time to seek health care, to attend health related media promotion like 'the first 1000 days' and probably to search health related information either, by consulting health care providers or by reading related papers.

According to this study, TT protective dose immunization was independently predicted by frequency of ANC visit during the recent pregnancy. Hence, mothers who had four or more number of ANC visit during the last pregnancy were more than five folds more likely to have been immunized with protective dose of TT than their counter parts. This implies that attending the recommended number of ANC visit is a good opportunity for valid TT immunization utilization. This was with regard to the study done in Peshawar, Pakistan [39] and in Kenya [38]. This could be due to the reality that the higher the frequency the mother visited health facilities, the higher the mothers received appropriate health care services and correspondingly, the valid the TT doses offered. Plus to that, as the contact time with health professional increased, the mother got more health related information and this in turn might change her health seeking behavior positively.

This study also elucidated that TT protective dose immunization was influenced by time of initiating ANC visit during the last pregnancy. Mothers with history of initiating ANC visit within the first trimester were nearly four folds more likely to have been immunized with this dose than those starting later. This suggests that if mothers started ANC visit in early gestation, they would get adequate time enough to take two or more TT vaccination based on the schedule prior to giving birth. This finding is in agreement with the study done in Lahore district, Pakistan [31].

Based on the current study, the odds of TT protective dose immunization was 2.20 times higher among mothers with perceived good quality of service than their counter parts. This suggested that no matter the real quality of service provided, simply client perception toward quality of service, matters receiving valid TT vaccination. This is consistent with the study conducted in Dormaa, Ghana [40]. This result also supported by study conducted in Hispanic and Houston, Texas [41].

Limitation of the study

The study was conducted solely in the urban area. As a result; it did not involve participants from rural areas. In addition, although using documented evidence for confirming protective dose immunization could be taken as strength, the finding of this study might be underestimated as compared to other studies which reported based on maternal verbal history alone.

Conclusion

The proportion of mothers who have been vaccinated with protective doses of TT immunization in the study area was below the national target. Formal education, planned last pregnancy, timely ANC visit, four or more ANC visit and perceived good quality of service were factors positively associated with protective doses of TT immunization. Thus; complete ANC visit, planned pregnancy and early initiation of ANC visit should be emphasized. Similarly; female education and correcting women perception toward quality of TT service is recommended.

Additional files

Additional file 1: English language copy of the questionnaire. English version of Questionnaire for the study conducted on tetanus toxoid protective dose immunization and associated factors among mothers who gave birth within one year prior to the study in Debre Tabor Town, Northwest Ethiopia, 2016.

Additional file 2: Interview Guide. Interview guide during the discussion with participants for the study conducted on tetanus toxoid protective dose immunization and associated factors among mothers who gave birth within one year prior to the study in Debre Tabor Town, Northwest Ethiopia, 2016.

Additional file 3: Study participant's consent sheet. English version of consent sheet for the study conducted on tetanus toxoid protective dose immunization and associated factors among mothers who gave birth within one year prior to the study in Debre Tabor Town, Northwest Ethiopia, 2016.

Abbreviations

ANC: Ante Natal Care; AOR: Adjusted Odds Ratio; COR: Crude Odds Ratio; EDHS: Ethiopian Demography and Health Survey; EPI: Expanded Program on Immunization; FMOH: Federal Ministry of Health; HEWs: Health Extension Workers; HH: House Hold; MNT: Maternal and Neonatal Tetanus; NNT: Neo Natal Tetanus; PAB: Protected at Birth; SPSS: Statistical Package for Social Science; TT: Tetanus Toxoid; TTTPDI: Tetanus Toxoid Protective Dose Immunization; WHO: World Health Organization

Acknowledgements

We would like to thank University of Gondar for ethical letter and financial support. We also like to forward our deepest and sincere appreciation to all data collectors and study participants. Our gratitude is also great to Debre Tabor town administration office for provision of support letter.

Competing interests

The authors declare that they have no competing interests.

Authors' contributions

MSM: designed the study, performed analysis and interpretation of data and drafted and revised the manuscript. MAB: designed and approved the proposal with some revisions, participated in data analysis, and revised subsequent drafts of the paper. TWG: designed the study, approved the proposal with some revisions, participated in data analysis and revised subsequent drafts of the paper, and developed and revised the manuscript. All authors read and approved the final manuscript.

References

1. Minisitry of Health: Ethiopia national Expanded Programme on Immunization. 2010.
2. Federal Republic of Ethiopia Minstry of Health: HMIS / M&E Indicator Definitions HMIS / M&E Redesign: Technical Standards: Area 1 version 1.0. 2007.
3. World Health Organization: Tetanus vaccine. Weekly epidemiological record 2006.
4. Thwaites CL, Farrar JJ. Preventing and treating tetanus -The challenge continues in the face of neglect and lack of research. Biomed J. 2003; 326(7381):117–8.
5. World Health Organization. Protection at birth (PAB) against tetanus. In: Global Health Observatory data; 2015.
6. World Health Organization. Expanded Programme on immunization Ethiopia. Ethiopia Country Office; 2014. http://www.who.int/countries/eth/areas/immunization/en/.
7. Blencowe H, Lawn J, Vandelaer J, Roper M, Cousens S. Tetanus toxoid immunization to reduce mortality from neonatal tetanus. Int J Epidemol. 2010;27:102–9.
8. Demicheli V, Barale A, Rivetti A. Vaccines for women for preventing neonatal tetanus. Cochrane Collaboration. Cochrane Database Syst Rev. 2015:1.
9. Thwaites CL, Loan HT. Eradication of tetanus. Oxford J British Med Bulletin. 2015;116(1):69–77.
10. World Health Organization. Neonatal tetanus (PAB)data by WHO region: Global health observatory data repository; 2015. http://www.who.int/gho/immunization/neonatal_tetanus/en/.
11. World Health Organization. Maternal and neonatal tetanus (MNT) elimination-the initiative and challenges. Immun Vaccin Biol. 2015;21:1–2.
12. Central Statistical A. Ethiopian demographic and health survey key indicators report. Rockville: The DHS Program, ICF; 2016.
13. Ethiopia Central Statistical Agency. Ethiopia Demographic and Health Survey 2011. Calverton: ICF International; 2012.
14. World Health Organization: Weekly epidemiological record. 2007;82:141–52. http://www.who.int/wer/2007/en/.
15. Verma R, Khanna P. Tetanus toxoid vaccine: elimination of neonatal tetanus in selected states of India: Human vaccines & immunotherapeutics; 2012. https://www.ncbi.nlm.nih.gov/pmc/articles/PMC3660763/.
16. World Health Organization. neonatal tetanus. Immun Vaccin Biol. 2015;512:1–4.
17. Khan R, Vandelaer J, Yakubu A, Raza AA, Zulu F. Maternal and neonatal tetanus elimination: from protecting women and newborns to protecting all. J Women's Health. 2015;171–180:7.
18. The Federal Democratic Republic of Ethiopia Ministry of Health: Health Sector Transformation Plan. 2015.
19. Kidane T, Yigzaw A, Sahilemariam Y, Bulto T, Mengistu H, Belay T, Bisrat F, Benti D, Mbakuliyemo N, Olusegum B. National EPI coverage survey report in Ethiopia, 2006. Ethiop J Health Dev. 2008;22:1–5.
20. WHO and UNICEF: Estimates of immunization coverage 2014.
21. Federal Democratic Republic of Ethiopia Ministry of Health: Health Sector Development Programme IV 2014.
22. Ethiopia Central Statistical Agency. Tetanus Toxoid Vaccination; 2005. p. 115–7.
23. Federal Democratic Republic of Ethiopia Population Census Commission. Summary and statistical report of the 2007 population and housing census :population size by age and sex. In: United Nations Population Fund; 2008.
24. Adugna E. factors influencing tetanus toxoid immunization and protection at birth coverage among child breang age women of Ambo town and its surrounding area. Ethiopia: Oromia regional state; 2011.
25. World Health Organization: Protection at birth against neonatal tetanus(PAB) data by WHO Region 2015.
26. Sule SS, Nkem-Uchendu C, Onajole AT, Ogunowo BE. Awareness, perception and coverage of tetanus immunisation in women of child bearing age in an urban district of Lagos, Nigeria. Niger Postgraduate Med J. 2014;21(2):107–14.
27. Nwokeukwu HI, Ukegbu AU, UE-U KCN, Nwankwo N, Osunkwo D, Ajuogu E. Tetanus Toxoid Immunization Coverage in Federal Medical Centre, Umuahia, Abia State,South East Zone, Nigeria. International journal of tropical disease & health. 2014;4(12):1268–77.
28. Maral I, Baykan Z, Aksakal FN, Kayikcioglu F, Bumin MA. Tetanus immunization in pregnant women: evaluation of maternal tetanus vaccination status and factors affecting rate of vaccination coverage. Public Health. 2011;115(5):359–64.
29. Orimadegun AE. Akinlolu a Adepoju, Olusegun O Akinyinka: prevalence and

socio-demographic factors associated with non-protective immunity against tetanus among high school adolescents girls in Nigeria. Ital J Pediatr. 2014; 40(29):1–8.

30. Diamenu SK, Bosnu G, Abotsi F, Tweneboa PO, Okoh-Owusu M, Amoh P, Yakubu A, Khan R. Introducing protection at birth (Pab) method of monitoring tetanus-diphtheria (td) vaccination coverage of mothers in Ghana. International Journal of Vaccines and Immunization. 2015;1:1.
31. Hasnain S, Sheikh NH. Causes of low tetanus toxoid vacccinatiuon coverage in pregnant women in Lahore District,Pakistan. East Mediterr Health J. 2007; 13(5):1142–52.
32. Hashmi FK, Islam M, Khan TA, Tipu MK. Vaccination coverage of mothers during pregnancy with tetanus toxoid and infants after Birth. Pakistan J Pharmacy. 2011;24(2):1–3.
33. Hager Awad Saeed Sultan: Assessment of tetanus toxoid coverage and protection at birth against neonatal tetanus in Khartoum state, Sudan. 2009.
34. Rahman M. Determinants of the utilization of the tetanus toxoid (TT) vaccination coverage in Bangladesh: evidence from a Bangladesh demographic health survey 2010. Internet J Health. 2010;8(2):3–5.
35. Guthmann JP, Fonteneau L, Antona D, Lévy-Bruhl D. Factors associated with tetanus vaccination coverage in adults in France and with knowledge of vaccination status. Medecine et maladies infectieuses. 2010;40(10):560–7.
36. Walle F, Kassa M. Coverage and factors associated with tetanus toxoid vaccination among private college students, Bahirdar, Ethiopia. J Vaccine. 2013;4:106.
37. Rahman M. Tetanus toxoid vaccination coverage and differential between urban and rural areas of Bangladesh. East African journal of public health. 2009;6(1):26–31.
38. Zelalem TH, Chertok IRA, Teweldeberhan AK. Determinants of utilization of sufficient tetanus toxoid immunization during pregnancy: evidence from the Kenya demographic and health survey, 2008–2009. J Community Health. 2013;38:492–9.
39. Naeem M, Khan MZ-U-I, Abbas SH, Adil M, Khan A, Naz SM, Khan MU. coverage and factors associated with tetanus toxoid vaccination among married women of reproductive age: a cross sectional study in Peshawar. J Ayub Med College. 2010;22(3):1.
40. Anokye M, John A, Mensah, Frank O, Frimpong, Emelia O, Aboagye, Acheampong N. Immunization coverage of pregnant women with tetanus toxoid vaccine in Dormaa East District-Brong Adaro region, Ghana. Mathematical Theory and Modeling. 2014;4:6.
41. Beel ER, Rench MA, Montesinos DP, Mayes B, Mary Healy C. Knowledge and attitudes of postpartum women toward immunization during pregnancy and the peripartum period. Human vaccines & immunotherapeutics. 2013; 9(9):1926–31.

10

Program assessment of efforts to improve the quality of postpartum counselling in health centers in Morogoro region, Tanzania

Amnesty LeFevre[1,2], Rose Mpembeni[3*], Charles Kilewo[3,4], Ann Yang[1], Selena An[1], Diwakar Mohan[1], Idda Mosha[3], Giulia Besana[5], Chrisostom Lipingu[5], Jennifer Callaghan-Koru[1], Marissa Silverman[1], Peter J. Winch[1] and Asha S. George[1,6]

Abstract

Background: The postpartum period represents a critical window where many maternal and child deaths occur. We assess the quality of postpartum care (PPC) as well as efforts to improve service delivery through additional training and supervision in Health Centers (HCs) in Morogoro Region, Tanzania.

Methods: Program implementers purposively selected nine program HCs for assessment with another nine HCs in the region remaining as comparison sites in a non-randomized program evaluation. PPC quality was assessed by examining structural inputs; provider and client profiles; processes (PNC counselling) and outcomes (patient knowledge) through direct observations of equipment, supplies and infrastructure ($n = 18$) and PPC counselling ($n = 45$); client exit interviews ($n = 41$); a provider survey ($n = 62$); and in-depth provider interviews ($n = 10$).

Results: While physical infrastructure, equipment and supplies were comparable across study sites (with water and electricity limitations), program areas had better availability of drugs and commodities. Overall, provider availability was also similar across study sites, with 63% of HCs following staffing norms, 17% of Reproductive and Child Health (RCH) providers absent and 14% of those providing PPC being unqualified to do so. In the program area, a median of 4 of 10 RCH providers received training. Despite training and supervisory inputs to program area HCs, provider and client knowledge of PPC was low and the content of PPC counseling provided limited to 3 of 80 PPC messages in over half the consultations observed. Among women attending PPC, 29 (71%) had delivered in a health facility and sought care a median of 13 days after delivery. Barriers to PPC care seeking included perceptions that PPC was of limited benefit to women and was primarily about child health, geographic distance, gaps in the continuity of care, and harsh facility treatment.

Conclusions: Program training and supervision activities had a modest effect on the quality of PPC. To achieve broader transformation in PPC quality, client perceptions about the value of PPC need to be changed; the content of recommended PPC messages reviewed along with the location for PPC services; gaps in the availability of human resources addressed; and increased provider-client contact encouraged.

Keywords: Postnatal care, Counselling, Postpartum care, Primary health care, Tanzania

* Correspondence: rcmpembeni@gmail.com
[3]School of Public Health and Social Sciences, Muhimbili University of Health and Allied Sciences, P.O. Box 65015, Dar es Salaam, Tanzania
Full list of author information is available at the end of the article

Background

While home to just 12% of the world's population, 56% of maternal deaths [1] and 50% of deaths in children under five years of age occur in sub-Saharan Africa [2]. Tanzania is the fifth most populous country in sub-Saharan Africa and one of 10 countries globally which together accounted for 59% of all maternal deaths in 2015 [3]. While declines in maternal and child deaths occurred throughout the last four decades, mortality continues to remain unacceptably high. In 2015, for every 100,000 live births, 398 maternal deaths occurred, and among children under 5, for every 1000 live births, 67 deaths occurred [1, 4].

The postpartum period, from birth to six weeks after birth represents a critical window of time where many maternal and child deaths occur – largely due to preventable causes [1, 4]. Postpartum care (PPC) services encompass prevention, early detection and management of complications for mothers and newborns, as well as provision of advice and services on breastfeeding, birth spacing, immunizations, nutrition and HIV services [5]. In Tanzania, the Ministry of Health and Social Welfare (MOHSW) recommends that mothers and children receive a minimum of 4 PPC consultations at the following times: within 48 h of delivery, between 3 and 7 days, 8–28 days, and 29 to 42 days (Table 1) [5, 6]. Despite these recommendations and near universal completion of at least one antenatal care visit (96%), only 50% of deliveries in 2015 occurred in facilities and only 35% of women with a live birth outcome received a PPC checkup following delivery [7].

Increasing access to and utilization of health services is necessary but alone may not be sufficient to improve maternal, newborn and child health (MNCH) [8]. Evidence is emerging that attention must be also placed on the quality of care [9]. In Tanzania, data on service quality are available from Maternal Child Health Integrated Program surveys, however, information specific to PPC counselling is limited [10].

In an effort to improve utilization and quality of facility-based PPC services, the Tanzanian MOHSW, with support from the USAID-funded Mothers and Infants, Safe Healthy, Alive (MAISHA) program facilitated by Jhpiego, conducted a 6-day in-service training of 2–4 health care providers in the Reproductive and Child Health (RCH) wards of nine Health Centers and one Regional Hospital in five districts of Morogoro in 2010 and 2011. In-service training drew upon national PPC guidelines and was complemented by the introduction of MOHSW-approved PPC registers to track service utilization, and quarterly supportive supervision from MOHSW and Jhpiego personnel. We sought to measure the quality of facility PPC and assess the effects of programmatic inputs to improve PPC service delivery in nine Health Centers that received additional training and supervision input with nine comparison Health Centers without such inputs.

Table 1 Ministry of Health and Social Welfare Guidelines for PPC Services in Tanzania

Timing and recommended service content for routine postpartum care visits
1. ≤24 h after delivery: • Clinical assessment of mothers and newborns within an hour after birth; • Infant feeding practices, skin-to-skin contact, and identification of danger signs for both mother and baby; • Prior to facility discharge providers to give counseling on danger signs, nutrition, family planning, self-care for the mother and child at home, as well as preventive measures such as bed nets and a supply of iron and vitamin A to the mother.
2. ≤7 days after birth: provider follow up with mother and baby about danger signs and continue health education.
3. 28 days after the birth: child immunization and examinations to check for continued recovery of mother and healthy development of child.
4. 42 days after the birth: child immunization and examinations to check for continued recovery of mother and healthy development of child.
5. Reproductive Child Health follow-up care for 1 year postpartum
6. Maternal and/or baby consultations as needed in event of complications
Basic PPC Care Package in Tanzania
Providers should:
• Discuss breastfeeding, breast care or alternate infant feeding options for HIV-positive women;
• Emphasize the Lactational Amenorrhoea Method (LAM) and later transition to other family planning methods;
• Provide nutritional support;
• Counsel on self-care and other healthy practices;
• Discuss mother and baby danger signs;
• Make complication readiness plans;
• Offer HIV counseling and testing;
• Provide immunizations;
• Offer preventive measures (i.e., iron/folate supplements);
• Provide antiretroviral medicine and cotrimoxazole prophylaxis as needed.

Assessing quality of postpartum care

Frameworks to assess quality of care trace back to Donabedian's [11] three dimensions: (1) *structure*, or settings within which care takes place, (2) *process* of providing care, and (3) *outcome* of care on health status [12–16]. These dimensions were supplemented by varying perspectives at different levels (care by practitioners, amenities, care undertaken by patients, and care received by community) [14]. The definition of quality was also broadened to include dimensions of effectiveness (delivering evidence-based care that results in improved health outcomes), efficiency (delivering health care in a manner which maximizes resource use and avoids waste), acceptability (care takes into account individual/

cultural preferences), and equity (care does not vary unfairly by social characteristics) [12]. In 2006, these dimensions were expanded by WHO to include accessibility (care is timely, geographically reasonable, and provided in a setting where skills and resources are appropriate to medical need) and safety (minimal risk/harm to users) [17–19].

Based on this trajectory of work on quality of care, we modified Donabedian's linear framework of *structure, processes* and *outcomes* to include both provider and client perspectives [20]. Figure 1 depicts the relationship between these domains, illustrating that attributes in the service environment (structural inputs) interact with client and provider profiles to influence delivery and receipt of care (processes), which correspond to changes in short- (patient knowledge) and long-term (careseeking and health status) outcomes. Consideration of the dynamic interaction between these dimensions provides a more comprehensive picture of quality of care in health facilities.

Methods

Study site, design and sampling

Located 200 km southwest of Dar es Salaam, Morogoro is the sixth most populous and second largest region (2.2 million population dispersed over 70,000 km; 73% in rural areas) of Tanzania's 30 regions [13]. Careseeking for PPC in Morogoro region (35%) mirrors the national average, while other indicators are slightly higher than national averages: antenatal care utilization (99% versus 98%), facility deliveries (75% versus 63%), and skilled birth attendance (78% versus 64%) [1, 4]. A non-randomized program assessment was carried out in 18 Health Centers (9 program and 9 comparison) located in nine districts (Gairo, Kilosa, Morogoro District Council, Mvomero and Ulanga) in late 2012. All health facilities provide the same core package of MNCH services. However, the nine program HCs were purposively selected by Jhpiego and the District Reproductive and Child Health Coordinator based on their higher utilization of Prevention of mother-to-child transmission services (program activities were funded by USAID using PEPFAR funding). The nine remaining HCs in these were selected for comparison purposes during the program assessment.

To assess quality of PPC services, we examined the following domains: 1. Structural inputs; 2. Provider profiles; 3. Client profiles; 4. Processes, including content of PPC counselling and accessibility; and 5. Outcomes, including short-term effects of care on patient knowledge (Fig. 1).

Structural inputs, including availability of PPC infrastructure, drugs, equipment, supplies, and testing services, were assessed through direct observations in all 18 HCs using standardized checklists of indicators drawn from the Service Provision Assessment tools [4] and the Maternal Child Health Integrated Program quality of care toolkit [21]. In the event of drug 'stock-outs,' the HC in-charge and/or attending pharmacist were asked to provide details on the duration and/or ever-availability of the

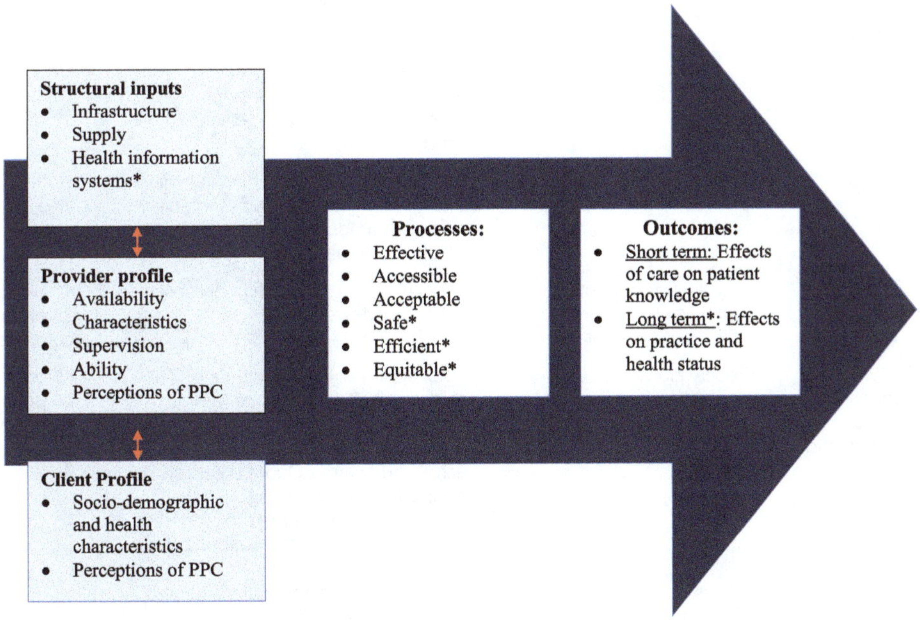

Fig. 1 Concepual Framework for assessing the context and Quality of PPC counseling in health centres in Morogoro Tanzania. ***Legend***: *Not measured in the current analysis. ***References***: 1. Donabedian A. The quality of care. How can it be assessed?1988, ARCH Pathol Lab Med 1997, 121 (11):Pg 1145-50. 2. Atherton F. G. Mbekem and I. Nyalusi. Improving service quality from thre Tanzania Family Health Project. Int J Qual Health Care. 3. WHO. Quality of care. A process for making strategic choices in health systems:2006, Worls Health Organization: France 4:p3

product in question. Data on the reported frequency of supervision were collected during provider interviews and stratified by source and content.

PPC providers were assessed according to their availability, knowledge, social profile, and perceptions of PPC. PPC health provider availability was determined through interviews with facility in-charges and compared with national guidelines. In addition, a structured questionnaire was administered to the sub-sample of RCH providers available during the research team's visit. Knowledge was assessed across five major domains: (i) postnatal danger signs, (ii) essential newborn care and care for low birth weight infants, (iii) maternal hygiene and recovery, (iv) infant and maternal nutrition, (v) family planning, HIV/ AIDS, and malaria. Data was drawn from the subset of RCH health workers who reported providing PPC services in the preceding seven days.

Client profile, including demographic and personal/ family characteristics, maternal health background, and PPC perceptions were assessed through exit interviews with PPC counselling recipients. Exit interviews included a quantitative survey to assess knowledge, demographic characteristics, travel and waiting times as well as semi-structured in-depth interview questions to capture perceptions of PPC.

Observations of the content of PPC counselling by data collectors during their two days visit of HCs were used to evaluate processes associated with giving care. Content of PPC counselling was evaluated using checklists containing over 85 group and individual counselling messages as per government guidelines. Additional data on job aids use and client/provider interaction were also collected. Longer-term effects of PPC on practice and health status fell beyond the scope of the current analysis (Table 2).

Data collection

A team of six research assistants, including two social scientists, two medical doctors, and two quantitative researchers, received training from MUHAS and Johns Hopkins School of Public Health (JHSPH) faculty over a one-week period in mid-September 2012. Training included two days of pilot testing in two HCs on the outskirts of Dar es Salaam and was immediately followed by the start of data collection in late September.

Table 2 PPC Data sources

Domains of Quality		Measurement Methods	Sampling	Final sample
Structural inputs	Supply and i nfrastructure availability	Observations of infrastructure, drugs, supplies, and commodities	100% of all health centers in 5 districts	18 health centers: 9 program, 9 comparison
	Supervision	PPC provider survey	• Interview with facility in-charge to determine available human resources (*n* = 18) • Sub-sample health center RCH providers (*n* = 88) available on day of visit • Sub-analysis of RCH service providers that reported providing PPC services in the preceding 7 days	18 health centers in-charges: 9 program, 9 comparison 62 PPC providers; 38 program area, 24 comparison
Provider profile	Health provider ability and availability			
	Perceptions of PPC	Qualitative in-depth provider interviews	Sub-analysis of PPC providers interviewed as part of qualitative in-depth interviews carried out among 57 RCH providers (mean of 3 per facility)	10 PPC Providers; 6 program area, 4 comparison
Client profile	• Social profile • Health profile	• Qualitative in-depth interviews • PPC client exit interviews	Of 45 PPC clients observed, 41 consented to exit interviews.	41 completed exit interviews; 25 program area, 16 comparison
Process	• PPC Counseling content • PPC Service accessibility and efficiency	Observations of PPC counseling sessions delivered	• Total approved target sample of 240 to detect a 30% difference (design effect of 2.0) in frequency of observed messages on postpartum family planning across study arms. Quota based on availability on day of visit. • 55 PPC Clients presented for services during 36 days of observation (2 days per facility). • Of 55 total PPC clients, 45 consented to observation; 9 departed prior to service delivery and 1 declined consent.	45 completed observations; 26 program area, 19 comparison
Outcome	Client knowledge	Quantitative PPC client exit interviews	Of 45 PPC clients observed, 41 consented to exit interviews.	41 completed exit interviews; 25 program area, 16 comparison

In Morogoro, data were collected over a two-day period in each HC. Prior to the start of data collection, study personnel visited the HC in-charges to brief them on data collection objectives, ascertain the days PPC services were provided, and coordinate the timing for data collection. Data collection included direct observations of equipment/supplies, observations of PPC counseling, and provider and client interviews. Observations of PPC counseling were carried out during outpatient clinical service provision – characteristically between 8 am and 1 pm – or at the time of patient discharge (a critical window for PPC counselling) among all consenting PPC clients during the two-day data collection window in each HC. PPC clients were approached prior to the start of counselling, and oral consent for observation and exit interview was obtained. Following observations, an exit interview of about one hour in duration was recorded on paper in a private area of the HC.

Quantitative provider interviews were carried out among consenting RCH providers available during the data collection shift of 8 am-6 pm. In each HC, of the approximately 20 total providers on the roster, 5–10 were present during the data collection shift of 8 am-6 pm and of these, 3–5 were RCH providers. Qualitative in-depth interviews were carried out among a sub-sample of about three RCH providers per facility and digitally recorded. Since the focus of this paper was on PPC, analyses focused on the sub-sample of health workers who reported providing PPC services.

Data analyses

Quantitative data were single entered and cleaned using Epi Info software, with statistical analyses performed using Stata 12.0 and 13.0. A target sample of 180 PPC observations was required to observe a 30% difference in the content of counselling on newborn danger signs between study arms. The total sample achieved of 45 PPC observations fell short of this, and thus descriptive analyses were carried out using basic cross-tabulations. For facility readiness and counselling content, summary composite scores were calculated by the probability-weighted average for each domain. To look for associations at the individual level in the duration of counselling and the scores for the different domains of counselling, we used non–parametric correlation methods (Spearman's rho).The Spearman statistic makes adjustments for ties by averaging ranks, with values ranging from – 1 (perfect negative association) to + 1 (perfect positive association) and with zero indicating the absence of association.

Qualitative elements of client exit interviews were recorded by hand, translated during data collection and coded manually, while the qualitative elements of provider interviews were recorded electronically, transcribed and translated into English, before being coded using Atlas.ti. Codes derived from the structure of the interview guide and from themes that emerged from daily, midpoint and endpoint team debriefings. Draft write-ups of the thematic analysis were circulated among co-investigators before finalization.

Preliminary findings from both the quantitative and qualitative analysis were shared with key decision makers in Tanzania belonging to the MOHSW and Jhpiego for their feedback and review prior to publications being drafted.

Results

Structural inputs

Physical infrastructure, equipment and supplies were comparable across program and comparison HCs (Fig. 2). An estimated 39% of facilities were observed to not have a functioning water source and 33% had no electricity in the newborn care/labor delivery ward. In qualitative interviews, across all HCs providers discussed the challenges imposed by limited space, particularly when juggling the needs of different MCH services, including ANC and PPC.

Program HCs were observed to have better availability of drugs, commodities and testing supplies for PPC (Fig. 2), including CD4 (89% versus 56%), adult HIV testing kits (78% versus 56%), early infant HIV diagnosis (89% versus 78%) and hemoglobin (89% versus 56%). The availability of HIV commodities was similar across both program and comparison HCs. Cotrimoxazole was observed in all HCs; however, stock-outs of Nevirapine (single dose and syrup), Zidovudine, and Lamivudine were noted in more than 25% of all HCs. Among family planning commodities, program HCs were observed to have a wider selection of contraceptives in stock (average of 4.9 of 6 total products versus 3.3 in comparison HCs).

Provider profiles

HCs were staffed by a median of 24 (range 11–54) providers, nearly half of whom (11, range of 3–24) reported providing MNCH services (Table 3). Only 63% of HCs met MOHSW recommended staffing requirements for MNCH cadres - Registered Nurses, Enrolled Nurses, and Medical Attendants. In addition, among the total MNCH providers listed on the rosters, 17% were reported by the HC In-Charge to be absent. Shortages in staffing, as a result of misallocation of staff and absenteeism, were reported by providers to make responding to diverse client needs challenging.

> *"But still the challenge is that there are few attendants...maybe at RCH perhaps people have arrived, maybe there are four for postpartum care, you need to thoroughly examine these [patients] and still there are pregnant women [coming for ANC visits]...so*

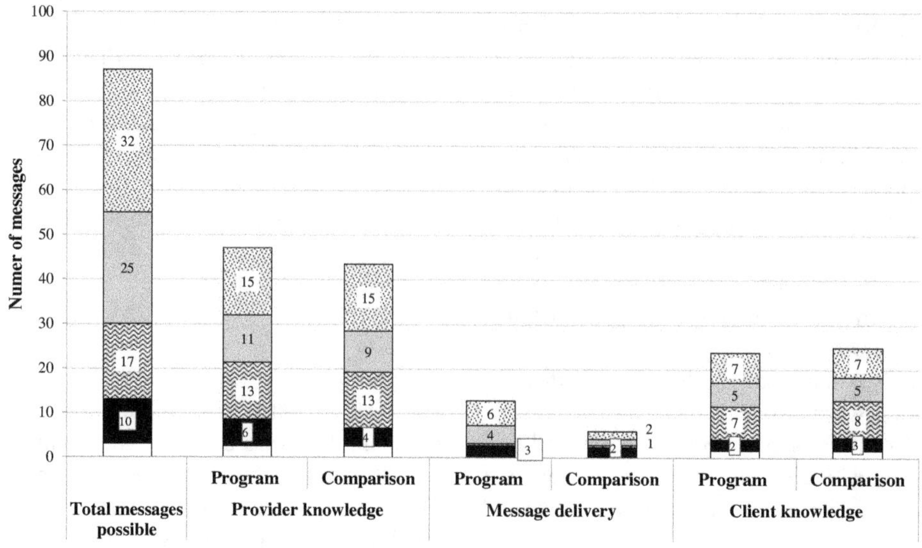

Fig. 2 Availability of essential PPC infrastructure, drugs, equipment, supplies and testings services in 18 health centres in Morogoro region, Tanzania in 2012: Mean composite scores. ***Legend: Physical Infrastructure*** (On call staff housing, electricity, water source, client toilet, waiting area, wash basin with running water in the PPC area). ***Drugs and Commodities***: (Iron/folic acid, vitamin A, tetracycline, polio vaccine, BCG vaccine, DPT vaccine, Condoms, Oral Contraceptive pills, depo provera, intra uterine devices, implants, cotrimoxazole, NVP for mother, NVP for child, AZT, 3TC, ARVs.) ***Equipment /supplies:*** (Tape measure, sterile clamps, thermometer, baby weighing scale, sterile gloves, syringes, vaccine thermometer, ice box, ice packs and fridge). ***Diagnostic tests:*** (CD4 count, HIV testing, DBS HIV for newborns)

there comes the challenge to observe every aspect [of PPC]." (Registered nurse, 10 years of experience, PPC training)

Among available RCH providers, nearly one-third reported providing PPC services to mothers, children, or both in the preceding seven days (Table 3). PPC providers included Enrolled Nurses (51%), Registered Nurses (16%), and Medical Attendants (14%) – a cadre of providers with limited to no clinical training. The majority of PPC providers were females (77%) who had been working in their current HC for a median of 4.3 years, and as a health care provider for 17 years.

Interviewed providers in both program and comparison areas were asked about their ability to provide PPC. Most felt that they had limited practice in providing PPC as a stand-alone service, as most women were seen soon after a facility delivery and few returned after that.

"We were studying it at school, but after studying it, practicing it here in working stations was so minimal, only maybe there at the labor room after delivery after they have delivered." (Enrolled nurse, 5 years of experience, no PPC training)

PPC training was provided to 4 of 10 (40%) of RCH providers in program HCs. Those trained were primarily female (82%) and enrolled (71%) or registered (24%) nurses. Nearly half of providers interviewed across all HCs reported receiving supervision visits at least once in the 12 months preceding the survey (Additional file 1: Table S1). While all providers interviewed received supervision from Child Health Management Teams (CHMT), regional and MoH supervisors equally, program areas received twice as much supervision from a non-government organization (NGO) (64% vs. 33%) and from district non-Child Health Management Teams (CHMT) (42% vs. 21%) than comparison areas.

Despite the training and supervision inputs provided to program areas, wide differences in provider knowledge of PPC counselling messages were not observed across HCs (Additional file 2: Table S2). The proportion of messages that providers reported knowing for each domain was lower for infant, newborn and maternal health, than for HIV, family planning and malaria, (Fig. 3). This waspartly related to the total number of messages to recall for each domain: infant and newborn health (32), maternal health (25), HIV (17), family planning (10) and malaria (3).

Client profiles

PPC women (26 women in program HCs, 19 women in comparison HCs) were between 20 and 35 years of age (median 24), with limited (48%) to no formal education (33%), mostly facility births (71%), uncomplicated vaginal deliveries (93%), and with deliveries one week prior to the interview (median 7 days) (Table 4).

Table 3 Characteristics of PPC providers interviewed ($n = 65$) and trained ($n = 19$) in 18 health centers in 4 districts of Morogoro region, Tanzania in 2012

	Total	Program	Control
All facility characteristics[a]			
Median number of providers reported per facility	24	28	21
Median number of providers reported providing MNCH per facility	11	10	11
Median number of providers trained in PPC per facility	1	4	0
Characteristics of interviewed RCH providers who reported providing PPC	($N = 63$)	($N = 37$)	($N = 26$)
Female provider	49 (77%)	28 (76%)	21 (79%)
Designation			
Enrolled Nurse	32 (51%)	19 (50%)	15 (58%)
Registered Nurse	10 (16%)	6 (16%)	4 (15%)
Medical Attendant	9 (14%)	7 (18%)	2 (8%)
Clinical officer/ Ass. Clinical officer	5 (8%)	3 (8%)	2 (8%)
Other[a]	6 (10%)	3 (8%)	3 (12%)
Years working as a health worker (Median)	13	13	12.5
Years working in this health facility (Median)	4	3	4.5
PPC providers whom have received PPC training	18 (29%)	17 (46%)	1 (4%)
Characteristics of interviewed RCH providers trained in PPC	($N = 19$)	($N = 17$)	(N) = 2
Female provider	16 (84%)	14 (82%)	2 (100%)
Designation			
Enrolled Nurse	14 (74%)	12 (71%)	2 (100%)
Registered Nurse	4 (21%)	4 (24%)	0%
Other[b]	1 (5%)	1 (6%)	0%
Years working as a health worker (Median)	17	15	29
Years working in this health facility (Median)	4.3	4	15

[a]Data obtained through facility in-charge interview
[b]Other here includes Assistant Medical Officer, Health Officer, and Health Assistant

Women sought PPC services because they felt that PPC was beneficial to ensure child health, particularly with regard to vaccinations and/or receipt of registration cards. Some women named specific diseases against which children are routinely immunized, including polio and tetanus. One woman emphasized the importance of PPC for her child over and above her own care:

"If I come here and I don't get any service for myself, I won't care. But if my child won't be given

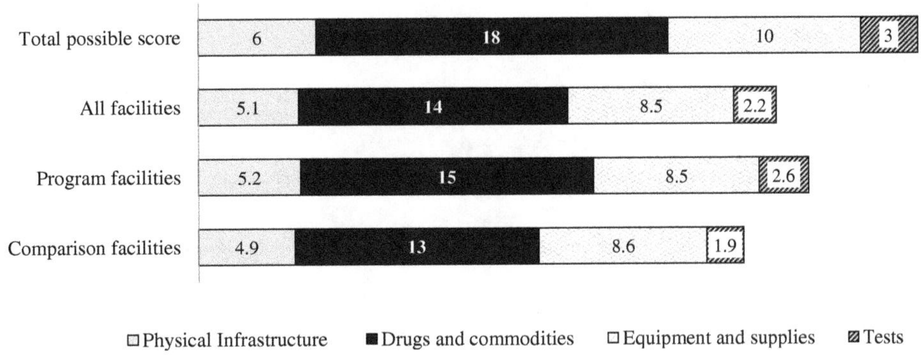

Fig. 3 Composite scores of provider knowledge ($N = 62$), observed message delivery ($N = 45$), and client knowledge ($N = 41$) of PPC messages in 18 health centers in 4 districts of Morogoro region, Tanzania in 2012

Table 4 Characteristics of PPC counseling sessions observed (n = 45) and clients interviewed (*n* = 41) in 18 health centers in 4 districts of Morogoro region, Tanzania in 2012

	Total	Program	Comparison
PPC Client Characteristics	*N* = 41	*N* = 25	*N* = 16
Age (median time in years)	24	23	28
Health facility delivery	29 (71%)	14 (55%)	12 (76%)
Days since delivery (median)	7.0	7.0	11
Mode of delivery			
Normal without episiotomy	38 (93%)	23 (92%)	15 (94%)
Normal with episiotomy	2 (5%)	1 (4%)	1 (6%)
Cesarean	1 (2%)	1 (4%)	0 (0%)
Years of Schooling			
No formal education	14 (33%)	12 (48%)	2 (12%)
Primary	20 (48%)	10 (40%)	9 (59%)
Secondary	6 (14%)	3 (12%)	3 (18%)
Others	1 (2%)	0 (0%)	2 (12%)
Number of times pregnant prior to delivery of last child (median)	1.5	1.0	2.0
Patient recalled visit characteristics	*N* = 41	*N* = 25	*N* = 16
Duration of travel time to get health facility (median time in minutes)	30	60	15
Duration of waiting time between arriving at clinic and being seen by provider (median time in minutes)	30	30	15
Client perceptions on waiting time			
Long / too long	17 (41%)	11 (43%)	6 (40%)
Acceptable	22 (53%)	13 (52%)	8 (53%)
Short	2 (6%)	1 (5%)	1 (7%)
Reason for PPC Visit			
Baby well-visit	25 (61%)	14 (56%)	11 (69%)
Mother well-visit	14 (34%)	11 (44%)	3 (19%)
Baby symptoms/ sickness	2 (5%)	2 (8%)	0 (0%)
Mother symptoms/ sickness	1 (2%)	1 (4%)	0 (0%)
Observed visit characteristics	*N* = 45	*N* = 26	*N* = 19
Duration of Individual PPC counseling (median time in minutes)	9.5	20	2.0
Counselling type			
Group	12 (30%)	5 (21%)	7 (44%)
Individual	14 (35%)	14 (54%)	1 (6%)
Both	14 (35%)	6 (25%)	8 (50%)
PPC visit number			
At discharge post delivery	9 (22%)	7 (27%)	3 (16%)
First follow up visit after delivery (within 7 days)	20 (49%)	14 (54%)	7 (42%)
Second visit (within 28 days)	9 (22%)	4 (15%)	5 (32%)
Third visit (within 42 days)	12 (29%)	1 (4%)	2 (11%)
PPC Visit recipient			
Child	1 (2%)	1 (4%)	0 (0%)
Mother	13 (31%)	1 (4%)	11 (68%)
Mother and child	27 (67%)	23 (92%)	5 (32%)
Provider used job aides	12 (29%)	1 (4%)	10 (63%)

Table 4 Characteristics of PPC counseling sessions observed (n = 45) and clients interviewed (*n* = 41) in 18 health centers in 4 districts of Morogoro region, Tanzania in 2012 *(Continued)*

	Total	Program	Comparison
Provider told client return visit date			
Sets a date for the next visit with the client	41 (100%)	25 (100%)	16 (100%)
Encourages her to return to the next planned visit	40 (98%)	24 (96%)	16 (100%)
PPC provider was the same as that who attended you during a previous visit to this health facility	11 (26%)	6 (23%)	5 (29%)

immunization or nothing is done to her, I will question." (28 years old, 15 days since delivery, PPC2)

PPC for women was largely seen as unnecessary, especially among women with prior healthy, complication-free pregnancy and delivery experiences that did not require them to return to a health facility. The few women that did mention seeking PPC services for themselves, did so largely for family planning. Women noted that they knew family planning would be available and, in some cases, reported being informed by providers to return for family planning counselling and supplies.

"Some of them [mothers], they come for further mother health examination, but honestly speaking, most of them they don't know if a mother should also be involved." (28 years old, 15 days since delivery, PPC2)

In addition, work demands and other domestic priorities also took precedence for women who had recently given birth. One woman commented:

"Other women do not come because they do not prioritize. They would rather do their chores at home than come for a clinic visit. She sees that her work is more important than the clinic visit." (29 years old, 14 days since delivery, PPC2)

Processes

In the program area, PPC consultations were a median of 20 min in duration as compared to two minutes in the comparison area. A Spearman's correlation coefficient determined that the number of messages observed during counselling was significantly associated with the total duration of PPC consultation (rho = 0.44, 95% CI: 0.17 to 0.6) (Table 5).

Additional file 2: Table S2 summarizes the frequency of PPC messages observed to be delivered and Fig. 3 depicts mean composite scores of observed PPC message delivery during individual counselling sessions ($n = 45$) in program and comparison areas. While infant, newborn and maternal health form the bulk of counselling messages delivered, the content delivered is still very limited. While this is somewhat higher in program areas, the frequency of observed messages fell below 25% for all domains assessed (Fig. 3).

In contrast to the low frequency of delivery of PPC messages, 100% of providers were observed to set a date for the next visit and 98% encouraged the woman to return for this scheduled visit.

PPC women reported traveling for a median of 30 min to get to the health facility and waiting for a median of 30 min prior to being seen by a provider. Cumulative travel (to and from), waiting and consultation time was an estimated 209 min for program area PPC women, as compared to 100 min in the comparison area. Women's perceptions of whether the time taken was acceptable (53%), too long (41%), or too short (6%) were the same in both program or comparison areas (Table 4).

Across program and comparison areas, geographic accessibility, measured by distance and the availability of transport, was cited frequently by women as a reason why women do not attend PPC services.

Table 5 Correlation between duration of PPC counselling and message delivery: Composite scores for observed PPC counselling (*n* = 45) in 18 health centers in 4 districts of Morogoro region, Tanzania in 2012. One a scale of 1 to −1, where 1 denotes strong positive correlation and – 1 strong negative correlation, findings suggest that the more time spent on counselling corresponds to more messages delivered

Domain	Total (*n* = 45)	Program (*n* = 26)	Comparison (*n* = 19)
Total Composite Score	0.44 (0.17, 0.65)*	0.46 (0.08, 0.72)*	0.27 (−0.21, 0.64)
Maternal Health	0.56 (0.31, 0.73)*	0.52(0.15, 0.76)*	0.48 (0.04, 0.77)*
Infant & child health	0.41 (0.13, 0.63)*	0.22(− 0.19, 0.57)	0.46(0.01, 0.76)*
HIV	0.27(− 0.03, 0.53)	0.1(− 0.31, 0.47)	0.37 (− 0.1, 0.71)
Family Planning	0.02 (− 0.28, 0.32)	0.51 (0.14, 0.75)*	− 0.34 (− 0.69, 0.14)

*Significant at $p < 0.05$

In addition, women's access to PPC was also hampered by gaps in the continuity of care. One woman noted that if a pregnant woman did not complete ANC and/or delivered at home, access to information about services after delivery might be limited.

> *"Many don't come for ANC visit and they deliver at home, so they don't get a chance to know the importance of PPC visits." (23 years old, 21 days since delivery, PPC3)*

PPC users also reported that when women who delivered at home do reach services, they were often treated harshly by providers and/or asked to pay out of pocket costs for PPC services.

> *"Sometimes, those who have delivered at home, they are mistreated...when they come for PPC and they have to pay some amount for them to start PPC visits. For example, I paid 3000 shillings so that I could get a card to start PPC services for myself and my child." (23 years old, 21 days since delivery, PPC3)*

> *"...saying the truth when they come here... We blame them, why did she decide to give birth at home." (Enrolled nurse, 3 years experience, no PPC training)*

Outcomes

Across program and comparison areas, exit interviews of PPC women following observations ($n = 41$) indicate that over 20% of users are able to recall (unprompted) at least one key message for each of the 10 domains (Fig. 3, Additional file 2: Table S2). Among critical danger signs, women recalled nearly half the 13 newborn danger signs assessed, including fever (55%), difficulty in breastfeeding (43%), pitched cry/irritability (40%), convulsions/fits (30%), and hypo/hyperthermia (20%). Similar trends were observed in women's recall for maternal danger signs, maternal/infant nutrition, and family planning. While counselling messages for HIV/AIDS were infrequently observed (< 5% for most indicators), women's knowledge of modalities of transmission, prevention and testing were moderate (32%) to high (64%) (Additional file 2: Table S2).

Discussion

Our study findings indicate that program HCs were better than comparison HCs with respect to availability of PPC drugs, commodities and testing supplies; reported higher PPC supervision and training; and higher duration and more comprehensive PPC counselling sessions. However, across both areas, physical infrastructure, equipment and supplies were similar, with notable limitations related to water supply and electricity. Deficits in human resources, attributed to poor staffing levels and absenteeism, contributed to the use of unqualified providers and were reported to hinder PPC service delivery across both areas.

The majority of PPC recipients were women with uncomplicated vaginal deliveries (93%) in a health facility (71%). This suggests that women most at risk, including those with complications or who deliver at home may not be seeking PPC. Across both program and comparison areas, PPC services were perceived by clients to be beneficial for child health, while services for women were largely seen as unnecessary. Findings on the overall content of observed counselling sessions, while focused on maternal and child health, were still far below program guidelines.

Evidence on the quality of PPC in low resource settings is emerging [22]. Qualitative interviews in Ghana with providers and women [9, 23, 24] and elsewhere in Tanzania with providers [23], first time fathers [25] and mothers [26], and broader support structures [27, 28] echo findings observed here. This suggests that PPC is not well recognized by women [29] and its value largely tied to the receipt of technical interventions, including immunizations for children and family planning for women. Elsewhere in sub-Saharan Africa, despite higher rates of reported PPC awareness, utilization also remains low [23]. To increase demand, women need to respected by providers and see value in PPC. In addition, efforts to increase availability and quality of PPC services at facility and community levels include introduction of PPC home visits, strengthening postpartum outreach services, integration of PPC with mother and child immunization clinics, distribution of PPC guidelines among health workers and upgrading PPC knowledge and skills through training [30].

While the program sought to improve PPC capacity through provider training and ongoing supportive supervision, only a median of 4 RCH providers per program HC received PPC training. Transparent criteria for selecting providers for training; a planned approach for building capacity among the remaining providers not selected; addressing transport and funding constraints that impede the frequency of supervision visits; and ensuring that providers have sufficient PPC women with which they can maintain their skills is critical to ensure that these training and supervision inputs translate into improved service delivery.

There is discordance between provider knowledge and observed delivery of counselling content across all major domains. This suggests that training and supervisory inputs alone may not be sufficient to improve the content of counselling. Increased duration of PPC consultations corresponded to more counselling messages delivered.

While this prolonged client waiting times, women across program and comparison HCs reported similar satisfaction levels. Unless efforts are made to address critical deficits in the availability of human resources (40% of HCs fell short of the minimum MOHSW standard for human resources); absenteeism (17% among MNCH providers); and the use of unqualified providers (medical attendants comprised 14% of PPC service providers) improvements in PPC service delivery are unlikely.

Prioritization of the over 80 PPC messages recommended by national PPC guidelines may ensure that women receive and retain the most critical messages. Increased delivery of core maternal health messages may also serve to overcome perceptions that PPC is for child health and of limited benefit to the mother. Finally, wider dialogue on what services should be delivered optimally at different levels of the health system is needed. Current activities underway by the MOHSW to support a national cadre of community health workers may provide a forum for PPC promotion and counselling at community level; allowing facility based cadres of providers to focus more on delivery of services requiring greater clinical or technical expertise. Further review of and inputs to services at dispensary level may provide a similar opportunity to improve and expand availability of PPC services.

Limitations

Studies on the quality of PPC conducted to date have largely gathered data through qualitative interviews with providers and/or women. Ours is one of the few studies to triangulate data from multiple sources using qualitative and quantitative methods including direct observations of facilities and service delivery, as well as provider and women's interviews. Despite these strengths, efforts to determine the quality of PPC were hampered by the infrequency of PPC service utilization and logistical challenges associated with achieving the sample size required to draw statistical inferences. Similarly the small numbers of trained providers meant that assessing knowledge and service delivery comparisons within facilities by training status would not be meaningful. Efforts to assess the differential quality of PPC were additionally limited by the purposive selection of HCs in a non-randomized design by program implementors. The program assessment was not commissioned until two years after the start of the program and thus modifications to the program design were not possible. Elsewhere, PPC quality of care assessments have assumed a pre/post study design [30] and thus better isolated the effect of training and program support activities.

The framework used in this analysis focused on the Health Center level. Inputs from the Regional or District level were not considered and processes related to improvements in efficiency not measured. The latter, defined by WHO as delivering health care in a manner which maximizes resource use and avoids waste [31], would best be measured through economic evaluation or assessments of inputs over outputs using Data Envelopment Analysis [20] or Frontier Analyses. These, along with measurement of health outcomes and impact, were all considered beyond the scope of this analysis.

Conclusions

Our study measured the quality of PPC and assessed the effects of program efforts at HC level to implement national PPC guidelines, and upgrade provider PPC knowledge and skills through PPC training and supervision in rural Tanzania. Study findings highlight deficits in the quality of PPC services in HCs in five districts of Morogoro region, Tanzania. While viewed favorably for ensuring child health, PPC services were not part of the women's conception of care as needed for themselves after delivery. Content of care was largely constrained to a few counselling messages on immunizations for newborns, benefits and sources of family planning. While this study is limited by the small sample size of observed PPC clients, findings demonstrate that PPC training and supervision inputs had modest effects on the content of counselling services but did yield improvements in the observed duration of consultation—a factor significantly associated with increased message delivery. Although increased provider-woman contact is needed to improve quality in counselling, these improvements are unlikely unless human resource shortages are addressed, provider capacity built, challenges with respectful maternity care addressed, and efforts to strengthen other levels of the health care system undertaken.

Additional files

Additional file 1: Table S1. Reported supervision provided to RCH providers ($n = 88$) from July 2011 to June 2012.

Additional file 2: Table S2. Provider knowledge ($N = 62$), delivery ($N = 45$) and client knowledge ($N = 41$) of PPC messages in 18 health centers in 4 districts of Morogoro region, Tanzania in 2012.

Abbreviations

ANC: Antenatal care; HC: Health Center; IEC: Information, education, communication; IP: Integrated Program; JHU: Johns Hopkins Bloomberg School of Public Health; MCHIP: Maternal and Child Health Integrated Program; MEP: Morogoro Evaluation Project; MNH: Maternal, newborn, health.; MOHSW: Ministry of Health and Social Welfare; MUHAS: Muhimbili University of Health and Allied Sciences; PMTCT: Prevention of mother to child transmission; PPC: Postpartum care; PPFP: Postpartum family planning; RCH: Reproductive child health; SSA: Sub-Saharan Africa

Acknowledgements

The authors wish to thank the health care providers and postpartum women in Morogoro for their time and insights. We additionally thank Drs. Japhet Kilewo and Abdullah Baqui – the study Principal Investigators – for their guidance and support. Inputs and support to study design, training, data collection, analysis and dissemination from David Urassa, Gasto Frumence of MUHAS; and Dr. Shivam Gupta, and Ms. Joy Chebet from JHSPH are acknowledged with gratitude.

Funding

This work was supported by the U.S. Agency for International Development (USAID), under the This study was supported by USAID through the Health Research Challenge for Impact (HRCI) Cooperative Agreement (#GHS-A-00-09-00004-00). The contents are the responsibility of Johns Hopkins School of Public Health (JHSPH) and Muhimbili University of Health and Allied Sciences (MUHAS) and do not necessarily reflect the views of USAID or the United States Government. Asha George is also supported by the South African Research Chair's Initiative of the Department of Science and Technology and National Research Foundation of South Africa (Grant No 82769). Any opinion, finding and conclusion or recommendation expressed in this material is that of the author and the NRF does not accept any liability in this regard.

Authors' contributions

AL, AG, RM, CK, AY, SA, IM, JCK, and PW developed data collection instruments with inputs from CL and GB. RM, AL and AG coordinated data collection and management. AY, SA, and IM supervised facility level data collection. Coding and analysis for qualitative analyses were carried out by SA, MS, and AG. AL, DM, and AY conducted quantitative analyses. AL wrote the first draft of the paper with AG and inputs from all other authors. All authors read and approved the final version of the manuscript.

Competing interests

The authors of this manuscript do not have competing interests.

Author details

[1]Department of International Health, Johns Hopkins Bloomberg School of Public Health, Baltimore, MD, USA. [2]School of Public Health and Family Medicine, Division of Epidemiology and Biostatistics, University of Cape Town, Cape Town, South Africa. [3]School of Public Health and Social Sciences, Muhimbili University of Health and Allied Sciences, P.O. Box 65015, Dar es Salaam, Tanzania. [4]Department of Obstetrics and Gynaecology, Muhimbili University of Health and Allied Sciences, P.O. Box 65001, Dar es Salaam, Tanzania. [5]Jhpiego Tanzania, Box 9170, Dar es Salaam, PO, Tanzania. [6]School of Public Health, University of the Western Cape, Bellville, South Africa.

References

1. WHO. Trends in maternal mortality: 1990 to 2015: estimates by WHO, UNICEF, UNFPA, World Bank Group and the United Nations Population Division. Geneva: World Health Organization; 2015.
2. Liu L, Oza S, Hogan D, Chu Y, Perin J, Zhu J, Lawn JE, Cousens S, Mathers C, Black RE. Global, regional, and national causes of under-5 mortality in 2000-15: an updated systematic analysis with implications for the sustainable development goals. Lancet. 2016;388(10063):3027–35.
3. WHO, UNICEF, Bank W, Division UNP. Trends in maternal mortality: 1990 to 2015. Geneva: Estimates by WHO, UNICEF, World Bank, and the United Nations Population Division; 2015.
4. Ministry of Health, Community Development, Gender, Elderely and Chilrden (MOHCDGEC) [Tanzania Mainland], Ministry of Health Zanzibar (MoH) [Zanzibar], National Bureau of Statistics (NBS), Office of the Chief Government Statistician (OCGS), and ICF International 2016. Tanzania Demographic and Health Survey and Malaria Indicator Survey (TDHS- MIS) 2015-16. Dar es Salaam, Tanzania and Rockville, Maryland, (MOHCDGEC), USA: MoHSW, MoH, NBS, OCGS, and ICF International.
5. WHO. Oportunities for African Newborns: Practical Data, Policy and Programmatic Support for newborn care in Africa. In. Edited by Lawn J, Kerber K; 2006.
6. Salam RA, Mansoor T, Mallick D, Lassi ZS, Das JK, Bhutta ZA. Essential childbirth and postnatal interventions for improved maternal and neonatal health. Reprod Health. 2014;11(Suppl 1):S3.
7. Tanzania MoHaSW, JHPIEGO. National Postnatal Care Guidelines. In: Dar es Salaam: Ministry of Health and Social Welfare; 2012.
8. Statistics NBo, Macro I. Tanzania Demographic and Health Survey 2010. In: Salaam D e, editor. Tanzania: NBS and ICF Macro; 2011.
9. Austin A, Langer A, Salam RA, Lassi ZS, Das JK, Bhutta ZA. Approaches to improve the quality of maternal and newborn health care: an overview of the evidence. Reprod Health. 2014;11(Suppl 2):S1.
10. van den Broek NR, Graham WJ. Quality of care for maternal and newborn health: the neglected agenda. BJOG : an international journal of obstetrics and gynaecology. 2009;116(Suppl 1):18–21.
11. Sitrin D, Guenther T, Murray J, Pilgrim N, Rubayet S, Ligowe R, Pun B, Malla H, Moran A. Reaching mothers and babies with early postnatal home visits: the implementation realities of achieving high coverage in large-scale programs. PLoS One. 2013;8(7):e68930.
12. Donabedian A. The quality of care. How can it be assessed? JAMA. 1988;260:1743–8.
13. Hulton L, Matthews Z, Williams Stones R. A framework for the evaluation of quality of care in maternity services. Highfield, Southampton: University of Southampton; 2000.
14. Donabedian A. Evaluating the quality of medical care. The Milbank Memorial Fund Quarterly. 1966;44(3):691–729.
15. Campbell S, Rolad M, Buetow S. Defining quality of care. Soc Sci Med. 2000;51(11):1611–25.
16. Atherton F, Mbekem G, Nyalusi I. Improving service quality: experience from the Tanzania Family health project. International journal for quality in health care : journal of the International Society for Quality in Health Care / ISQua. 1999;11(4):353–6.
17. Donabedian A. The seven pillars of quality. Archives of pathology & laboratory medicine. 1990;114(11):1115–8.
18. Maxwell R. Quality assessment in health. Br Med J. 1984;288
19. Maxwell R. Dimensions of quality revisited: from thought to action. Quality in Health Care. 1992;1:171–7.
20. WHO. Quality of care : a process for making strategic choices in health systems. France: World Health Organization; 2006.
21. Statistics NBo: Tanzania Service Provision Assessment 2006; 2007.
22. Plotkin M, Tibaijuka G, Makene C, Currie S, Lacoste M. Quality of Care for Prevention and Management of Common Maternal and Newborn Complications: A study of 12 regions in Tanzania. In: Salaam D e, editor. Tanzania: USAID, MCHIP, MAISHA; 2013.
23. Hill Z, Okyere E, Wickenden M, Tawiah-Agyemang C. What can we learn about postnatal care in Ghana if we ask the right questions? A qualitative study. Glob Health Action. 2015;8:28515.
24. Tesfahun F, Worku W, Mazengiya F, Kifle M. Knowledge, perception and utilization of postnatal care of mothers in Gondar Zuria District, Ethiopia: a cross-sectional study. Matern Child Health J. 2014;18(10):2341–51.
25. Mrisho M, Obrist B, Schellenberg JA, Haws RA, Mushi AK, Mshinda H, Tanner M, Schellenberg D. The use of antenatal and postnatal care: perspectives and experiences of women and health care providers in rural southern Tanzania. BMC pregnancy and childbirth. 2009;9:10.
26. Mbekenga CK, Lugina HI, Christensson K, Olsson P. Postpartum experiences of first-time fathers in a Tanzanian suburb: a qualitative interview study. Midwifery. 2011;27(2):174–80.
27. Mbekenga CK, Christensson K, Lugina HI, Olsson P. Joy, struggle and support: postpartum experiences of first-time mothers in a Tanzanian suburb. Women and birth : journal of the Australian College of Midwives. 2011;24(1):24–31.
28. Mbekenga CK, Pembe AB, Darj E, Christensson K, Olsson P. Prolonged sexual abstinence after childbirth: gendered norms and perceived family health risks. Focus group discussions in a Tanzanian suburb. BMC international health and human rights. 2013;13:4.
29. Mbekenga CK, Pembe AB, Christensson K, Darj E, Olsson P. Informal support to first-parents after childbirth: a qualitative study in low-income suburbs of Dar es salaam, Tanzania. BMC pregnancy and childbirth. 2011;11:98.
30. Duysburgh E, Kerstens B, Kouanda S, Kabore CP, Belemsaga Yugbare D, Gichangi P, Masache G, Crahay B, Gondola Sitefane G, Bique Osman N, et al. Opportunities to improve postpartum care for mothers and infants: design of context-specific packages of postpartum interventions in rural districts in four sub-Saharan African countries. BMC pregnancy and childbirth. 2015;15:131.
31. Warren C, Mwangi A, Oweya E, Kamunya R, Koskei N. Safeguarding maternal and newborn health: improving the quality of postnatal care in Kenya. International journal for quality in health care : journal of the International Society for Quality in Health Care / ISQua. 2010;22(1):24–30.

11

Limits to the scope of non-invasive prenatal testing (NIPT): an analysis of the international ethical framework for prenatal screening and an interview study with Dutch professionals

A. Kater-Kuipers[1], E. M. Bunnik[1*], I. D. de Beaufort[1†] and R. J. H. Galjaard[2†]

Abstract

Background: The introduction of non-invasive prenatal testing (NIPT) for foetal aneuploidies is currently changing the field of prenatal screening in many countries. As it is non-invasive, safe and accurate, this technique allows for a broad implementation of first-trimester prenatal screening, which raises ethical issues, related, for instance, to informed choice and adverse societal consequences. This article offers an account of a leading international ethical framework for prenatal screening, examines how this framework is used by professionals working in the field of NIPT, and presents ethical guidance for the expansion of the scope of prenatal screening in practice.

Methods: A comparative analysis of authoritative documents is combined with 15 semi-structured interviews with professionals in the field of prenatal screening in the Netherlands. Data were recorded, transcribed verbatim and analysed using thematic analysis.

Results: The current ethical framework consists of four pillars: the aim of screening, the proportionality of the test, justice, and societal aspects. Respondents recognised and supported this framework in practice, but expressed some concerns. Professionals felt that pregnant women do not always make informed choices, while this is seen as central to reproductive autonomy (the aim of screening), and that pre-test counselling practices stand in need of improvement. Respondents believed that the benefits of NIPT, and of an expansion of its scope, outweigh the harms (proportionality), which are thought to be acceptable. They felt that the out-of-pocket financial contribution currently required by pregnant women constitutes a barrier to access to NIPT, which disproportionally affects those of a lower socioeconomic status (justice). Finally, professionals recognised but did not share concerns about a rising pressure to test or discrimination of disabled persons (societal aspects).

(Continued on next page)

* Correspondence: e.bunnik@erasmusmc.nl
†I. D. de Beaufort and R. J. H. Galjaard contributed equally to this work.
[1]Department of Medical Ethics and Philosophy of Medicine, Erasmus MC, University Medical Centre Rotterdam, Room 24.17, Wytemaweg 80, 3015 CN Rotterdam, The Netherlands
Full list of author information is available at the end of the article

(Continued from previous page)

Conclusions: Four types of limits to the scope of NIPT are proposed: NIPT should generate only test outcomes that are relevant to reproductive decision-making, informed choice should be (made) possible through adequate pre-test counselling, the rights of future children should be respected, and equal access should be guaranteed. Although the focus of the interview study is on the Dutch healthcare setting, insights and conclusions can be applied internationally and to other healthcare systems.

Keywords: Prenatal screening, Non-invasive prenatal testing (NIPT), Reproductive autonomy, Informed consent, Public health ethics, Ethical framework, Qualitative interview study

Background

Non-invasive prenatal testing (NIPT) is based on the analysis of cell free foetal DNA for chromosomal abnormalities [1]. Non-invasiveness refers to the way the foetal DNA sample is obtained: not from the placenta or amniotic fluid, which requires an invasive procedure, but from a blood sample of the mother. NIPT for chromosomal abnormalities was first offered in 2011, in the United States of America, Western-Europe and China [2]. In the Netherlands, prenatal screening for untreatable disorders is subjected to licensing under the Population Screening Act. NIPT has been offered to high-risk women, exclusively within the context of the TRIDENT-1 study (Trial by Dutch laboratories for Evaluation of Non-Invasive Prenatal Testing) since early 2014 [3]. When a woman received a high-risk outcome (chance ≥1:200) from the first trimester combined test (FCT) and wanted further testing, she was offered the choice between NIPT or invasive testing [3]. Low-risk pregnant women who wanted NIPT could not access NIPT in the Netherlands, and went abroad. Since April 2017, NIPT is also offered within the TRIDENT-2 study to low-risk pregnant women, who are given a choice between FCT and NIPT. The current NIPT-based prenatal test includes detection of trisomy 21 (Down syndrome), trisomy 18 (Edwards syndrome) and trisomy 13 (Patau syndrome). Compared to the FCT the sensitivity, the specificity and the positive predictive value of NIPT are remarkably high for those trisomies [3]. The positive predictive value is slightly lower in low-risk pregnant women but still higher than the positive predictive value of the FCT [1, 4, 5]. However, NIPT is not a diagnostic test. This is because of several factors. First, cell free foetal DNA circulating in maternal blood originates from the placenta, not the foetus. The presence of a chromosomal anomaly can be limited to the placenta in case of confined placental mosaicism without affecting the foetus, thus resulting in a false positive NIPT outcome. Furthermore, the presence of maternal chromosomal anomalies, including those originating from a maternal tumour, low foetal DNA fraction in maternal blood, and a vanishing twin [6, 7], may still lead to inconclusive, false positive or false negative results [8]. Yet NIPT leads to fewer unnecessary invasive follow-ups tests - through amniocentesis and chorionic villus sampling - than the FCT. These invasive tests have a 0.1–0.2% risk, respectively, of miscarriage [3]. To minimize the need for invasive testing – and the associated risk of miscarriage – has been one of the major reasons for implementing NIPT in current screening programmes.

When genome-wide sequencing techniques are used to perform NIPT, they allow for the detection of chromosomal abnormalities other than trisomy 13, 18 and 21, and thus for an expansion of the current scope of prenatal screening [3, 9]. Several studies have indicated that additional findings could include other full trisomies, sex-chromosomal abnormalities, and sub-chromosomal aberrations, associated with rare diseases [3, 10–12]. However, the possibility to find more abnormalities has raised questions, notably the policy question whether the screening offer should be expanded to include all those abnormalities. When discussing the question whether or not to include additional conditions, experts have brought up considerations of clinical utility and concerns related to the consequences of a broader test for informed choice [13–15]. These concerns were raised 10 years ago, when genome-wide arrays were introduced in prenatal diagnosis, and are raised again with renewed urgency in the context of the introduction of NIPT [16].

Various statements and position papers about prenatal screening, issued by governmental organisations and ethical committees, have addressed ethical issues of prenatal screening [15, 17–24]. Together with scholarly studies of ethical issues in prenatal screening [25–30] these statements and position papers could be seen as an – unofficial, but broadly shared and often referred to – international ethical framework for prenatal screening. An ethical framework can be defined as a specification of general principles in a specific context, through which the scope of general principles is narrowed by spelling out why and how actions should be undertaken or avoided [31]. The aim of an ethical framework is to "provide practical guidance for public health professionals and to highlight the defining values of public health" [32].

The aim of this article is firstly to reconstruct and analyse the main tenets of the ethical framework for prenatal screening and then to compare these with the practice of prenatal screening, through interviews with professionals in the field of prenatal screening. Secondly, this article examines whether and how the ethical framework can guide an expansion of the scope of prenatal screening.

Methods

For this study we used a combination of methods, a literature study and a qualitative interview study. We conducted a comparative analysis of ethical statements about requirements for (non-invasive) prenatal testing formulated by national and international organisations or committees. Also, we conducted in-depth interviews with Dutch professionals in the field of prenatal screening. The interviews serve to illustrate how the ethical framework for prenatal screening is translated into practice, and to offer insight into professionals' moral views on recent developments in prenatal screening.

Document analysis

To identify important documents that represent an ethical framework we started with an authoritative article of the European Society of Human Genetics (ESHG) and the American Society of Human Genetics (ASHG), which offers a consensus view of responsible innovation in prenatal screening, which is also endorsed by the Human Genetics Society of Australasia and other related professional associations in Europe [15]. We built on this consensus view and postulated four pillars of an ethical framework: the aim of prenatal screening, proportionality of testing, justice, and societal aspects. Other studies and documents – notably from the World Health Organisation (WHO), UNESCO International Bioethics Committee (IBC), German Ethics Council (Ethikrat) and the Dutch Health Council (GR) – were reviewed to corroborate, adapt and complement the ethical framework. We selected these four other documents for our analysis because – in contrast to other publications we have reviewed – these documents contain discussions of issues related to all four pillars.

Interviews

For the qualitative interview study, professionals in the field of prenatal screening and follow-up diagnostic testing from six academic centres in the Netherlands were invited. In total 15 individual in-depth interviews were conducted with two midwives, seven medical specialists (three gynaecologists, four clinical geneticists specialised in prenatal diagnosis), two lab specialists working with NIPT, two test developers and two policy makers. The interviews were conducted at the respondents' work places or at Erasmus MC. A semi-structured interview guide was used. This guide included five themes: informed decision-making, proportionality, access to NIPT, societal aspects and the scope of prenatal screening. Interviews were digitally recorded, transcribed verbatim and analysed with Atlas.ti using thematic analysis, based on the five indicated themes.

Results

The documents each point at the four pillars - the aim of screening, the proportionality of the test, justice, and societal aspects - but differ in some aspects of their interpretations. Table 1 presents an overview of interpretations of the four pillars in the five documents. Below we present the four pillars of the ethical framework for the practice of prenatal screening, complemented with results from the interviews.

Aim of prenatal screening

The first pillar of the ethical framework for prenatal screening pertains to the aim of prenatal screening for foetal abnormalities. Prenatal screening differs from other areas of public health, where the aim is reduction of morbidity and mortality associated with disorders in the population [15]. Translating this aim to prenatal screening might imply that the success of a prenatal screening programme would be defined in terms of maximisation of the termination rate of foetuses with abnormalities, which would be problematic, as abortion is often a point of controversy [15, 17, 19, 20]. Besides, prenatal screening is thought to imply discriminatory messages about the value of the lives of people living with the relevant conditions [15, 17–19]. The widely supported view therefore is that governments can only justifiably offer prenatal screening when the aim is to enable pregnant women and their partners to make autonomous reproductive choices [15, 17, 19].

Although interviewed professionals recognised informed choice as the aim of prenatal screening, some of them pointed out that prenatal screening also provides the opportunity to prepare for the birth of a disabled child and to improve the care for it. Several respondents thought that the latter should be emphasised more during pre-test counselling and that it should be made clear that prenatal screening is not exclusively aimed at offering women the opportunity to terminate an affected pregnancy.

The right not to know about the options of prenatal screening is considered very important. In the Netherlands, this has been formalised in the obligation of professionals to present women with an 'information offer' first [33], in order to stress the fact that prenatal screening for aneuploidies is not mandatory. When a pregnant woman visits the midwife or obstetrician, the professional must first ask whether the woman wants to be informed about prenatal screening at all. The woman is free to decline this information offer. Not all professionals agreed with this policy, and some argued - contra current policy - that this first question should be

Table 1 An ethical framework for prenatal screening

	ESHG/ASHG (2015)	WHO (2003)	Ethikrat (2013)	Dutch Health Council (2013)	UNESCO (2015)
Aim of prenatal screening	The aim is to enable autonomous reproductive choices, i.e. meaningful choices, related to serious health problems. The aim is achieved when women are enabled to make informed choices. Prenatal screening has a different goal than other forms of screening, because of the 'morally sensitive practice' of (selective) abortion and the stigmatisation of disabled people.	The aim is to obtain information and to promote freedom of choice and autonomy. Being able to prepare for the birth of a child with a disability is also seen as a way to exercise reproductive autonomy. Free choice requires: 1) adequate, unbiased information; 2) availability of relevant alternatives, including availability of healthcare services for disabled children or the (legal) possibility of abortion.	The aim is not specified, but prenatal screening is linked to self-determination and autonomy: "If a pregnant woman makes decisions about her pregnancy, these must be seen inter alia in the context of her right to reproductive self-determination." Reproductive decisions affect the unborn child and are thus not unlimited.	The aim is to enable and promote choice concerning terminating or continuing the pregnancy. "Informed choice is not a condition for, but the aim of prenatal screening." The aim is not to maximise reproductive choice as such. If informed choice is not reached, the aim is not achieved.	The aim is "not health gain but to decide (…) whether to carry a pregnancy to term." Furthermore, "it allows those involved to prepare for the birth of a sick or disabled child." There is controversy about the limits of reproductive autonomy in the light of a child's right to an un-manipulated genetic make-up. Prevention, focused on "reducing care costs for people with congenital conditions or disabilities, cannot be the goal of such screening. That would imply a discriminatory practice that sends the message that these people are unwelcome in society."
Proportionality	Proportionality is defined as a balancing of benefits and harms. Benefits of NIPT include reassurance, assistance in making informed reproductive decisions, and less invasive testing. Harms of prenatal screening generally include false reassurance, stress and anxiety, and risk of miscarriage in follow-up diagnostic testing. Balancing of benefits and harms includes consideration of quality aspects of the test and adequate counselling.	Proportionality is not discussed. Benefits and burdens are included in a cost-benefit analysis. Benefits are the chance to prepare for the birth of a child that will need medical treatment or a relief of maternal anxiety. Burdens include selective abortion of a wanted pregnancy.	Proportionality is not discussed, although it is stated that quality assurance is a precondition to meeting the aim of prenatal screening. Balancing benefits and harms is difficult: "The effect of a differentiated prenatal diagnosis is ambivalent. It may relieve the pregnant woman of fears, but on the other hand there is the danger that the (...) associated burden of deciding make[s] the couple affected (…) and may even overstrain them." It is seen as a great risk that women may be insufficiently aware of the consequences of testing and subsequent decisions they will have to make.	Proportionality is a central requirement for prenatal screening. Screening is only justified when the value or utility of the offer is established and the benefits outweigh the disadvantages. Benefits of NIPT include reassurance, informed reproductive decisions and less invasive testing. 'Disadvantages' of screening include false reassurance, test-related stress and anxiety and risk of miscarriage.	Proportionality and proven usefulness are preconditions for a justified prenatal screening offer. The advantages should outweigh the disadvantages. Benefits are having freedom to choose and fewer invasive tests. Disadvantages are "routinization and institutionaliza tion of choice of not giving birth to an ill or disabled child." If a test becomes self-evident women might feel pressured to test or stigmatised when they will not test.
Justice	Justice refers to the distribution of costs: "As health budgets are	Justice refers to the "equitable distribution of genetics services,	Justice refers to equal access to prenatal screening and to the	Justice refers to an appropriate use of healthcare resources.	Justice refers to the organisation of healthcare systems,

Table 1 An ethical framework for prenatal screening *(Continued)*

	ESHG/ASHG (2015)	WHO (2003)	Ethikrat (2013)	Dutch Health Council (2013)	UNESCO (2015)
	inevitably limited (…), opportunity costs will have to be taken into account as well." The requirement of just distribution of healthcare costs will demarcate the scope of prenatal screening.	including prenatal diagnosis, is owed first to those with the greatest medical need, regardless of ability to pay, or any other considerations." Relief of maternal anxiety has lower priority than medical indications for prenatal screening, in the just distribution of healthcare resources.	danger of "discrimination and stigmatization of people with particular genetic characteristics."	Prenatal screening can be used appropriately by couples wishing to prepare for the birth of an affected child, which is considered a justified aim of screening. Justice is also mentioned in the context of equal access to an expanded scope of prenatal screening: screening for abnormalities other than trisomy 21, 18 and 13 should not only be available for high-risk women (through invasive follow-up testing).	so that innovations are shared with society as a whole, without becoming a new source of inequality and discrimination. Justice also pertains to education: people should be actively enabled to exercise their freedom and autonomy. Finally, it refers to proper distribution of costs and investments in various fields within the healthcare system (e.g. care for people with disabilities).
Social aspects	As a public health programme, prenatal screening might have "consequences for other individuals and groups (including those living with the relevant conditions)". To avoid discriminatory messages, the aim of screening (reproductive autonomy) should be stressed. NIPT might be seen as a routine procedure, which might lead to routinisation of prenatal screening, affecting the informed choices of pregnant women.	Prenatal screening may have negative effects for people with disabilities, but does not lead to the birth of fewer people with disabilities, as long as chromosomal and single gene disorders account for only a minority of disabilities present at birth. Healthcare for people with disabilities will and should not be reduced, also to prevent 'economic eugenics' which would hinder voluntary decision-making. Although "cultures or medical settings may be implicitly coercive," these problems are seen as part of the general sociocultural context and not attributed to prenatal screening specifically.	Prenatal screening generates genetic information and could have social consequences including stigmatisation and discrimination. There is a (shared) duty to create a society without discrimination, which will be a result of interactions between people and does not depend on the presence or absence of one test. Routine offer of prenatal screening might have negative consequences for reproductive freedom and put pressure on women to test: the idea that pregnant women should take their parental responsibility and opt for testing should be avoided.	Prenatal screening programmes may have social impact but are not necessarily discriminatory, because they aim at reproductive choice and not at prevention. However, concerns related to the social impact of screening on people with a disability are realistic. Therefore ongoing ethical monitoring of screening practices is necessary. Also, the state should guarantee good-quality care for people with a disability. A simple and safe test could possibly lead to routinisation, including pressure to test. This might affect reproductive autonomy.	Prenatal screening is often not a therapeutic intervention but likely to lead to abortion and it might lead to discrimination and stigmatisation. "The adding up of a lot of individual choices to the 'acceptability' of aborting certain kinds of embryos (…) brings forward a societal phenomenon, which resembles a kind of eugenics in the search for a 'perfect child'." Non-discrimination should be emphasised and guaranteed. Prenatal screening as a 'routine measure' might negatively affect society's perception of disability and societal solidarity with disabled people and the women who give birth to them.

skipped, *"because many people actually do not know what it [prenatal screening] entails. How could you say 'yes' or 'no' to this question when you do not exactly know what this test is for?"* (I3 medical specialist)

In order to reach the aim of prenatal screening, it is of paramount importance that pregnant women or couples can make informed choices for or against a screening offer [15, 17–20]. Informed choice is often defined as "a choice that is based on relevant knowledge, consistent with the decision maker's values and behaviourally implemented" [34, 35]. This means that women should understand the purpose of the test and its potential risks and implications [36], because they may be confronted with "a large number of further decisions which [they] might have wished to avoid if [they] had been aware of the consequences before screening" [18]. To help women make informed choices pre-test counselling is offered. During pre-test counselling women are presented with information about the purpose, nature, scope and validity [18] and complete information about diseases, including e.g. "name(s) and general characteristics of the major disorder(s)," possible treatments, possible unexpected or unclear findings of the test and kinds of test-outcome [20]. Furthermore, pre-test counselling for first-trimester prenatal screening should be conducted at a designated moment, clearly separated from information provision about other aspects of antenatal care, such as lifestyle, health aspects (e.g. screening for HIV) and birth planning [15].

Many professionals noticed that when women talked about their reasons for choosing prenatal screening, they often mentioned wanting to be reassured about the health of their child. Professionals thought that women sometimes do not realise in advance what kinds of outcomes they might face and difficult choices they might have to make: women *"have to realise that if [they] opt for NIPT and a congenital disorder is found, [they] kind of jump on a train on which [they] might not want to be. [... I] hear people say that they are in a rollercoaster."* (I8, medical specialist).

Some professionals thought that especially in the case of NIPT this might be a problem. The previous screening programme in the Netherlands was step-wise: the first step was a FCT, which provided only a risk estimate for aneuploidies. Then women had to think carefully about invasive follow-up testing, taking into account the risk of miscarriage. Women could choose whether or not to undergo invasive testing to obtain a diagnostic result. Professionals thought that this step-wise process gradually prepared women for the obtaining of an abnormal test result. They thought that, with NIPT, by contrast, women will opt for an easy test and – in one single step – may be confronted with an almost 'diagnostic outcome' at once. NIPT *"gives the idea of a decisive outcome."* (I10, midwife) As said, this idea is not accurate, as diagnostic follow-up testing is required also with NIPT. The odds that the result turns out false positive, however, are much lower.

In order to protect women from the negative consequences of uninformed choices, professionals emphasised that counselling plays a crucial role. Counselling serves to explain women's options and to correct misunderstandings of tests and disabilities, but should also explore the norms and values and the attitudes of women towards having a child with a disability. During counselling women should be encouraged to think about their views about testing, about having a child with a disability and termination of pregnancy: *"Yes, I think, that with a few standard questions [the counsellor] will [be able to] achieve a lot. Just to trigger [women], let's say [to think about the consequences of NIPT]. That does not necessarily take a lot of time. [... As a counsellor, you could ask women:] What does Down syndrome mean to you?"* (I3, medical specialist).

Respondents took the view that the current quality of counselling in the Netherlands is moderate, and needs improvement: professionals should pay more attention to and spend more time on pre-test counselling. Dedicated counselling sessions will help women understand that the aim of prenatal screening for chromosomal abnormalities is different from the aims of antenatal care (i.e. maintaining and/or improving the health of the pregnant woman and the foetus). Some respondents, who were medical specialists, feared that professionals underestimate the importance of (non-directive) counselling for NIPT and should be aware that the ease of the test, requiring only a maternal blood sample, and its high reliability may lead to less informed choices. One study suggested that professionals might indeed attach less importance to informed consent for a non-invasive test compared to an invasive test [37].

To conclude, in order to reach the aim of prenatal screening - reproductive autonomy - informed choice is of crucial importance. Counselling should be non-directive and of high quality, and include deliberation on personal values of women, in order to achieve informed choice and promote this aim.

Proportionality

In the identified ethical framework, the pillar of proportionality of screening programmes entails balancing benefits and harms, following the original screening criteria for population screening formulated by Wilson and Jungner, complemented with additional criteria from the WHO [15, 19, 38]. To assess benefits and harms, the quality of the test and the test offer, including the laboratory procedures, counselling and education of professionals should be evaluated [15]. According to the ESHG/ASHG and the Dutch Health Council, the benefits and harms or costs depend on the way NIPT will be offered, as a first-tier screening test or second-tier screening test, after FCT [15, 17]. When NIPT would replace FCT as a first-tier test, it might have the benefit of fewer false positive results for trisomy 21, 18, and 13, but on the other hand might also lead to a loss of other findings that can be identified on ultrasound as part of FCT. Experts must decide whether the benefits of a better test performance of NIPT regarding the three trisomies will outweigh this loss of diagnostic yield when the first-trimester ultrasound is removed from the screening programme.

For pregnant women or couples, prenatal screening for foetal abnormalities has the benefit of offering reproductive choices regarding an affected pregnancy, including termination of pregnancy or being able to prepare for the birth of an affected child, relief from anxiety in case of a negative test result and the reduction of invasive follow-up tests [15, 17–20]. Harms for pregnant women are related to false reassurance, burden of decision making and anxiety in case of false-positive outcomes and incidental findings, which can be of unclear clinical significance and might cause needless worries [15]. Respondents held that these harms are inevitable but acceptable. Yet the possibility of incidental findings needs to be explained during pre-test counselling. It has been suggested that making the choice to terminate a desired pregnancy after receiving an abnormal test result may be harmful, as well [20].

According to professionals, women might be faced with unwanted choices they have to make, because they may not have been fully aware of the consequences of prenatal screening beforehand, as some medical specialists indicated in the interviews: *"But sometimes I see people saying: 'I never would have wanted this choice. This is a horrible choice you're giving me. I don't want it. This is a wanted pregnancy. If I had not known that this child has Down syndrome I would go for [continuation of this pregnancy], I am sure. But now I have a choice and I am going to hesitate'."* (I7, medical specialist).

Justice

The third pillar of the ethical framework is justice. The principle of justice in prenatal screening relates to equal access to prenatal screening for all pregnant women, to policy questions concerning reimbursement of prenatal screening, and to equal distribution of healthcare resources [15, 17–20]. Equal access to prenatal screening means that differences in personal resources may not cause disparities in access to prenatal screening programmes: women's choices not to participate in screening should not be based upon a lack of financial resources [15, 17–20]. That would imply that prenatal screening should be offered especially to women with limited financial resources, either free of charge or against a small fee. On the other hand, it could be argued that a (small) payment might serve the aim of reproductive autonomy as it may "increases awareness that there is truly a choice to be made" [15].

Professionals recognised this dilemma concerning the reimbursement of prenatal screening. Respondents mentioned the impact of payment on the uptake of prenatal screening. A midwife suggested that the fee that is currently asked for FCT in the Netherlands (165 euros) has much impact and might explain the large difference in the uptake of FCT as compared to the 20-week ultrasound, which is offered free of charge: *"I am curious, when [NIPT] will be reimbursed and [as a counsellor] you explain to people the possibility of having a NIPT, whether they would say: 'If it is reimbursed and it gives information about the health of my child, of course I want [to use NIPT].' They do the same for the 20-week scan. I really wonder whether the difference [in uptake for the FCT and the 20-week ultrasound] is that big because people say: 'I [do want to] give birth to a child with Down syndrome but not to a child with spina bifida'. I do not believe that [differences in attitudes explain the] difference between 30% [the uptake of the FCT] and 95% [the uptake of the 20-week ultrasound]."* (I10, midwife)

Some professionals suggested that a financial contribution by women might serve as a helpful barrier, making women aware of the importance of the choice. It could prevent women from opting for a test 'just because it is possible and does not cost any money', and thus protect them against ill-considered testing. On the other hand, respondents mentioned two objections to payment as a barrier for test uptake. Firstly, professionals thought that some women refrain from screening because of lack of money: *"There are a lot of people for whom [165 euros] is a lot of money that can buy a lot of baby clothes."* (I13, medical specialist) They thought that lack of money is not a good reason to decline screening. Professionals think that when screening is offered, it should be reimbursed to guarantee unhindered access. Secondly, asking a contribution is in contradiction with equality in healthcare: *"Yes, it is a barrier, but for whom are you creating a barrier? For a specific group of people who cannot pay for it."* (I3, medical specialist)

Experts should understand that while requiring a personal financial contribution may serve a purpose (i.e. improving informed choice), it may also, and more importantly, create disparities in access to prenatal screening, which is undesirable and contrary to one of the moral pillars of prenatal screening: justice.

Societal aspects

Self-determination is not only a matter of individual freedom, but also has a societal dimension, and it may be threatened by for example group pressure or societal views about testing [18, 19]. One of the concerns related to group pressure is that it might lead to less-autonomous choices among pregnant women. This would be problematic, it is argued, because the aim of prenatal screening, reproductive autonomy, will not be reached when women fail to make informed choices [15, 17–20].

Furthermore, it is thought that the offer of prenatal screening for chromosomal abnormalities might also imply a discriminatory message to individuals and groups living with specific diseases [15, 17–20]. This objection is known as the 'disability rights critique' of prenatal screening and holds that discriminatory messages are inseparable from prenatal screening [15, 17]. This critique may apply both to the sheer societal availability of prenatal screening programmes and to individual women's choices. In response, it is underlined that the aim of prenatal screening is not preventing the birth of disabled people, but promoting reproductive autonomy [17]. Also, studies have shown that women's reasons for the selective termination of their pregnancies include prevention of a life of severe suffering and not being able to create the best conditions to care for a child with a disability [17, 39–43], which does not support this critique. However, with the introduction of NIPT, the uptake of first-trimester screening might increase and the number of persons with disabilities might decrease. This is not in itself problematic, but it might become problematic if a low prevalence of disabilities will negatively affect the position of persons with disabilities, and render the option to continue an affected pregnancy less attractive. Therefore the practice of prenatal screening should be evaluated continuously in comparison to its aim [17]. Moreover, a negative perception of people with a disability can be redressed with public information and education [19]. The WHO concludes that just non-discriminatory societal settings are important for making a free choice: "It is important to prevent discrimination and to provide improved support services for individuals and families with genetic conditions. The absence of adequate services for people with hereditary disabilities undermines the principle of free choice for couples at risk of having children with such disabilities" [20].

Professionals did not think that the uptake of prenatal screening would increase dramatically, although they suggested that an easier test is less likely to be declined and might become self-evident. They observed however that the need to participate in prenatal screening is not as self-evident to many pregnant women as the need for other tests in pregnancy. Besides, *"there will always be people who do not want to know [about health risks of their foetus], who just want a care-free pregnancy, and [who feel that] every child is welcome."* (I13 medical specialist) Moreover, professionals think that women will not choose to terminate pregnancies more often because women who participate in prenatal screening generally have desired pregnancies, and do not wish to undergo termination of pregnancy for trivial reasons [18]. Also, according to respondents, specific cultural aspects in the Netherlands might in part explain the low uptake of NIPT, as compared to other countries. In the Dutch prenatal screening programme, midwives play important roles in pre-test counselling, rather than medical specialists [44]. Among midwives, there is a tendency to avoid medical interference in the pregnancy. Also, in society, a rather positive public image of Down syndrome prevails. Professionals held the opinion that the fear that fewer people with Down syndrome will be born when NIPT is introduced, is not justified. Respondents thought that people with a disability are accepted in the Netherlands and that there is good care available for handicapped people. However, they agreed that care and support should be guaranteed to counteract possible negative consequences of prenatal screening, including discrimination.

In sum, societal aspects and concerns such as an increase in test uptake and a decrease in people born with disabilities are recognized, but disputed in the literature as well as among professionals. However, it is acknowledged that arrangements should be made (i.e. ensuring quality of care for the disabled) to counteract possible negative consequences.

Discussion

The four pillars of the ethical framework can be used to evaluate the potential expansion of the scope of NIPT. Below, four limits are proposed to the responsible expansion of the scope of NIPT in the future. These limits provide ethical guidance for professionals and policy-makers who are working in the field of NIPT and will be shaping its development and further implementation in the future.

Limits set by the aim of prenatal screening

In the five documents it is explicitly stated that although the aim of prenatal screening is not to maximise reproductive choice indefinitely, there is room for expansion of the screening offer [15, 17, 20]. In the interviews several professionals indicated that a broader test will contribute to the aim of prenatal screening because an expanded NIPT allows for detecting more disorders than trisomy 21, 18 and 13: *"People do not want a test for Down syndrome, but a test for a healthy child."* (I15)

However, an expanded scope might affect informed choice as a precondition of reproductive autonomy. When NIPT includes a high number of diseases, it will be difficult in pre-test counselling to discuss all possible test outcomes in detail, "including the full range of variability in the manifestations" of these diseases [15]. Testing for more abnormalities might thus "paradoxically undermine rather than serve or enhance reproductive autonomy." [15] A clinical professional feared that *"people have no idea what the results [of NIPT] can be and what these could mean to them. I am sure about this, because for Down syndrome it is already the case [that people do not understand what the outcome means to them]."* (I7, medical specialist)

This raises the question how to best inform pregnant women prior to the test. It has been suggested in documents and by some of our respondents that information about the possible outcomes of prenatal screening should be presented as categories of disorders: the scope of NIPT can be narrow or broad, with results pertaining to severe or non-severe disorders and early- or late-onset disorders. When the scope of NIPT expands to such an extent that it becomes impossible to describe in detail all possible test outcomes during pre-test counselling, the counsellor "should describe the general characteristics of the categories of disorders tested for (e.g., mental disability or neurological impairment). Women will receive intensive counselling after a foetal diagnosis." [20] This model of informed choice is sometimes referred to as 'generic consent', which is thought to be a solution for complex counselling and has already been discussed in the context of genetic screening. Generic consent aims to prevent 'information overload' and to avoid the provision of information that is "pointless or counterproductive" [45]. The question arises whether generic consent offers enough information to enable people to make a truly informed choices [46, 47]. The ESHG/ASHG and the Dutch Health Council have their reservations about generic consent [15, 17], because "the feasibility of this model has not yet been empirically tested in the prenatal context" and it remains unclear how *informed* generic consent would be [15]. The extent to which generic consent can be informed consent should be studied in line with previous studies on informed choice in the context of prenatal screening. These studies showed highly variable percentages of women having made informed choices: 89%, 77,9%, 51% and 44% [35, 48–50]. Some of that variation might be explained by variation in the nature and the quality of pre-test counselling practices, which will likely affect the 'informedness' of women's choices to a great extent, also in the context of an expanded NIPT. In practice, it is not clear whether a sufficient number of professionals will be available to counsel large numbers of pregnant women and their partners, and whether they will have enough time to explain the details of the test and facilitate informed decision-making. In some countries, measures have been put in place to counter this problem, including the use of decision aids and the additional training of midwives in NIPT counselling [51]. Another solution might be a change in the *focus* of counselling, from technical-medical aspects to women's values or goals related to screening. As respondents suggested, too, counselling is more than providing information; women should be triggered to think about why they would want prenatal screening and what they would do in case of an abnormal test result, to make them more aware of their attitude towards undergoing prenatal screening. Attitude is defined as the general feeling of 'favourableness' or 'unfavourableness' for testing [34]. Triggering women to think about testing might lead to a process of deliberation and evaluation of pros and cons, which, according to several authors, should be part and parcel of an informed choice [49]. Professionals could play a role in this deliberation and help women to formulate their values, for instance in accordance with the interpretive model of the physician-patient relationship, as described by Emanuel and Emanuel [52]. This model entails that the healthcare professional helps to elicit the norms and values of a patient.

We would suggest that in this process, the necessary technical information about the test could support or influence the attitude, but is not sufficient or even essential to the quality of decision-making. Shifting the focus of counselling from 'conveying knowledge about screening' to 'exploring women's attitude towards screening' might improve women's and their partners' decision-making processes, even in the context of an expanded scope of screening and, in combination with decision aids, takes away the time pressure to explain all clinical and technical details of NIPT.

Professionals differed in their opinions about whether women should be given a say in decisions regarding the scope of the screening offer. Some professionals suggested that a list of options should be offered from which women could choose, whereas others believed that experts should determine which (categories of) disorders should be included in the test. The main reason for preferring a predetermined offer was that women might not have the information – or the capacity to understand the information – required to make a decision about the adequate scope of NIPT. Another study of opinions of professionals showed that a majority of respondents preferred a predetermined offer or a fixed list of disorders to be tested [53].

A second category of problems arises with the dual aim of prenatal screening within antenatal care systems [15]. Some routinely offered prenatal screening tests are used to improve pregnancy outcomes or the health condition of the mother or the baby, such as the blood test for rhesus status in RhD-negative women. The rhesus test is currently offered as a separate test but could – for reasons of efficiency – be combined in one test with NIPT for autosomal aneuploidies. An objection to a combination of this test with screening for aneuploidies is the possible confusion in women about what test they should accept or decline, and for what reasons. Prenatal screening for aneuploidies is aimed at reproductive autonomy and requires non-directive counselling [15]. The term 'non-directiveness' refers to the absence of coercion or the withholding of advice, in order to respect the autonomy of a patient [54]. According to Ten Have, as cited in Oduncu, non-directiveness means that the expert who provides information about genetic conditions "should not, in any respect, try to influence the decision made by the persons who are counselled or screened. (...) his aim is merely to provide information and to help the patients or clients to work through possible options." [54] For prevention-aimed screening in antenatal care (e.g. screening for hypertension or rhesus status), it may not be objectionable for health professionals to recommend or insist on participation, because this type of screening promotes the health of the mother and the foetus, but for autonomy-aimed screening, directive counselling is not appropriate [15, 55]. In sum, one (expanded) NIPT that combines two aims and two - opposed - modes of counselling is not desirable.

NIPT is meant to offer reproductive options, but not to screen foetuses for all kinds of medical problems. For instance, children are usually not allowed to undergo predictive testing for (untreatable) late-onset diseases because this might affect their right to an open future and their right not to know unwanted predictive information [15, 17–20]. The principle to defer testing until adulthood applies to unborn children as well. Prenatal screening is not meant as a medical screening of future children: its scope should thus be limited to those conditions for which expecting parents may consider terminating the pregnancy. To protect the unborn child's right not to know, 'conditional access' models have been proposed for women who want information about late-onset diseases: testing for late-onset diseases, including some sex chromosomal aneuploidies, will only be offered if women "expressed the clear intention to choose abortion if a predisposition for a late-onset diseases is found." [56] However, as termination of a pregnancy is, and should continue to be, the result of a voluntary decision, women who change their minds about an earlier expressed intention cannot be forced to terminate an affected pregnancy. Therefore, it cannot be excluded that children may be born in the knowledge of carrying a mutation for a late-onset disease. Further research should focus on the consequences of living with this information for both parents and children and on its effects on their relationship [18, 19].

NIPT may contribute to the aim of prenatal screening: the promotion of reproductive autonomy. On the basis of the first pillar of the ethical framework for prenatal screening, however, limits can be set to the morally responsible expansion of the scope of NIPT: NIPT should generate only test outcomes that are relevant to reproductive decision-making, and informed choice should be (made) possible through adequate pre-test counselling.

Limits set by proportionality

The expansion of the scope of NIPT also raises questions concerning proportionality. According to the Dutch Health Council, proportionality is an important requirement of prenatal screening, and benefits of each 'test' (for each condition) to be included in the screening offer should outweigh the harms [17]. Professionals noted that it may be beneficial to include more disorders in a test because that means that more reproductive choices can be made: *"There are children who are born with a severe disorder. Then we do an exome analysis to see what the cause is. Then we find, say, in 40% of the cases, a new mutation, in a crucial gene, which the parents do not have. In the future it may be possible to detect that [mutation] in maternal blood."* (I15, lab specialist) Several professionals gave the example of the 22q11 deletion, which is associated with a severe phenotype. Studies on the attitudes of pregnant women towards an expanded scope of prenatal screening showed that women thought that it may be valuable especially to include severe disorders with no or short life expectancy in a screening test [57, 58]. Women also wanted to learn about sex chromosomal aneuploidies [59, 60] and about specific other aneuploidies, but were hesitant about learning about conditions with unknown or variable phenotypic expression. They were uncertain about what the benefit would be of knowing about such conditions [59].

Proportionality concerns might limit the expansion of the scope, on at least three points. Firstly, when genome-wide analyses are used in NIPT, it might be difficult to assess the clinical validity of many among the huge number of abnormalities that can be detected. Offering a test for disorders without knowing the validity might lead to false positives and false negatives, cause harm to pregnant women, and challenge the proportionality of including the disorders [17]. Professionals mentioned that outcomes should be actionable for pregnant women. When tests are not reliable (i.e. clinically valid), they provide few actionable options. Moreover, uncertain test outcomes might lead to unnecessary anxiety or insecurity in pregnant women, which is objectionable: *"I think that, when you introduce uncertainty in the pregnancy, it will become difficult. If you [can say that you] are sure that the child is disabled, then this is understandable for people, and they will be able to prepare [for the birth of a disabled child] or to decide that they do not want this. But if you say, 'we actually do not know what it means exactly; (...) it can turn out better than expected, but the child can also turn out severely disabled.' Well, what should you do, as parents?"* (I3, medical specialist) Several other professionals stated that in practice this should not pose a big problem, as only a small number of abnormalities that are currently being detected in labs are of unknown or little-known clinical validity. These will need to be discussed between expecting parents and clinical geneticists specialised in prenatal diagnosis.

A second point that several respondents stressed is that NIPT has shortcomings: NIPT is not a diagnostic test, and it still requires invasive follow-up. An expanded scope might lead to an increasing number of positive test results for a wide range of disorders, which will include false positive results that need confirmation by (unnecessary) invasive diagnostic testing. This is problematic, because a reduction of invasive tests as compared to FCT is seen as one of the important benefits of NIPT [15, 18, 19].

A third point that might limit the scope of NIPT is the burden of the decision to terminate a pregnancy. Some disorders may not be sufficiently severe to justify their inclusion in the NIPT; they may not meet the first screening criterion of Wilson and Jungner: "The condition sought should be an important health problem." [61] However, professionals mentioned that it is hard to define what 'serious' or 'non-serious' diseases are. In the documents it is stated, for instance, that severity should not be determined at all: "It would be dangerous to create medical, legal, or social definitions of 'serious', because these could infringe on couples' lives in several ways." [20] Expecting parents are the ones who should indicate whether they consider a disorder to be serious or not, in their life situation [20]. Although it will be difficult in practice to draw the lines, the seriousness of disorders can serve as an (arguable) limit to the expanding scope of NIPT.

From the pillar of proportionality a few additional limits can be derived for the expansion of the scope of NIPT: in order for tests to be included in an expanded scope of NIPT, they should be clinically valid. Especially the positive predictive value should be high, as confirmatory testing through invasive procedures will still be required and is associated with risks, costs and burdens. NIPT should not be offered for trivial conditions.

Limits set by justice aspects

When using the ethical framework to evaluate an expansion of the scope NIPT, the pillar of justice is less prominent than the other three pillars. However, there are three issues that arise from the pillar of justice. Firstly, when NIPT is offered as an expanded test, it should be available equally for every pregnant woman [17]. Equal access to healthcare is considered to be a fundamental right that should preclude the exclusion of specific groups from healthcare services [62]. Women should not face restrictions to having reproductive options. Ideally, all women should have access to the same information about their foetus, and the scope of first-trimester prenatal screening should be equal for all women. When expanded NIPT is made available only to women who have an increased risk of trisomy 21, 18 or 13 as a second-tier test after FTC, for instance, low-risk pregnant women will not have access to information about the foetus other than the three more common trisomies detected through FCT, whereas high-risk women will [17]. For this reason, justice would require making NIPT available as a first-tier test to all women (or restricting the scope of NIPT as a second-tier test). Also, it is important to note that diagnostic follow-up testing should be made available to women who have undergone NIPT, in line with the criterion of Wilson and Jungner that in screening programmes, diagnostic follow-up testing should be available to those found to be at risk [38]. This is of special importance in countries in which access to follow-up testing is not self-evident.

A second aspect, according to the International Bioethics Committee, is that education is a matter of justice: "Persons with a lower education level and lower health literacy are denied the information which is required to exercise their freedom and autonomy." [19] Some women may not be able to understand all relevant information pertaining to the screening offer, which is necessary to make an informed choice. The expansion of NIPT will only exacerbate this inequality [19], it is feared, as the test becomes more elaborate and more complex, and decision-making places higher demands on women's health literacy.

A third concern is that an expanded NIPT could challenge a justifiable distribution of healthcare resources. As resources are scarce and should be distributed equally, efforts must be taken to demarcate the scope of prenatal screening tests to prevent unnecessary follow-up of clinically insignificant findings. Besides, when prenatal screening is offered within the context of a public health programme and is upheld by taxpayers, there should be transparency with regard to the utility of the test [15]. This also underlines the importance of ensuring the proportionality of a test.

When considering the costs of prenatal screening it should be noted that a widespread implementation and uptake of prenatal screening programmes is likely to lead to the birth of fewer affected children, which reduces the costs associated with their healthcare and support. Although this should not be an aim of prenatal screening, these long-term costs savings are undeniably part of a cost-effectiveness analysis of new screening tests [15].

From the pillar of justice another limitation can be derived: expanded NIPT should be available for all pregnant women, which may increase the costs of the programme. This limitation may change over time as the technology improves and becomes cheaper.

Limits set by societal aspects

In discussions on the expansion of the scope of NIPT, concerns are reiterated that have already been raised in the context of earlier prenatal screening programmes, such as discrimination and stigmatisation of people with chronic diseases. New societal aspects, unique to expanded NIPT, are raised as well. Professionals noted in the interviews, for instance, that a benefit of an expanded scope could be a removal of the focus of prenatal testing on Down syndrome. Down syndrome is the most common of the three trisomies and in the Netherlands first-trimester screening for chromosomal abnormalities is often referred to as a 'test for Down syndrome'. By expanding the scope of prenatal screening this focus could shift, which might reduce concerns related to discriminatory messages conveyed by the screening programme. This benefit of the expansion is also acknowledged by parents of children with Down syndrome, who experience the focus on Down as stigmatising for their children [63]. On the other hand, the Dutch Health Council mentioned that expanded NIPT is not free from the allegation of stigmatisation either, as, for instance, a list of selected disorders can be thought of as 'subjective' and vulnerable to stigmatisation of specific groups, too [17]. According to some professionals, an expanded scope might reduce the acceptance of children with a disability: "*With 22q11 deletion, [children] can be mentally retarded, etc. When people hear a story like that, they tend to terminate [the pregnancy]. I find it very hard. Everybody wants a healthy child; I understand that. So it is good to have these options. On the other hand, I am afraid that, when more [screening] becomes possible, what space is there for children with a disability? I find it terrible that there may be no respect or no care [for these children].*" (I10, midwife).

Adverse societal consequences of an expanded scope are also mentioned by pregnant women and parents of children with Down syndrome, who fear a loss of diversity in society and a 'slippery slope', implying that people might want to start testing for increasingly trivial abnormalities [57, 63]. However, respondents questioned whether these consequences of an expanded scope will occur and denied that society will eventually be without children with a disorder or disability. Although it is difficult to predict the societal consequences (if any) of NIPT or how these would limit the expansion of its scope, it is clear that negative consequences for people with disabilities should be mitigated, and the practice of prenatal screening should be monitored continuously, not only with a focus on the risks and benefits for individuals, but also for its wider societal implications.

Conclusion

An expansion of the scope of NIPT fits the aim of prenatal screening, as it contributes to more reproductive options for pregnant women and couples. However, drawing on the broadly shared ethical framework for prenatal screening as well as on the findings of our qualitative study of professionals' opinions and experiences of the translation of the pillars of this framework in practice, we conclude that expansion of the scope of NIPT is not unlimited. Four moral limits can be set to demarcate a responsible expansion of the scope of NIPT. Firstly, informed choice as a central precondition for prenatal screening should limit its scope: when NIPT is expanded to include more chromosomal or sub-microscopic abnormalities, and relevant pre-test information about the test becomes more elaborate and more complex, counsellors will need to improve pre-test counselling to uphold its quality. This requires new models for counselling, with a special focus on generic information about possible test outcomes and on expecting parents' attitudes and values in relation to prenatal screening. Secondly, any expansion of NIPT should be proportionate: the test should be clinically valid and useful to women. Findings that generate mainly anxiety and for which no courses of action are available, do not meet the criterion of proportionality. Thirdly, respect for the right of the future child to an open future excludes testing for late-onset disorders when women or couples know beforehand that they will not terminate the pregnancy based on the results. Finally, healthcare resources should be justly distributed: when possible, NIPT should be made available to all pregnant women either free of charge or for a small sum. At the same time, any expansion of the scope of NIPT should be based upon a favourable assessment of the benefits of including additional 'tests' for additional disorders in proportion to the costs and burdens. Both in the literature and in our interview study of professionals' opinions, we observed differences in the sense of urgency or importance that is attributed to each of the four limitations. We contend that the criterion of reproductive autonomy as the aim of prenatal screening as well as that of proportionality – or a positive balance between the benefits and burdens for pregnant women and their future children – should together be guiding in decisions whether particular disorders should be tested or communicated to women or couples. This means that for example, depending on the test performance, disorders that are comparable to trisomies 13, 18 and 21 in terms of severity could be included in the NIPT. Over the next decade, those working in the field of NIPT may strive to maximise the potential benefits of NIPT and include more abnormalities in the screening test, keeping these moral limits to a justified scope of NIPT in mind.

Abbreviations

ASHG: American Society of Human Genetics; ESHG: European Society of Human Genetics; FCT: First trimester combined test; IBC: UNESCO International Bioethics Committee; NIPT: Non-Invasive Prenatal Test; TRIDENT-1: Trial by Dutch laboratories for Evaluation of Non-Invasive Prenatal Testing; WHO: World Health Organisation

Acknowledgements

The authors wish to thank the professionals who participated in the study.

Funding

This study is a result of a research project 'To report or not to report? The ethics of broadening the scope of (non-) invasive prenatal testing ((N)IPT)', which was funded by through Erasmus MC Grants (Mrace). The funding body had no role in the design of the study, in the collection, analysis, interpretation of data, or in writing or reviewing the manuscript.

Authors' contributions

All authors contributed to the design of the study and the interpretation of data. AKK collected and analysed the data. AKK and EMB drafted the manuscript. IDB and RJHG critically revised the manuscript for important intellectual content. All authors have read and approved the final manuscript.

Competing interests

The authors declare that they have no competing interests.

Author details

[1]Department of Medical Ethics and Philosophy of Medicine, Erasmus MC, University Medical Centre Rotterdam, Room 24.17, Wytemaweg 80, 3015 CN Rotterdam, The Netherlands. [2]Department of Clinical Genetics, Erasmus MC, University Medical Centre Rotterdam, Wytemaweg 80, 3015 CN Rotterdam, The Netherlands.

References

1. Norton ME, Jacobsson B, Swamy GK, Laurent LC, Ranzini AC, Brar H, et al. Cell-free DNA analysis for noninvasive examination of trisomy. N Engl J Med. 2015;372(17):1589–97.
2. Chandrasekharan S, Minear MA, Hung A, Allyse M. Noninvasive prenatal testing goes global. Sci Transl Med. 2014;6(231):231fs15.
3. Oepkes D, Page-Christiaens GC, Bax CJ, Bekker MN, Bilardo CM, Boon EMJ, et al. Trial by Dutch laboratories for evaluation of non-invasive prenatal testing. Part I—clinical impact. Prenat Diagn. 2016;36(12):1083–90.
4. Bianchi DW, Parker RL, Wentworth J, Madankumar R, Saffer C, Das AF, et al. DNA sequencing versus standard prenatal aneuploidy screening. N Engl J Med. 2014;370(9):799–808.
5. Meck JM, Kramer Dugan E, Matyakhina L, Aviram A, Trunca C, Pineda-Alvarez D, et al. Noninvasive prenatal screening for aneuploidy: positive predictive values based on cytogenetic findings. Am J Obstet Gynecol. 2015;213(2):214.e1–5.
6. Van Opstal D, Srebniak MI. Cytogenetic confirmation of a positive NIPT result: evidence-based choice between chorionic villus sampling and amniocentesis depending on chromosome aberration. Expert Rev Mol Diagn. 2016;16(5):513–20.
7. Bianchi DW, Wilkins-Haug L. Integration of noninvasive DNA testing for aneuploidy into prenatal care: what has happened since the rubber met the road? Clin Chem. 2014;60(1):78–87.
8. Van Opstal D, Srebniak MI, Polak J, de Vries F, Govaerts LCP, Joosten M, et al. False negative NIPT results: risk figures for chromosomes 13, 18 and 21 based on chorionic villi results in 5967 cases and literature review. PLoS One. 2016;11(1):e0146794.
9. Benn P. Expanding non-invasive prenatal testing beyond chromosomes 21, 18, 13, X and Y. Clin Genet. 2016;90(6):477–85.
10. Helgeson J, Wardrop J, Boomer T, Almasri E, Paxton WB, Saldivar JS, et al. Clinical outcome of subchromosomal events detected by whole-genome noninvasive prenatal testing. Prenat Diagn. 2015;35(10):999–1004.
11. Lau TK, Cheung SW, Lo PSS, Pursley AN, Chan MK, Jiang F, et al. Non-invasive prenatal testing for fetal chromosomal abnormalities by low-coverage whole-genome sequencing of maternal plasma DNA: review of 1982 consecutive cases in a single center. Ultrasound Obstet Gynecol. 2014; 43(3):254–64.
12. Wapner RJ, Babiarz JE, Levy B, Stosic M, Zimmermann B, Sigurjonsson S, et al. Expanding the scope of noninvasive prenatal testing: detection of fetal microdeletion syndromes. Am J Obstet Gynecol. 2015;212(3):332.e1–9.
13. Brady P, Brison N, Van Den Bogaert K, de Ravel T, Peeters H, Van Esch H et al. Clinical implementation of NIPT–technical and biological challenges. Clin Genet. 2015;89(5):523–30.
14. Lo KK, Karampetsou E, Boustred C, McKay F, Mason S, Hill M, et al. Limited clinical utility of non-invasive prenatal testing for subchromosomal abnormalities. Am J Hum Genet. 2016;98(1):34–44.
15. Dondorp W, De Wert G, Bombard Y, Bianchi DW, Bergmann C, Borry P, et al. Non-invasive prenatal testing for aneuploidy and beyond: challenges of responsible innovation in prenatal screening. Eur J Hum Genet. 2015;23(11):1438–50.
16. Shuster E. Microarray genetic screening: a prenatal roadblock for life? Lancet. 2007;369(9560):526–9.
17. Gezondheidsraad. NIPT: dynamiek en ethiek van prenatale screening. Den Haag: Gezondheidsraad; 2013.
18. Deutscher Ethikrat. The future of genetic diagnosis from research to clinical practice; opinion. Berlin: Deutscher Ethikrat; 2013.
19. UNESCO. Report of the IBC on updating its reflection on the human genome and human rights. Paris: United Nations Educational Scientific and Cultural Organization; 2015.
20. Wertz DC, Fletcher JC, Berg K. Review of ethical issues in medical ethics: report of consultants to WHO. Geneva: World Health Organization; 2003.
21. Swedish National Council on Medical Ethics. Prenatal diagnosis: the ethics. 2006. Socialdepartemetet. http://www.smer.se/wp-content/uploads/2012/04/Prenatal-diagnosis-the-Ethics.pdf. Accessed 23 Aug 2017.
22. Nuffield Council on Bioethics. Critical care decisions in fetal and neonatal medicine: ethical issues: a guide to the report; 2007.
23. Skirton H, Goldsmith L, Jackson L, Lewis C, Chitty L. Offering prenatal diagnostic tests: European guidelines for clinical practice [corrected]. Eur J Hum Genet. 2014;22(5):580–6.
24. Superior Health Council of Belgium. Implementation of non-invasive prenatal genetic screening for trisomy 21 (Down Syndrome) in the practice of health care in Belgium. 2014. https://www.health.belgium.be/en/advise-8912-nipt#anchor-20611. Accessed 15 Oct 2018.
25. Minear MA, Alessi S, Allyse M, Michie M, Chandrasekharan S. Noninvasive prenatal genetic testing: current and emerging ethical, legal, and social issues. Annu Rev Genomics Hum Genet. 2015;16:369–98.
26. Allyse M, Minear MA, Berson E, Sridhar S, Rote M, Hung A, et al. Non-invasive prenatal testing: a review of international implementation and challenges. Int J Womens Health. 2015;7:113–26.
27. de Jong A. Prenatal screening à la carte?: ethical reflection on the scope of testing for foetal anomalies. Maastricht: Maastricht University; 2013.
28. Gates EA. Ethical considerations in prenatal diagnosis. West J Med. 1993; 159(3):391–5.
29. Vanstone M, King C, de Vrijer B, Nisker J. Non-invasive prenatal testing: ethics and policy considerations. J Obstet Gynaecol Can. 2014;36(6):515–26.
30. Gekas J, Langlois S, Ravitsky V, Audibert F, van den Berg DG, Haidar H, et al. Non-invasive prenatal testing for fetal chromosome abnormalities: review of clinical and ethical issues. Appl Clin Genet. 2016;9:15–26.
31. Beauchamp TL. Methods and principles in biomedical ethics. J Med Ethics. 2003;29(5):269–74.
32. Kass NE. An ethics framework for public health. Am J Public Health. 2001; 91(11):1776–82.
33. Gezondheidsraad. Juridische aspecten van prenatale screening: achtergronddocument bij prenatale screening. Den Haag: Gezondheidsraad; 2016.
34. Marteau TM, Dormandy E, Michie S. A measure of informed choice. Health Expect. 2001;4(2):99–108.
35. Lewis C, Hill M, Skirton H, Chitty LS. Development and validation of a measure of informed choice for women undergoing non-invasive prenatal testing for aneuploidy. Eur J Hum Genet. 2016;24(6):809–16.
36. Biesecker BB, Schwartz MD, Marteau TM. Enhancing informed choice to undergo health screening: a systematic review. Am J Health Behav. 2013;37(3):351–9.
37. van den Heuvel A, Chitty L, Dormandy E, Newson A, Deans Z, Attwood S, et al. Will the introduction of non-invasive prenatal diagnostic testing erode informed choices? An experimental study of health care professionals. Patient Educ Couns. 2010;78(1):24–8.
38. Andermann A, Blancquaert I, Beauchamp S, Déry V. Revisiting Wilson and Jungner in the genomic age: a review of screening criteria over the past 40 years. Bull World Health Organ. 2008;86(4):317–9.
39. van den Berg M, Timmermans DR, Kleinveld JH, Garcia E, van Vugt JM, van der Wal G. Accepting or declining the offer of prenatal screening for congenital defects: test uptake and women's reasons. Prenat Diagn. 2005;25(1):84–90.
40. García E, Timmermans DRM, van Leeuwen E. The impact of ethical beliefs on decisions about prenatal screening tests: searching for justification. Soc Sci Med. 2008;66(3):753–64.
41. Crombag NM, Bensing JM, Iedema-Kuiper R, Schielen PCJI, Visser GH. Determinants affecting pregnant women's utilization of prenatal screening for Down syndrome: a review of the literature. J Matern Fetal Neonatal Med. 2013;26(17):1676–81.

42. Crombag NMTH, van Schendel RV, Schielen PCJI, Bensing JM, Henneman L. Present to future: what the reasons for declining first-trimester combined testing tell us about accepting or declining cell-free DNA testing. Prenat Diagn. 2016;36(6):587–90.
43. Ternby E, Axelsson O, Annerén G, Lindgren P, Ingvoldstad C. Why do pregnant women accept or decline prenatal diagnosis for Down syndrome? J Community Genet. 2016;7(3):237–42.
44. Vassy C, Rosman S, Rousseau B. From policy making to service use. Down's syndrome antenatal screening in England, France and the Netherlands. Soc Sci Med. 2014;106:67–74.
45. Elias S, Annas GJ. Generic consent for genetic screening. N Engl J Med. 1994;330(22):1611–3.
46. de Wert GMWR. Met het oog op de toekomst: voortplantingstechnologie, erfelijkheidsonderzoek en ethiek. Rotterdam: Erasmus University; 1999.
47. de Jong A, Dondorp WJ, de Die-Smulders CEM, Frints SGM, de Wert GMWR. Non-invasive prenatal testing: ethical issues explored. Eur J Hum Genet. 2009;18(3):272–7.
48. van Schendel RV, Page-Christiaens GC, Beulen L, Bilardo CM, de Boer MA, Coumans ABC, et al. Trial by Dutch laboratories for evaluation of non-invasive prenatal testing. Part II—women's perspectives. Prenat Diagn. 2016; 36(12):1091–8.
49. van den Berg M, Timmermans DRM, ten Kate LP, van Vugt JMG, van der Wal G. Informed decision making in the context of prenatal screening. Patient Educ Couns. 2006;63(1–2):110–7.
50. Gourounti K, Sandall J. Do pregnant women in Greece make informed choices about antenatal screening for Down's syndrome? A questionnaire survey. Midwifery. 2008;24(2):153–62.
51. Oxenford K, Daley R, Lewis C, Hill M, Chitty LS. Development and evaluation of training resources to prepare health professionals for counselling pregnant women about non-invasive prenatal testing for Down syndrome: a mixed methods study. BMC Pregnancy Childbirth. 2017;17(1):132.
52. Emanuel EJ, Emanuel LL. Four models of the physician-patient relationship. JAMA. 1992;267(16):2221–6.
53. Tamminga S, van Schendel RV, Rommers W, Bilardo CM, Pajkrt E, Dondorp WJ, et al. Changing to NIPT as a first-tier screening test and future perspectives: opinions of health professionals. Prenat Diagn. 2015;35(13):1316–23.
54. Oduncu FS. The role of non-directiveness in genetic counseling. Med Health Care Philos. 2002;5(1):53–63.
55. Bianchi DW. From prenatal genomic diagnosis to fetal personalized medicine: progress and challenges. Nat Med. 2012;18(7):1041–51.
56. de Jong A, Dondorp WJ, Frints SGM, de Die-Smulders CEM, de Wert GMWR. Advances in prenatal screening: the ethical dimension. Nat Rev Genet. 2011; 12(9):657–63.
57. van Schendel RV, Kleinveld JH, Dondorp WJ, Pajkrt E, Timmermans DRM, Holtkamp KCA, et al. Attitudes of pregnant women and male partners towards non-invasive prenatal testing and widening the scope of prenatal screening. Eur J Hum Genet. 2014;22(12):1345–50.
58. van der Steen SL, Diderich KE, Riedijk SR, Verhagen-Visser J, Govaerts LC, Joosten M, et al. Pregnant couples at increased risk for common aneuploidies choose maximal information from invasive genetic testing. Clin Genet. 2015;88(1):25–31.
59. Agatisa PK, Mercer MB, Leek AC, Smith MB, Philipson E, Farrell RM. A first look at women's perspectives on noninvasive prenatal testing to detect sex chromosome aneuploidies and microdeletion syndromes. Prenat Diagn. 2015;35(7):692–8.
60. Lau TK, Chan MK, Salome Lo PS, Chan HYC, Chan WK, Koo TY, et al. Non-invasive prenatal screening of fetal sex chromosomal abnormalities: perspective of pregnant women. J Matern Fetal Neonatal Med. 2012;25(12):2616–9.
61. Wilson JMG, Jungner G. Principles and practice of screening for disease. Geneva: World Health Organization; 1968.
62. Office of the United Nations High Commissioner for Human Rights. The Right to Health. Geneva: Office of the United Nations High Commissioner for Human Rights; 2008.
63. van Schendel RV, Kater-Kuipers A, van Vliet-Lachotzki EH, Dondorp WJ, Cornel MC, Henneman L. What do parents of children with Down syndrome think about non-invasive prenatal testing (NIPT)? J Genet Couns. 2017;26(3):522–31.

12

Magnitude of postpartum depression and associated factors among women in Mizan Aman town, Bench Maji zone, Southwest Ethiopia

Tigistu Toru[1*], Fantaye Chemir[2†] and Susan Anand[2†]

Abstract

Background: The first 12 months after childbirth may represent a high-risk time for depression. In Ethiopia there is a paucity of evidence about its magnitude and associated factors during that period. So, the aim of this study was to assess the magnitude of depression and associated factors among postpartum women in Mizan Aman town, Bench Maji Zone, Southwest Ethiopia 2017.

Methods: A community based cross- sectional study design was employed from March 15 to April 15, 2017. Four hundred sixty women were selected using multistage random sampling technique. Face to face interview were conducted using structured questionnaires and standardized scales. Bivariate logistic regression analysis was done to see crude association between each independent variable and outcome variable. Variables with p value < 0.25 in bivariate analysis were entered to multivariable logistic regression analysis to control for confounding. Adjusted odd ratios with 95%CI were calculated to identify independent predictors of postpartum depression.

Result: Four hundred fifty-six postpartum women participated in the study giving a response rate of 99%. The magnitude of postpartum depression among the study population was 102 (22.4%, 95% CI: 19.84–24.96). Postpartum depression is relatively higher in the first 6 weeks after birth. Postpartum depression is higher among mothers with age range between 18 and 23 years (aOR 3.89 95%CI: 1.53–9.90), unplanned pregnancy (aOR 3.35 95% CI: 1.701–6.58), child having sleeping problems (aOR 3.72 95%CI: 1.79–7.72), domestic violence (aOR 2.86 95%CI 1.72–8.79), unsatisfied marital relation (aOR 2.72 95% CI 1.32–5.62), poor social support (aOR 4.30 95% CI 1.79–10.30), history of previous depression (aOR 7.38 95% CI 3.12–17.35) and substance use (aOR 5.16 95% CI 2.52–10.60).

Conclusion: The magnitude of postpartum depression was high. This underlines health care planners' needs to incorporate screening strategies for depression following childbirth.

Keywords: Postnatal, Depression, Magnitude, Mental health, Ethiopia

Background

Depression is a significant contributor to the global burden of disease and affects people in all communities across the world [1]. Major depressive disorder is among the top ten causes of years lived with disability (YLDs) in every country [2].

The postpartum period is well established as an increased time of risk for the development of serious mood disorders [3]. Postpartum depression can be defined as a non-psychotic depression that happens during the first 12 months after childbirth. The symptoms are no different from depression which anyone can have [4]. It is a type of depression that affects about one in 10 new mothers within the first year after childbirth and has the potential to negatively impact a new mother's health and her ability to nurture her infant [5].

* Correspondence: tigistutoru112@gmail.com
†Fantaye Chemir and Susan Anand contributed equally to this work.
[1]Mizan Aman college of health science, Mizan Aman, Ethiopia
Full list of author information is available at the end of the article

The prevalence of postpartum depression in African American women ranges from 10 to 15% [6].

A synthesis of evidence in a systematic review on common perinatal mental disorders in women in low and middle income countries revealed a pooled prevalence of postpartum common mental disorders to be higher than in high-income countries with an average prevalence rate of 19.8%. However, perinatal mental health of women living in low and middle income countries has only recently become the subject of research since the priority is given to preventing pregnancy related complications [7].

Despite the fact that postpartum depression is the major maternal mental health problem following childbirth, little was known about the magnitude of the problem and contributing factors in Ethiopia in general and it was not investigated in the study area in particular; therefore, this study was aimed to fill this gap.

Methods

Study area and period

This study was conducted in Mizan-Aman town from March 15 2017 to April 15 2017. Mizan Aman is Bench Maji zonal town, one of the 13th zones in the Southern Nations Nationalities and People's Regional Government (SNNPRG). The town is located 561 Km away from Addis Ababa and 832 Km away from Hawassa (capital of SNNPRG). Mizan Aman Town is administratively structured by five kebeles and has an estimated total population of 50,113 of which 23,721 were females. Out of all females, 11,679 were women of reproductive age (15–49 yr.). The town has one teaching hospital, one health center and five health posts and all are runned by the government. On the other hand, there were nine private clinics and eight drug stores.

Study design

Community based quantitative cross-sectional study.

Source and study population

The source populations for the study were all postpartum women who gave birth within 12 months before data collection. Randomly selected women who gave birth within 12 months prior to data collection and who fulfilled the eligibility criteria were included. Women who gave birth within the last 12 months prior to data collection irrespective of type of delivery and outcome of delivery were included in the study.

Sampling procedure

Sample size was determined by using single population proportion formula based on the assumptions of 19% proportion of women who developed postpartum depression from a previous study in Tigray region, Northern part of Ethiopia [8] with precision (margin of error) 5% between sample and population parameter and 95% confidence level. The final sample of 460 postpartum women was included in the study after considering finite population correction, design effect of two and 10% non-response rate.

Three among five kebeles in the town were selected using lottery method. Then, the sample was proportionally allocated to the three kebeles and simple random sampling technique was used to get 460 participants from 1720 postpartum mothers by taking the community health extension workers' postpartum registration book as a frame.

Measurement

An interviewer-administered structured questionnaire containing socio-demographic, obstetric, pediatric, psychosocial, substance use, psychiatric and medical illness history was adopted from previously published studies. Moreover, 9- items Patient Health Questionnaire, 3-item Kansas Marital Satisfaction Scale and 3-item Oslo Social Support Scale were used to assess the magnitude of postpartum depression, level of marital satisfaction and level of social support respectively (Additional file 1).

The questionnaire is prepared in English and then translated to local language (Amharic) as well as back to English by bilingual experts in order to check consistency. Pretest was done by taking 5% of the sample in 'Kometa' kebele which was not included in the actual data collection phase to assess the face validity of the questionnaire.

Data collection

Six trained diploma nurses collected the data while three BSc nurses closely supervised data collection procedures. The principal investigator followed the overall data collection procedure plan. Face to face interviewer administered method of data collection was employed using structured questionnaires. Actual data collection was conducted after minor modification was made on tools based on pre-test findings. To assure the quality of the data, data collectors and supervisors were trained for two days on the clarity of tools and overall data collection procedures to standardize interview procedures and reduce interviewers' bias.

Data analysis

Data was entered to Epi- Data version 3.1 and then exported to SPSS version 21 for analysis purpose. Before analysis, missing values were checked and new categories created as needed. Descriptive statistics (frequencies, percentages) were performed. Bivariate logistic regression analysis was employed to determine the crude association between the dependent variable with each independent variable. Those exposure variables with p-values < 0.25 were entered into multivariable logistic regression analysis to control for confounders. Adjusted odds ratios with 95% CI were used to identify statistically significant associations between dependent and independent variables.

Operational and term definitions

Postpartum depression

In this study, postpartum depression was measured by using the Patient Health Questionnaire scale with 9 items and total sum score of 27. PD was categorized in to depressed (total sum score ≥ 10) and not depressed (total sum score < 10) [9].

Infant sleeping problem

Infants sleeping problem was defined based on maternal response of infants sleep duration as irregular or not sufficient.

Baby blues

Were measured by mother's experience of mood instability, depressed mood, sadness, irritability, anxiety, lack of concentration and/or feelings of dependency within two weeks following childbirth.

Level of marital satisfaction

Was assessed using Kansas Marital Satisfaction scale with 3 items and total sum score of 21. Total sum score of 17 and above was used as a cutoff point to identify women satisfied with their marital relation. Total sum score below 17 indicates dissatisfaction with marital relation [10].

Domestic violence

Is any behavior within an intimate relationship that causes physical, psychological or sexual harm and reported by mothers with yes or no items. Mothers were categorized as a victim of domestic violence when they experienced any of the harms (physical, psychological and sexual) in their intimate relationship.

Social support

Measures of available support that women perceive or believe that people in their social network would provide in times of need. Measured by 3- Items Oslo Social Support Scale with total sum score of 15 and categorized as; a score of 3–8 is poor support, 9–11 is moderate support and 12–15 is strong support [11].

Women substance use history

Is history of using any kind of substances such as fabricated or local alcohol, chat chewing, cigarette or tobacco smoking and other such addictive substance during pregnancy or after childbirth measured by yes or no items with at least one yes response.

Husband substance use

Husband's history of using any kind of substances such as fabricated or local alcohol, chat chewing, cigarette or tobacco smoking and other such addictive substance and measured by at least one yes response.

Result

From four hundred sixty women, 456 women completed the interview which gives a response rate of 99%.

Socio demographic characteristics of participants

All the study participants age ranged from 18 years to 39 years with majority 192 (42.1%) between 18 and 23 years. Four hundred forty-three (97.1%) of women were married, 163 (35.7%) were from Bench Ethnic group, 179 (39.3%) participants followed Orthodox religion, and 211 (46.3%) had attended up to diploma level and above. Regarding husband's educational level and occupation, 152 (34.3%) had diploma and above and 229 (51.7%) were merchants. One hundred fifty-three (33.6%) participants reported that their average family monthly income from all sources was less than 1000 ETB (~ 35 USD) (Table 1).

Magnitude of postpartum depression

According to this study, the maximum sum score which was recorded by participants was 16. The overall prevalence of postpartum depression among the study participant was found to be 102 (22.4%) (Fig. 1). Among those depressed, the prevalence of depression was more or less similar during the first six weeks 38 (37.3%), during 6 weeks to 6 months 33(32.4%) and above 6 months' postpartum period 31(30.4%).

Factors associated with postpartum depression

Among all the explanatory variables entered to bivariate binary logistic regression analysis, nineteen of them with p-value < 0.25 entered into multivariable analysis to control for confounding. These variables include age, marital status, women' occupation, family monthly income, gravidity, status of recent pregnancy, complication after childbirth, difficulty of child feeding, child sleeping problem, domestic violence, marital satisfaction, social support level, previous depression, family mental illness, recent medical illness and substance use. Eight independent predictor variables for occurrence of postpartum depression were identified in the multivariable binary logistic regression model.

Accordingly, mothers prone to postpartum depression were likely to be those with; history of previous depression (aOR: 7.38, 95%CI: 3.12–17.35), substance use (aOR: 5.17, 95%CI: 2.52–10.60), poor social support (aOR: 4.30, 95%CI: 1.79–10.30), age range between 18 and 23 years (aOR: 3.89, 95%CI: 1.53–9.90), infant sleeping problems (aOR: 3.72, 95%CI: 1.79–7.72), unplanned pregnancy (aOR: 3.35, 95%CI: 1.70–6.58), domestic violence (aOR: 2.86 95% CI

Table 1 Socio-demographic characteristics of postpartum women in Mizan Aman Town, Bench Maji Zone, SNNPR, Ethiopia from March 15, 2017 to April 15, 2017 (*n* = 456)

Variables	Category	Frequency	Percentage
Age	18–23	192	42.1
	24–29	167	36.6
	> = 30	97	21.3
Marital status	Married	443	97.1
	Others	13	2.9
	Others: divorced, widowed, separated		
Ethnicity	Bench	163	35.7
	Amhara	99	21.7
	Keffa	79	17.3
	Oromo	46	10.1
	Gurage	24	5.3
	Tigre	24	5.3
	Others	21	4.3
Religion	Orthodox	179	39.3
	Protestant	162	35.5
	Muslim	94	20.6
	Catholic	21	4.6
Women education	Unable to read and write	16	3.5
	Elementary	147	32.2
	Secondary	82	18.0
	Diploma and above	211	46.3
Women occupation	Government employee	199	43.6
	Housewife	166	36.4
	Merchant	61	13.4
	Private employee	25	5.5
	Student	5	1.1
Husband education	Unable to read and write	33	7.4
	Elementary	147	33.2
	Secondary	111	25.1
	Diploma and above	152	34.3
Husband occupation	Merchant	229	51.7
	Government employee	117	26.4
	Private employee	75	16.9
	Others	22	5
	Others: student, farmer, contractor, carpenter		
Average family monthly income(ETB)[a]	< 1000	153	33.6
	1000–2000	179	39.2
	> 2000	124	27.2

[a]1 USD = ~28ETB

1.72,8.79), and unsatisfied marital relation (aOR: 2.72, 95%CI 1.32–5.62) (Table 2).

Discussion

The magnitude of postpartum depression in this study was 22.4% (95% CI: 19.84–24.96). This was higher when compared with findings from Southern India (12%) [12], Sudan (9.2%) [13], Greenland (8.6%) [14] and Northern part of Ethiopia (19%) [8]. The variation might be due to differences in study setting (facility based in India), or measurement scale (Edinburgh depression screening tool in most of the studies). The higher postpartum depression prevalence in this study may also be explained by low living standards in the study setting where ¾ (72.8%) of the mothers had low socio-economic status. This finding was in agreement with the findings from Sudan [13] and Egypt [15] where mothers with low household income were more likely to develop PPD.

The magnitude of postpartum depression in this study was found to be lower than findings from Egypt (49.5%) [15], South Africa (50.3%) [16] and Nigeria (28%) [17]. The discrepancy might also be attributed to differences in sampling methods utilized since we used 12-month period while the comparable studies used less than 6 months which may make sample size smaller. Social desirability bias is most likely since we have employed interviewer administered method of data collection technique. This could have made them not feeling safe and therefore not willing to express their true feelings and ideas. The presence of a different measurement scale for measuring depression might also contribute to the discrepancy in the prevalence in both directions.

Postpartum depression was more common among women age between 18 and 23 years compared with thirty years and above. This might be due to younger women being more exposed to emotional distress as they experience childbirth for the first time and extra burden was added for caring infants as well as the whole family in this particular period. This finding is consistent with findings in Sudan and North America [13, 18].

Women who did not plan their pregnancy were nearly three times more likely to experience PPD when compared with their counter parts. This is in line with findings in South Africa [16] and Cameroon [19]. This might be explained as inadequate preparation for pregnancy, childbirth, and nursing, leading to mothers to feel anxious, helpless and have less (or no) ability to cope with all the changes and challenges babies bring.

Mothers whose infants had sleeping problems were nearly four times more likely to be depressed when compared with mothers whose infants sleep regularly. The findings are consistent with findings in Cameroon [19] and Egypt [15]. This could be explained as sleeping problems in the early years would cause maternal sleep

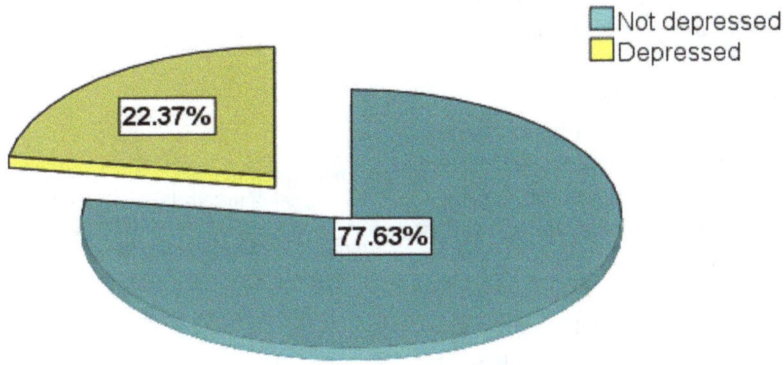

Fig. 1 Prevalence of postpartum depression among women in Mizan Aman Town, Bench Maji Zone, Southwest Ethiopia 2017

loss and feelings of fatigue contributing to maternal depressive symptoms. The current study also identified that the odds of postpartum depression among women who experienced domestic violence from their partner was nearly four times higher than those who did not. This is in line with findings in Egypt [15], Sudan [13] and Japan [20]. Violence of any kind has a devastating physical, psychological, behavioral and developmental effect on the victims.

The occurrence of postpartum depression was high among women who were previously diagnosed for depression. This is explained in studies conducted in China and Canada [21, 22]. Women with unsatisfied marital relations and poor social support were more likely to experience postpartum depression. This finding was supported by findings in Cameroon [19], Pakistan, Iran [23] and South Asia [24]. Lack of support, love, affection and guidance of husband on top of a stressful childbirth event could make women vulnerable to PPD. Women who have a history of substance use were nearly five times more likely to have postpartum depression than non-users. Similarly, this is supported by findings from a systematic review [25]. Postpartum substance use could limit a mother's ability to stay emotionally connected to

Table 2 Predictors of postpartum depression in multivariable analysis among postpartum women in Mizan Aman Town, Bench Maji Zone, Southwest Ethiopia March to April, 2017

Variables	Category	Depressed *N* (%)	Not depressed N (%)	aOR(95% CI)
Age	18–23	71(37)	121(63)	3.89(1.5,9.9)[a]
	24–29	19(11.4)	148(88.6)	0.72(0.2,2.1)
	> = 30	12 (12.4)	85 (87.6)	1
Recent pregnancy status	Unplanned	71(33)	126(67)	3.35(1.7,6.6)[a]
	Planned	31(15)	228(85)	1
Child sleeping problem	Yes	54(55)	45(45)	3.72(1.8,7.7)[a]
	No	48(13)	309(87)	1
Domestic violence	Yes	40(42.5)	54(57.5)	2.86(1.7,8.8)[a]
	No	62(20)	299(80)	1
Marital satisfaction	Dissatisfied	70(36.5)	129(63.5)	2.72(1.3,5.6)[a]
	Satisfied	26(10)	221(90)	1
Social support	Poor	53(54)	41(46)	4.29(1.8,10.3)[a]
	Moderate	24(17)	137(83)	2.00(0.8,4.9)
	Good	25(12)	176(88)	1
Previous depression	Yes	40(71)	27(29)	7.38(3.1,17.4)[a]
	No	62(12)	327(88)	1
Substance use	Yes	52(49)	57(51)	5.16(2.5,10.5)[a]
	No	50(12)	297(88)	1

[a]Statistically significant association, 1 reference group

her infant, adjust to his or her rhythms and behaviors, and anticipate or follow his or her development.

Strengths and limitations of the study

The study used a community based design which helped to address those mothers who were unable to visit health care facilities enhancing generalizability of the findings. Standardized tools which were tested for their validity according to Ethiopian context were employed to diagnose depression. Women may commit social desirability bias in order to avoid discrimination that could follow after stating that they have mental health problems. The cross-sectional nature of the study limits the capacity to draw any causal implications.

Conclusion

The magnitude of postpartum depression among women in the study was significantly higher requiring better strategies to integrate maternal mental health care packages during prenatal and postpartum periods. The study also reported different factors that contribute to the occurrence of postpartum depression such as unplanned pregnancy, presence of domestic violence, unsatisfied marital relation, poor social support and substance use history. Increasing awareness and access to contraceptive options during the preconception period will enhance maternal pregnancy planning. Health institutions should devise a strategy to create and strengthen support groups that create opportunities for positive interpersonal exchanges and emotional support for the mothers during pregnancy and after childbirth. In the community, health extension workers could provide anticipatory guidance for new mothers, such as organizing peer-support group fora and facilitating vicarious experience, as it is recognized as a parental self-efficacy enhancement strategy.

Abbreviations

aOR: Adjusted odds ratio; CMD: Common mental disorders; ICD-10: International classification of diseases, 10th revision; IPV: Intimate partner violence; LICs: Low- income countries; PND: Postpartum depression; WHO: World Health Organization

Acknowledgements

We would like to acknowledge Jimma University for giving financial support to do this research. We also acknowledge the data collectors, supervisors and study participants.

Funding

This study was funded by Jimma University in partial fulfillment of the requirement for masters of Science degree in maternity health nursing.

Authors' contributions

TT involved in designing of the study, data collection, data analysis, drafting and critically reviewing the manuscript. FC and SA involved in designing of the study, analysis of the data and critically reviewing the manuscript. All authors read and approved the final manuscript.

Authors' information

TT is lecturer of maternal health nursing in Mizan Aman College of Health Science; FC is lecturer of maternal health nursing in institute of health, Jimma University and SA is professor of psychiatry in institute of health, Jimma University. All authors are currently staff members in their respective school in aforementioned institutions.

Competing interests

The authors declare that they have no competing interests.

Author details

[1]Mizan Aman college of health science, Mizan Aman, Ethiopia. [2]School of nursing and midwifery, Jimma University, Jimma, Ethiopia.

References

1. World Health Organization. Depression- a global public health concern. 2012. http://www.who.int/mental_health/management/depression/who_paper_depression_wfmh_2012.pdf. Accessed 15 Oct 2016.
2. Global Burden of Disease Study. Global, regional, and national incidence, prevalence, and years lived with disability for 301 acute and chronic diseases and injuries in 188 countries, 1990–2013: a systematic analysis for the Global Burden of Disease Study 2013. Lancet. 2015;386:743–800.
3. Stewart, D.E., Robertson, E., Dennis, C-L., Grace, S.L., & Wallington, T. Postpartum depression: literature review of risk factors and interventions 2003 http://www.who.int/mental_health/prevention/suicide/lit_review_postpartum_depression.pdf. Accessed 20 Jan 2017.
4. Guille CN, Fryml R, et al. Management of postpartum depression. J Midwif Women's Health. 2013;58:643–53 (PUBMED).
5. Oklahoma State Department of Health. Recognizing Postpartum Depression. Oklahoma City; 2011. https://www.ok.gov/health2/documents/PPDepression%205.23.11.pdf. Accessed 22 Oct 2016.
6. Moses-Kolko E, Roth EK. Antepartum and postpartum depression: healthy mom, healthy baby. J Am Med Wom Assoc. 2004;59:181–91 (PUBMED).
7. Fisher JRW, et al. Prevalence and determinants of common perinatal mental disorders in women in low- and lower-middle-income countries: a systematic review. Bull World Health Organ. 2012;90:139–49.
8. Mersha AG, Abebe SA, Sori LM, Abegaz TM. Prevalence and associated factors of perinatal depression in Ethiopia: a systematic review and meta-analysis. Depress Res Treat. 2018;2018:8 Article ID 1813834, (PUBMED).
9. Gelaye, et al. Validity of the patient health Questionnaire-9 for depression screening and diagnosis in East Africa. Psychiatry Res. 2013;210:653–61 (PUBMED).
10. Crane D, Middleton C, Kenneth A, Bean R. Establishing criterion scores for the Kansas marital satisfaction scale (KMSS) and the revised dyadic adjustment scale (RDAS). Am J Fam Ther. 2000;28:53–60 (Cross Ref).
11. Bøen, et al. The importance of social support in the associations between psychological distress and somatic health problems and socio-economic factors among older adults living at home: a cross sectional study. BMC Geriatr. 2012;12:27 (PUBMED).
12. Hirani D, Bala DV. A study of postnatal depression and its determinants in postnatal women residing in rural areas of Ahemdabad district, Gujarat, India. IOSR-JDMS. 2015;14(7):10–5 http://www.iosrjournals.org/iosr-jdms/papers/Vol14-issue7/Version-7/C014771015.pdf.
13. Khalifa et al. Postnatal depression among Sudanese women: prevalence and validation of the Edinburgh postnatal depression scale at 3 months postpartum Int J Women's Health 2015; 7: 677–84. (PUBMED).

14. Iben Motzfeldt, et al. Prevalence of postpartum depression in Nuuk, Greenland- a cross sectional study using Edinburgh postnatal depression scale. Int J Circumpolar Health. 2013;72:21114 (PUBMED).
15. Mohammed ES, et al. Predictors of postpartum depression among rural women in Minia, Egypt: an epidemiological study. Public Health. 2014; 128(9):817–24 https://doi.org/10.1016/j.puhe.2014.06.006.
16. Stoltenberg EL, Abrahams JM. Prevalence of and factors influencing postnatal depression in a rural community in South Africa. Afr J Prm Health Care Fam Med. 2015;7(1) (PUBMED).
17. Danasabe M, Elias Bt N. Postpartum depression among Hausa ethnic women in Abubakar Tafawa Balewa University teaching hospital, north East Nigeria. IMPACT: international journal of research in humanities. Arts Literat (IMPACT: IJRHAL). 2016;4(3):55–64 http://oaji.net/articles/2016/488-1460366334.pdf. Accessed 1 Apr 2017.
18. Brett K, Barfield W, Williams C. Prevalence of self-reported postpartum depressive symptoms (2004-2005). MMWR. 2008;57(14):361–6 https://www.cdc.gov/mmwR/preview/mmwrhtml/mm5714a1.htm. Accessed 3 Nov 2016.
19. Adama, et al. Prevalence and risk factors of postpartum depression in Yaounde, Cameroon. Open J Obst Gynecol. 2015;5:608–17 http://file.scirp.org/Html/6-1431004_59760.htm. Accessed 15 Sept 2016.
20. Miura A, Fujiwara T. Intimate partner violence during pregnancy and postpartum depression in Japan: a cross-sectional study. Front Public Health. 2017;5:81 (PUBMED).
21. Chi, et al. Screening for postpartum depression and associated factors among women in China. Front Psychol. 2016;7:3–8 (PUBMED).
22. Lanes, et al. Prevalence and characteristics of Postpartum Depression symptomatology among Canadian women. BMC Public Health. 2011; (PUBMED).
23. Jahromi MK, et al. A study of marital satisfaction among non-depressed and depressed mothers after childbirth in Jahrom, Iran. Global J Health Sci. 2015; 7(3):140 (PUBMED).
24. Abdollahi F, Lye MS, Md Zain A, Shariff Ghazali S, Zarghami M. Postnatal depression and its associated factors in women from different cultures. Iran J Psychiatry Behav Sci. 2011;5(2):5–11 (PUBMED).
25. Ross L, Dennis C. The prevalence of postpartum depression among women with substance use, an abuse history, or chronic illness: a systematic review. J Women's Health. 2009;18(4):1–13 (PUBMED).

/

13

Effect of antenatal care and social well-being on early neonatal mortality in Bangladesh

Sanjit Roy and Md. Aminul Haque*

Abstract

Background: Bangladesh has achieved MDG 4, but although post neonatal and child mortality have shown impressive declines, neonatal mortality is still lagging behind. More efforts have to be made to improve this state of affairs. The objective of this paper is to identify the effect of proper antenatal care and social wellbeing on early neonatal mortality in Bangladesh.

Methods: The data used for this study is the Bangladesh Multiple Indicator Cluster Survey. This study used several independent variables such as mother's school attendance, receiving antenatal care, receiving TT injection, place of residence and wealth quintile. Here both bivariate and multivariate analysis have been used. At bivariate level, simple cross tabulation and appropriate measures of association have been used to find out the statistical association between dependent and independent variables. In this study the outcome/dependent variable is early neonatal mortality (children who died within 7 days after birth) which is a binary variable. If early neonatal mortality occurs among the respondents then it is considered as 1, otherwise it is considered as 0. Logistic regression was used to identify the factors which are involved in reducing this early neonatal mortality.

Results: Women who received antenatal care during their time of pregnancy are likely to have 18% lower odds of experiencing early neonatal mortality (OR = 0.82, CI = (0.71–0.95)) compared to groups who did not receive antenatal care during pregnancy. In terms of social well-being, the woman who comes from the richest family are likely to have 45% lower odds of experiencing early neonatal mortality (OR = 0.55, CI = (0.42–0.720) compared to the poorest one.

Conclusion: The outcomes of this paper suggest that the women's antenatal care and social well-being has a significant effect on early neonatal mortality.

Keywords: Early neonatal mortality, Antenatal care, Social well-being, Effect, Bangladesh

Background

Reduction of child mortality was one of the major goals of MDGs and its target was to reduce childhood mortality rate up to 66% within the year 2015 [1]. With the target of sustainable development goals (SGD) for achieving universal health coverage, neonatal mortality must decline in tandem with child mortality. Childhood mortality is a very prominent factor in the public health sector of any country (Mustafa and Odimegwu 2008). As a cause of childhood mortality, including early neonatal mortality, different socio-economic factors, socio-demographic factors, nutritional factors of the mothers are involved [2] and other factors may also be responsible [3].

The infant mortality rate was 94/1000 live births and the under-five child mortality was 151/1000 live births in the year 1990 [4]. But just after 6 years both infant mortality rate and under five child mortality rate have declined with IMR at 46/1000 live births and under-5 mortality rate at 58/1000 live births in the year 2015 [5]. According to the Health Bulletin 2017 of DGHS, the neonatal mortality rate is reported as 19 per 1000 live births (SVRS 2016) and 28 per 1000 live births (BDHS 2014) [6]. The neonatal period (first 28 days of life) is the most vulnerable time for a child. But recently the neonatal mortality is decreasing worldwide as well as in

* Correspondence: aminul.haque@du.ac.bd
Department of Population Sciences, University of Dhaka, Dhaka 1000, Bangladesh

Bangladesh, where the neonatal mortality rate has decreased from 36 to 19 deaths per 1000 live births [7]. However, the decreasing rate of neonatal mortality is slower compared to post-neonatal mortality rate. So, more emphasis has to give to improve this state of affairs.

The most significant indicator of child well-being is the under-five child mortality rate including good health and nutritional status of the children across the world [8].

The rate of child mortality is decreasing globally. For example, during the year 1990, the rate of child mortality has declined across all the regions under WHO with the exception of Western Pacific Regions [8]. Despite this decreasing pattern, child survival remains an urgent concern. In spite of the subsequent development of health sectors, still a significant percentage of children (i.e. 17,000/per day) die before reaching their fifth birthday and this rate of childhood mortality is significantly higher in the low income countries compared to high income countries [9]. According to UNICEF, in 2013 the rate of under-five child mortality for low income countries was 76/1000 live births and this rate was approximately twelve times higher than high income countries [10].

Overall it has been found that across the globe the neonatal mortality is decreasing but this rate of decline is slower compared to post neonatal mortality. In the total life span for a human being the first 28 days of life are the most vulnerable time period for his survival. For that reason, more efforts should be made to reduce early neonatal mortality. Bangladesh is not an exception to this trend of childhood mortality. So, by considering all these issues, this paper aims to find out the effect of antenatal care and social well-being on early neonatal mortality in the context of Bangladesh.

Methods

Source of data

In this study the Bangladesh Multiple Indicator Cluster Survey [5] data was used which was conducted from December 2012 to March 2013 with the collaboration of the Bangladesh Bureau of Statistics (BBS) and Ministry of Planning. The survey used the multistage stratified sampling method for collecting data. Both technical and financial support for conducting this survey was provided by UNICEF, Bangladesh. The number of respondents who were both ever married and ever given birth was 44,207 and belonged to the reproductive age group.

Model specification

Here, early neonatal mortality has been defined as neonates who died before reaching age 7 days after birth. In this study, early neonatal mortality has been considered as the dependent variable. On the other hand the independent variables are: Maternal related factors: School attendance or literacy, Received antenatal care, Received TT injection, Socioeconomic factors: Place of residence and Wealth index.

The proposed hypothesis of this study includes:

> Hypothesis 1: The mothers who are receiving sufficient antenatal care have lower probability of early neonatal mortality (ENM).
> Hypothesis 2: The mothers with higher socio-economic status have lower probability of ENM.

Statistical methods

In this study both bivariate and multivariate analyses have been used. At bivariate level, simple cross tabulation and appropriate measures of association have been applied i.e. chi-square test have been used to find out the statistical association (which are considered statistically significant at 5% level) between dependent and independent variables. Here, the outcome/dependent variable is early neonatal mortality (ENM) and it is considered as a dichotomous variable indicating 1 (if occurred) and 0 (if not occurred). Logistic regression was used to identify the factors which involved reducing this early neonatal mortality. The entire analyses have been conducted using the statistical software STATA.

Results

In this study, around 17.0% respondents reported that they ever had experience of early neonatal mortality in their reproductive life-span (Fig. 1).

The average age of the study population is 29 years. Women's school attendance is an important factor to reduce early neonatal mortality. In this study around 72.2% respondents reported that they had ever attended school and the remaining 27.8% stated that they never attended school. In terms of place of residence, only 17.3% respondents came from urban areas and 82.7% from the rural areas. In terms of wealth index of the respondents, 22.7% are poorest, 20.8% are poorer, 20.1% are less poor, 19.6% are richer and the remaining 16.7% comes from the richest family. Among the respondents around 65.2% reported that they received antenatal care during their time of pregnancy and the remaining 34.9% did not. Approximately 59.1% respondents reported that they received TT injection during their pregnancy, whereas 40.9% did not (Table 1).

The early neonatal mortality is influenced by many factors. According to the findings of this study women's school attendance shows a significant association ($p < 0.001$) with early neonatal mortality. This study found that the women who ever attended school has lower percentage of early neonatal mortality (11.8%) compared to women who never attended school (26.8%).Women who received antenatal care during their pregnancy has significantly ($p < 0.001$)

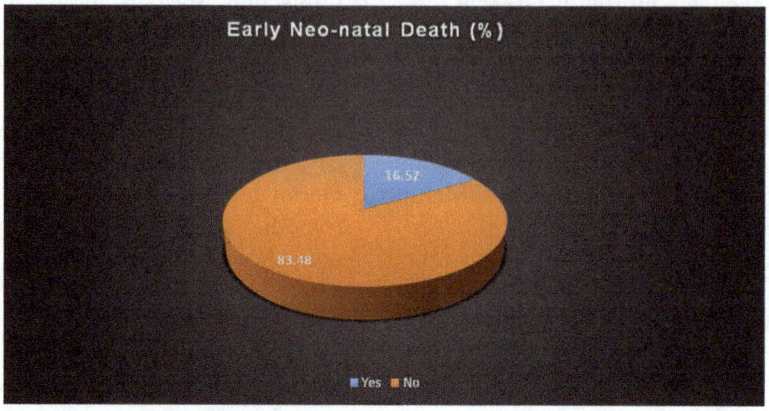

Source: Data Analysis of MICS 2012-2013

Fig. 1 Early Neo-natal Death (%)

lower percentage of early neonatal mortality (ENM) (10.2%) compared to women who never received antenatal care during their pregnancy (15.6%). The study also found significant association ($p < 0.001$) between receiving TT injection and early neonatal mortality. According to the findings of this study around 10.7% women reported early neonatal mortality although they had received TT injection, in comparison to 14.0% women who had never received TT injection.

Table 1 Socio-demographic characteristics of the respondents

Background characteristics	Number of respondents (%)
Average Age of the Respondent	Mean (SD) 29.72 (9.46)
Ever Attended School	
Yes	37,315 (72.22)
No	14,357 (27.78)
Total	51,627 (100.00)
Received Antenatal Care	
Yes	5051 (65.15)
No	2702 (34.85)
Total	7753 (100.00)
Received TT Injection	
Yes	4581 (59.09)
No	3172 (40.91)
Total	7753 (100.00)
Place of Residence	
Urban	8925 (17.27)
Rural	42,747 (82.73)
Total	51,672 (100.00)
Wealth Index	
Poorest	11,744 (22.73)
Second	10,769 (20.84)
Middle	10,392 (20.11)
Fourth	10,118 (19.58)
Richest	8649 (16.74))
Total	51,627 (100.00)

In terms of place of residence, women who live in rural areas have significantly higher ($p < 0.001$) early neonatal mortality (17.2%) compared to the women living in urban areas (13.0%).Wealth index has also statistically significant impact ($p < 0.001$) on early neonatal mortality (ENM). This study found that ENM is higher in the poorest groups (20.8%) compared to the richest groups (10.1%) (Table 2).

Logistic regression was used to determine the effect of antenatal care and social well-being on ENM. According to the findings of logistic regression model, women who received antenatal care are likely to have 18.0% lower odds of ENM (OR = 0.82, CI = (0.71–0.95)) compared to women who did not and this difference is statistically significant. The odds of experiencing ENM for the respondents who received TT injection during pregnancy is significantly 21.0% lower (OR = 0.79, CI = (0.69–0.91)) compared to unvaccinated respondents. This study found significant impact of school attendance of the women on ENM compared with women who ever attended school having 54.0% lower odds of ENM (OR = 0.46, CI = (0.39–0.53)) compared to women who never attended school. In terms of place of residence, the urban respondents reported that they experienced 20.0% lower odds of ENM (OR = 0.80, CI = (0.64–0.99) compared to rural women. In terms of wealth quintile, woman from the richest families are at 45.0% lower odds of experiencing ENM (OR = 0.55, CI = (0.42–0.72) compared to the poorest, with the difference being statistically significant (Table 3).

Discussion

Along with other socioeconomic factors, the antenatal period is significantly important for the health of mother

Table 2 Percentage of Childhood mortality/Early stage neo-natal mortality by different factors

Childhood mortality/ early stage neo-natal mortality			
Factors	Yes N (%)	No N (%)	P-value
Ever Attended School (*N* = 44,207)			
Yes	3554 (11.76)	26,667 (88.24)	0.000
No	3750 (26.81)	10,236 (73.19)	
Received Antenatal Care (*N* = 7753)			
Yes	513 (10.16)	4538 (89.84)	0.000
No	422 (15.62)	2280 (84.38)	
Received TT Injection (*N* = 7753)			
Yes	491 (10.72)	4090 (89.28)	0.000
No	444 (14.00)	2728 (86.00)	
Place of Residence (*N* = 44,207)			
Urban	968 (13.02)	6466 (86.98)	0.000
Rural	6336 (17.23)	30,437 (82.77)	
Wealth Index(*N* = 44,207)			
Poorest	2193 (20.75)	8375 (79.25)	0.000
Second	1743 (18.61)	7625 (81.39)	
Middle	1479 (16.68)	7390 (83.32)	
Fourth	1184 (14.08)	7227 (85.92)	
Richest	705 (10.08)	6286 (89.92)	

Table 3 Odds ratios of selected explanatory variables to predict Childhood mortality/Early stage neo-natal mortality

Predictor variables	Childhood mortality/early stage neo-natal mortality	
	Odds ratio	CI (*p* value)
Received Antenatal Care		
Yes	0.82	0.71–0.95 (0.009)
No	1.00	
Received TT Injection		
Yes	0.79	0.69–0.91 (0.001)
No	1.00	
Ever Attended School		
Yes	0.46	0.39–0.53 (0.000)
No	1.00	
Place of Residence		
Urban	0.80	0.64–0.99 (0.050)
Rural	1.00	
Wealth Index		
Richest	0.55	
Poorest	1.00	0.42–0.72 (0.000)
Constant	0.34	
Model chi-square	205.72	
p-value	0.000	
N	7753	

and her future offspring. Child survival can be improved by improving care during antenatal period. The present study examined the effects of antenatal care and social well-being on early neonatal mortality (ENM) in Bangladesh. In this study the Bangladesh Multiple Indicator Cluster Survey data was used which was conducted from December 2012 to March 2013 with the collaboration of the Bangladesh Bureau of Statistics (BBS) and Ministry of Planning. The survey used the multistage stratified sampling method for collecting data. This is one of the few studies that focus on the impact of antenatal care and social well-being on early neonatal mortality using a large scale secondary data set.

The results of this study give an overall idea about how proper antenatal care and social well-being can reduce the early neonatal mortality in Bangladesh. The study population of this research was 15–49 years aged group women and among these 51,627 women 44,207 were ever married and had ever given birth. Among these ever married women, 17.0% had history of ENM in their entire reproductive age. To find out the causes of death this study examined several possible factors that could contribute majorly.

The multivariate analysis has been applied to determine the effect of antenatal care and social well-being on early neonatal mortality. Findings from logistic regression model showed that women who received antenatal care, compared to those who did not, experienced 18.0% lower odds of early neonatal mortality; similar findings have been reported by other researchers [11–17]. In terms of wealth quintile, women from the richest family are likely to have 45.0% lower odds of ENM than their poorest counterparts. This finding is consistent with that of other researchers [12, 17–19].

Receiving proper vaccination is an important factor to reduce early neonatal mortality. Findings of this study shows that odds of experiencing ENM for the respondents who received TT injection during pregnancy is significantly 21.0% lower compared to unvaccinated respondents. This finding related to immunization is consistent with that of other researcher [4]. Similar to other socio-demographic factors, place of residence also creates an effect in experiencing early neonatal mortality. In terms of place of residence, based on the findings of this study, the urban respondents reported that they experienced 20.0% lower odds of ENM compared to rural women; similar findings have been reported by other researchers [1, 20, 21].

School attendance is also a significant factor affecting the respondents' risk of experiencing early neonatal mortality. This study found significant impact of school attendance of the women on ENM with women who ever attended school having 54.0% lower odds of ENM compared to women who never attended school; this finding related to educational attainment is consistent with that of other researchers [1, 14, 22]. So, education is an important factor to reduce early neonatal mortality because having proper education will encourage all pregnant mothers to engage in effective health care seeking behavior that will ultimately reduce neonatal deaths.

Conclusion

Findings of this paper suggest that women's antenatal care, social well-being and TT vaccination have a significant role in lowering ENM. This study recommends that for reducing early neonatal mortality (ENM) we should ensure proper antenatal care during pregnancy. Another issue is that the people who are richest and educated will be able to prevent early neonatal mortality by taking the necessary proper actions. So, socio-economic development is also important to address this issue properly. If all the measures taken sufficiently and with alacrity, it will be possible lower ENM which will impact child mortality favorably.

Limitations

There are several limitations of the present study, i.e. the analysis of the study had to depend on the variables available in the MICS 2012–2013. The issue under study is very complicated and difficult to measure. For that, we had to use indirect and proxy indicators to complete the analysis. However, we were careful in constructing proxy indicators, conducting analysis and interpretation of the data.

Abbreviations

BBS: Bangladesh Bureau of Statistics; CI: Confidence interval; ENM: Early neonatal mortality; MDGs: Millennium development goals; MICS: Bangladesh multiple indicator cluster survey; OR: Odds ratio; SDGs: Sustainable development goals; WHO: World Health Organization

Acknowledgements

The authors are thankful to Bangladesh Multiple Indicator Cluster Survey for providing us with the raw data. We are also grateful to all the families who contributed directly and indirectly to the study.

Funding

No fund was received from any source to conduct the research.

Authors' contributions

SR: Had the original idea for the study, planned the study, drafted the manuscript, revised it critically for important intellectual content, handled supervision of overall work, and final approval of the version to be submitted. Helped in data cleaning, analyzed the data, and drafted the manuscript. MAH: Revised critically for important intellectual content, helped in statistical interpretation, and final approval of the version to be submitted. Both authors read and approved the final manuscript.

Competing interests

The authors declare that they have no competing interest.

References

1. Mustafa HE, Odimegwu C. Socioeconomic determinants of infant mortality in Kenya: analysis of Kenya DHS 2003. J Humanit Soc Sci. 2008;**2**(8):1934–722.
2. Gage TB, et al. Maternal education, birth weight, and infant mortality in the United States. Demography. 2013;50(2):615–35.
3. Aquino R, et al. Impact of the family health program on infant mortality in Brazilian municipalities. Am J Public Health. 2009;99(1):87–93.
4. Sayem AM, et al. Achieving the millennium development goal for under-five mortality in Bangladesh: current status and lessons for issues and challenges for further improvements. J Health Popul Nutr. 2011;29: 92–102.
5. GoB, B., SID, UNICEF. Multiple Indicator Cluster Survey, 2012–2013. 2015.
6. Health Bulletin. Government of the People's Republic of Bangladesh, Ministry of Health and Family Welfare, MIS. Bangladesh: DGHS; 2017.
7. UNICEF. Neonatal Mortality. Online (Access on 12 July 2017). https://data.unicef.org/topic/child-survival/neonatal-mortality/.
8. Ahmad OB, et al. The decline in child mortality: a reappraisal. Bull World Health Organ. 2000;78:1175–91.
9. Kim D, Saada A. The social determinants of infant mortality and birth outcomes in Western developed nations: a cross-country systematic review. Int J Environ Res Public Health. 2013;10(6):2296–335.
10. UNICEF. World bank; United Nations. Levels & trends in child mortality report 2014: estimates developed by the UN InterAgency Group for Child Mortality Estimation (cited 2015 Feb 17). 2014
11. Van Eijk AM, et al. Use of antenatal services and delivery care among women in rural western Kenya: a community based survey. Reprod Health. 2006;3(1):1.
12. Hollowell J, et al. The effectiveness of antenatal care programmes to reduce infant mortality and preterm birth in socially disadvantaged and vulnerable women in high-income countries: a systematic review. BMC Pregnancy Childbirth. 2011;11(1):1.
13. Zafari M, et al. A study the factors affecting under the age of 5 years child mortality. Int J Prev Treat. 2012;1(3):49–52.
14. Owais A, et al. Maternal and antenatal risk factors for stillbirths and neonatal mortality in rural Bangladesh: a case-control study. PloS One. 2013;8(11): e80164.
15. Singh A, et al. Do antenatal care interventions improve neonatal survival in India? Health Policy Plan. 2013:czt066.
16. Trujillo JC, et al. Relationship between professional antenatal care and facility delivery: an assessment of Colombia. Health Policy Plan. 2013: czt033.
17. Shera HMMJ, Dar IS. Addressing Corner Solution Effect for Child Mortality Status Measure: An Application of Tobit Model. Int J Acad Res Bus Soc Sci. 2014;4(12):218.
18. Kembo J, Van Ginneken JK. Determinants of infant and child mortality in Zimbabwe: Results of multivariate hazard analysis. Demog Res. 2009; 21:367–84.
19. Belizán JM, et al. Neonatal death in low-to middle-income countries: a global network study. Am J Perinatol. 2012;29(08):649–56.
20. Fottrell E, Osrin D, Alcock G, Azad K, Bapat U, Beard J, et al. Cause-specific neonatal mortality: analysis of 3772 neonatal deaths in Nepal, Bangladesh, Malawi and India. Arch Dis Child Fetal Neonatal Ed. 2015, 2014.
21. Nahar J, Zabeen B, Akhter S, Azad K, Nahar N. Neonatal morbidity and mortality pattern in the special care baby unit of BIRDEM. Ibrahim Med Coll J. 2007;1(2):1–4.

14

Postnatal care service utilization and associated factors among women who gave birth in Debretabour town, North West Ethiopia

Kihinetu Gelaye Wudineh*, Azezu Asres Nigusie, Shumiye Shiferaw Gesese, Azimeraw Arega Tesu and Fentahun Yenealem Beyene

Abstract

Background: World health organization stated that postnatal care is defined as a care given to the mother and her newborn baby immediately after the birth of the placenta and for the first six weeks of life. Majority of maternal and neonatal deaths occur during childbirth and the postpartum period. Scaling up of maternal and newborn health through proper postnatal care services is the best way of reducing maternal and neonatal mortality.

Method: A community based cross sectional study was conducted among 588 mothers who gave birth in the last one year from March 1–21; 2017. Systematic random sampling technique was used to select study participants. A pre-tested and structured questionnaire was used to collect the data. Data was entered in EPI info version 7 and analyzed using SPSS version 21. Logistic regression was applied to identify association between explanatory variables and the outcome variable. An adjusted odds ratio with 95% confidence interval and *p*-value less than 0.05 was computed to determine the level of significance.

Result: A total of 588 participants were included in the analysis which was the response rate of 100%.
The prevalence of postnatal care service utilization in this study was 57.5%.
Maternal educational status of secondary school and above (AOR = 3.29, 95%CI: 1.94–5.57), family monthly income of above 1500 ETB (AOR = 2.85, 95%CI: 1.21–6.68), alive birth outcome of last pregnancy (AOR = 5.70, 95%CI: 1.53–21.216), planned and supported last pregnancy (AOR = 3.94, 95%CI: 1.72–9.01) and institutional delivery of last pregnancy (AOR = 3.08, 95%CI: 1.24–7.68) were positively associated with PNC service utilization.

Conclusion: This study showed that the overall utilization of PNC service in Debretabour town is low. Mothers' education, monthly income, last pregnancy birth outcome, wantedness of the pregnancy and place of delivery were significantly associated with postnatal care service utilization. To enhance PNC service utilization and reduce maternal and neonatal mortality women should obtain appropriate education. Furthermore all pregnant women should give birth in the health facilities.

Keywords: Utilization, Postnatal care, Maternal death

* Correspondence: kihinetugelaye031@gmail.com
Department of Midwifery, College of Medicine and Health Sciences, Bahir Dar University, Bahir Dar, Ethiopia

Background

The world Health Organization (WHO) stated that postnatal care (PNC) is defined as a care given to the mother and her newborn baby immediately after the birth of the placenta and for the first 42 days of life [1].

Majority of maternal and neonatal deaths occur during childbirth and postnatal period [2, 3].

The estimated maternal mortality ratio (MMR) declined across all MDG regions between 19,990 and 2015, although the magnitude of reduction varies substantially between regions [4].

According to 2015, the two regions with highest MMR are sub-Saharan Africa and Oceania. The MMR in developing regions was 19 times higher than in developed regions. Sub-Saharan Africa has the highest regional MMR (546) per 100,000 live births [4].

The 2016 Ethiopian Demographic and Health Survey (EDHS) showed that the MMR was 412 deaths per 100,000 live births. In other words for every 1000 live births about four women (4.12) died during pregnancy, childbirth or within six weeks of childbirth.

According to EDHS 2016, only 17% of women receive at least one postnatal care service from a health institution in the first 48 h after birth and Amhara region is the 3rd least region in postnatal care service utilization [5].

Utilization of maternal health care services decreases maternal and child mortality.

Postnatal care particularly prevents most maternal and child morbidity and mortality. Care given in the postpartum period assists health care providers to detect post-delivery problems and to give treatments timely [3, 6]. Shortage of care during this period could result in ill health, disabilities and deaths [3]. Around 65% of maternal deaths and 75% of newborn deaths occur in the first seven days after birth, and around half of these deaths occur in the first one day. A newborn is about 500 times more likely to die in the first day of life than at one month of age [7].

Appropriate postnatal care could save up to 60,000 newborn lives a year. In Ethiopia, if all new born receives appropriate postnatal care in the recommended time, neonatal mortality could be reduced by 10–27% [7].

Globally, there were an estimated 303,000 maternal deaths from complications related to pregnancy and childbirth in 2015 which is a decline of 43% from 1990. Majority of the maternal deaths occur in developing regions. It accounts for approximately 99% of the global maternal deaths in 2015, with Sub- Saharan Africa alone accounting for roughly 66% followed by southern Asia 22% [4].

Less attention was given for postnatal period in developing countries; women and their newborns don't receive postnatal care services from a skilled birth attendant during the first days after childbirth [2].

Great majority of maternal and neonatal deaths occur during the first 2 days after childbirth. Hence, postnatal care for the women and the child is important in detecting and treating complications occur during the delivery as well as providing information for the mother on her and her newborn health [5].

To assess the extent of postnatal care utilization, EDHS 2016 asked respondents for their last birth in the 2 years preceding the survey, whether they had received a check up after delivery and the timing of the first checkup and it was found that the level of postnatal care coverage was low in Ethiopia. Only 17% of women reported having received a PNC checkup in the first 2 days after birth. In the case of the Amhara region percentage of women with a postnatal checkup in the first two days after birth was18.4% [5].

Methods

Study area and period

This study was conducted from March 1st to 21th, 2017, at Debretabour town. Debretabour, the city of South Gondar zone is found in the northern part of Amhara regional state 98 Kilometers from Bahirdar, the main city of Amhara regional state and 666 Kilometers away from Addis Ababa, the capital city of Ethiopia. According to the 2015 population projection estimate, there were 55,596 residents and around half of them were females. There are 3 health centers, 4 health posts, and 1 general hospital providing postnatal care services in the town.

Study design and population

A quantitative research involving community based cross-sectional study was conducted among randomly selected reproductive age group of mothers who gave birth in the past one year preceding the data collection period.

Mothers who lived less than six months in the study area at the time of interview and who had communication problem were excluded from the study.

Sample size calculation and sampling procedure

The single population proportion formula was used to calculate the sample size considering the following assumptions: proportion of women using postnatal care services 33.5% [8], 95% confidence level, 4% margin of error (absolute level of precision).

$$\text{Thus, } n = [Z\,\alpha/2^{*}\ P\ (1-P)]$$
$$/d2 = 1.96^{2*}\ 0.335(1-0.335)$$
$$/0.04^{2} = 535$$

Adding 10% non-response rate, a total sample size of 588 women were included.

Debretabour town intentionally was selected as a study site by considering the health status of women in the town and lack of previous researches related to maternal health care services. Systematic sampling technique was used to select the study units. From the four kebeles all kebeles were selected. The calculated sample size was distributed across the four kebeles proportionally to the size of the households in each kebele. Then the proportion of eligible mothers those who gave birth in the last one year prior to this study were identified. Based on this assumption the available data from registry of the local health extension workers they recently conducted the survey for immunization program was used. The sampling interval of households in each kebele was determined by dividing the total number of households to the allocated sample size. The initial household to be interviewed was selected randomly from the kebele house number registry using a number between 1 and the sample interval. The subsequent household to be included in the study was identified systematically through house-to-house visit. For households with more than one eligible woman, interview was done for one of the mothers using simple random sampling technique. Revisits of two to three times were made in case where eligible respondents were not available at the time of the survey by asking the neighbors whether an eligible women in that house was present or not, after all they were considered as non-respondents.

Data collection tools and procedures

Data was collected by face to face interview using a structured and pre-tested questionnaire. The questionnaire first prepared in English and translated to Amharic, and then back to English. Four 3rd year diploma midwife students were used to collect data. Two BSC midwives were assigned to supervise the data collection process. Both the data collectors and supervisors were given one day training before the actual work about the aim of study, procedures and collection techniques going through the questionnaires question by question, art of interviewing and ways of collecting the data.

Data quality control

The quality of data was assured by proper designing and pre-testing of the questionnaires in one of the Kebeles other than Debretabour, in Woreta town on 30 participants. Every day after data collection, questionnaires were reviewed and checked for completeness by the supervisor and principal investigator and the necessary feedback was offered to data collectors in the next morning and before ending all session incomplete questions were completed using precoded for controlling errors during data analysis.

Data processing and analysis

The entire questionnaire were checked, coded and entered into EPI Info version 7 and exported to SPSS version 21 software. For analysis descriptive statistical procedures were utilized. Descriptive statistics like percentage, mean and standard deviation were used for the presentation of demographic data and magnitude of post natal care service utilization. Tables and graphs were also used for data presentation.

Binary logistic regression was used to identify factors associated with PNC service utilization on mothers. Variables with *P*-value less than or equal to 0.2 were selected in to multiple logistic regression models for controlling the possible effect of confounders and finally variables which had independent association with PNC service utilization were identified on the basis of AOR, with 95%CI and *p*-value less than 0.05.

Ethical consideration

Ethical clearance was obtained from institutional Ethical Committee of Bahirdar University. Formal letter of cooperation was written for Regional Health Bureau, Debretabour health office and respective kebeles and permission was obtained. Written informed consent was obtained from each study subjects, each respondent was informed about the objective of the study that it contribute to improve maternal health. Any mother who was not willing to participate in the study has not been forced to participate. They were also informed that all data obtained from them would be kept confidential by using codes instead of any personal identifiers and is meant only for the purpose of the study. Health education on postnatal care service and related complication and other information was given for the participants during interview.

Results

Socio demographic characteristics of the participants

The total of 588 women participated in the study making the overall response rate 100%. More than half 330(56.1%) of the respondents were in the age group 20–29 with the mean ± SD 27.35 ± 5.48 years. Five hundred twenty one (88.6%) of them were married and 564(95.9%) of them were Orthodox Christian followers. Nearly one-six, 102(17.3%) of the respondents were unable to read and write and 260(44.2%) of them attend secondary school and above. Concerning their husbands' educational status, 337(57.3%) of them were attended secondary school and above, and 269(45.7%) of respondents' husband were government employed by occupation. The total monthly household's income was ranging from 100 to 16,000 ETB while 74% of the participants had earned above 1500 ETB per month. Majority, 530 (90%) of the respondents had either TV and/or Radio in their houses (Table 1).

Table 1 Socio-demographic characteristics of study participants at Debretabour town, March 2017($n = 588$)

Variables	Frequency	Percent
Age		
< 20	61	10.4
20–29	330	56.1
30–39	173	29.4
40–49	24	4.1
Marital status		
Married	521	88.6
Single	32	5.4
Divorced	25	4.3
Widowed	10	1.7
Religion		
Orthodox	564	95.9
Muslim	18	3.1
Protestant	6	1.0
Ethnicity		
Amhara	580	98.6
Agew	8	1.4
Education		
Cannot read and write	102	17.3
Can read and write	68	11.6
Elementary education	158	26.9
Secondary and above	260	44.2
Occupation		
House wife	288	49
Government employed	139	23.6
Merchant	92	15.6
Daily laborer	42	7.1
Farming	5	0.9
Private employ	22	3.7
Husband education ($n = 521$)		
Cannot read and write	22	4.22
Can read and write	41	7.87
Elementary education	121	23.22
Secondary and above	337	64.68
Husband occupation (n = 521)		
Merchant	150	28.8
Farming	20	3.84
Government employed	269	51.63
Daily laborer	58	11.13
Driver	24	4.61
Average monthly income		
< 500 Eth birr	31	5.3
500–1500 Eth birr	121	20.6
> 1500 Eth birr	436	74.1

Obstetric characteristics of respondents

Among the total respondents, 347 (59.0%) mothers were categorized as Para two to Para four. Of these, 18(3.1%) of mothers faced stillbirth while they gave the last birth.

Three hundred ninety- six (67.3%) of the current pregnancy were planned and supported. Almost all, 567(96.4%) of the mothers had antenatal care follow-up during the last pregnancy while 559(95.1%) of mothers gave their last birth at health institution.

Regarding to the mode of delivery, most respondents 432(77.28%) delivered by spontaneous vaginal delivery (Table 2).

Proportion of postnatal care utilization

From total respondents, 338(57.5%) mothers were utilized postnatal care services with confidence interval of (53.4–61.6). Regarding to the frequency of postnatal care visit, 228(67.5%) of participants had visited once, 63(18.6%) women had two times, and the remaining 47(13.9%) were having three or more. The proportion of postnatal care visit within 24 h, at 3–7 days and at six weeks of postpartum were 103(30.5%),104(30.8%) and 162(47.9%) respectively.

Concerning types of service utilization during the postnatal visit, one-hundred sixty seven (28.4%) of the respondents utilized family planning, nearly half (44.9%) of them received immunization, 22.6% of them were tested and counseled for HIV and 106(18%) of them was counseled on breast feeding.

Reasons for nonutilization of PNC services

Different reasons were given by the participants for not attending postnatal care services. The most common reason mentioned by the participants for none utilization of postnatal care service was being apparently healthy (Fig. 1).

Associated factors of postnatal care utilization

During bivariable logistic regression analysis, those variables that had significant association were marital status, respondents educational level, monthly income, decision making style of the women on her health, decision making style of the women on her child health, parity, birth outcome of the last baby, nature of the last pregnancy and place of delivery.

In multiple logistic regression analysis all variables with p values less than 0.2 were entered. Only educational status of the respondents, monthly income, birth

Table 2 Obstetric characteristics of the women who gave birth in the last 12 months in Debretabour town, Northwest Ethiopia, March 2017(n = 588)

Variables	Frequency	Percent
Parity		
1	203	34.5
2–4	347	59.0
5 and above	38	6.5
Outcome of birth		
Alive	570	96.9
Still birth	18	3.1
Nature of last pregnancy		
Planned and supported	396	67.3
Unplanned but supported	155	26.4
Unplanned and unsupported	37	6.3
Place of delivery		
Home	29	4.9
Health institution	559	95.1
Mode of delivery (*n* = 559)		
Spontaneous vaginal delivery	432	77.28
Instrumental delivery	83	14.85
Cesarean section	44	7.87
Advise for any danger signs before discharge (*n* = 559)		
Yes	375	67.08
No	184	32.92
ANC visit during last pregnancy(n = 588)		
Yes	567	96.4
No	21	3.6
Awareness about PNC service		
Yes	379	64.5
No	209	35.5

outcome of the last pregnancy, nature of the last pregnancy and place of delivery were had significant association with postnatal care service utilization.

Accordingly, those women whose educational status secondary school and above were 3 times (AOR = 3.29, 95% CI: 1.94–5.57) more likely to utilize PNC service than those women who couldn't read and write. Those mothers who had monthly household income greater than 1500 ETB were 2.8 times more likely to utilize PNC services than those women who earned less than 500 ETB (AOR = 2.85, 95%CI:1.21–6.68).Mothers who gave birth alive neonate were 5.7 times more likely to get postnatal care services than mothers who gave still birth(AOR = 5.70,95%CI:1.53–21.21).

The odds of having postnatal care visit for those women whose pregnancy were planned and supported were 3.9 times more likely to have PNC visit than those women whose pregnancy were unplanned and unsupported(AOR = 3.96,95%CI:1.72–9.01).

Those mothers who gave birth to their latest child at the health institution were 3 times (AOR = 3.08, 95%CI: 1.24–7.68) more likely to get postnatal care service utilization when compared with those mothers who gave birth to their latest child at home (Table 3).

Discussion

This study indicated that more than half, 338(57.5%) of the participants had received PNC services with confidence interval of (53.4–61.6).

The utilization of postnatal care service in this study is lower than a study done in Bahi District, Tanzania 70.8% [9]. The possible explanation for this difference may be due to social context variation.

This result is also lower than the previous Ethiopian studies: Addis Ababa, 65.6% [10], Gondar Zuria District, 66.83% [11] and Adwa town 78.3% [12]. The possible explanation for this difference might be due to those communities with a low concentration of educated and poor women lead to the lower attention of the need for postnatal care service utilization. The other suggestion might be due to sample size determination differences. Lastly it might be due to lack of information about postnatal care, low maternal knowledge about danger signs of postnatal care and low attention of health professionals in counseling the women to came back for postnatal care.

According to this study the utilization of postnatal care service is higher than a study conducted in rural area of Western Rajasthan, India 35.86% [13], Nepal 43.2% [14], Palestine 36.6% [15], Soroti district Eastern Uganda 15.4% [16], Africa 36% [17] developing countries 36% [18], a study done in four Sub-Saharan African countries: Burkina Faso 25%, Kenya 33%, Malawi 41% and Mozambique 40% [19].The possible reason to the discrepancies might be due to cultural differences, time differences of study socioeconomic status, geographical factors, heterogeneity of study population and political concern of governments. The other possible explanation for the difference might be due to the unique nature of Ethiopia utilizing health extension workers.

This finding is also higher than the 2016 EDHS national and Amhara regional report [5].The possible reason for this difference may be the study area where EDHS included both women who lives in urban and rural areas of the country while our study includes only urban residents. Hence, women who live in urban areas are at a greater advantage of getting education opportunity and maternal health care services. Additionally, women in the urban areas may get easy access to health facility and health professionals as compared to their counterparts.

Postnatal care utilization of this study is higher than the research carried out in Sidama zone (Southern Ethiopia) 37.2% [20], Debre Markos town 33.5% [8], Abuna

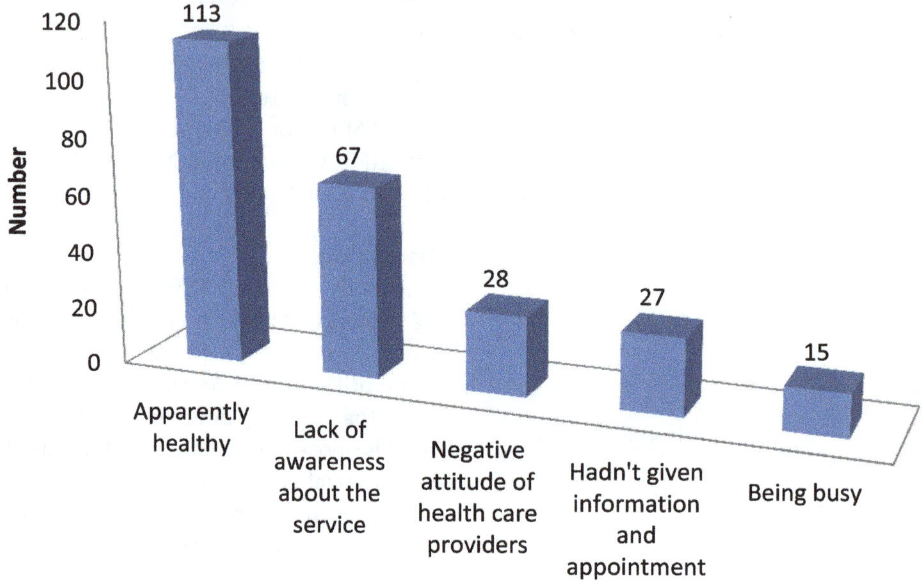

Fig. 1 Reasons for not attending postnatal care services given by the study participants at Debretabour town, North West Ethiopia, March 2017($n = 250$)

Gindeberet District, Oromiya 31.7% [21],Hadiya zone, South Ethiopia 22.7% [22], Dembecha District 34.8% [23], baseline and end line postnatal care surveys in Amhara and Oromia region [24], Jabitena district, Amhara regional state, 20.2% [25] and Lemo Woreda 51.4% [26].This difference may be due to time difference between these studies, socioeconomic status, and cultural factor. The Other possible explanation for these differences may be increased governmental focuses from year to year in order to improve maternal and neonatal healths.

According to this study, the odds of PNC service utilization among women with secondary school and above by education were 3 times than those who couldn't read and write. This finding is consistent with the study done in Nepal [14], Cambodia [27], rural area of Western Rajasthan, India [13], developing countries [18], Africa [17], Nigeria [28], Bahi District, Tanzania [9], rural India [29], Entoto Fana health center, Addis Ababa [30], rural Haramaya District, Eastern Ethiopia [31], southern Ethiopia [20], Abi-Adi Town, Tigray [32], Jabitena district, Amhara region [25] and Dembecha District, North West Ethiopia [23].The possible reasons for this similarity might be due to the fact that once a women is educated, her autonomy and decision making skill on her health and maternal health care services utilization is high [32].Similarly, uneducated mothers have no chance to participate in different social and economic positions, decision making and women's empowerment. Additionally, education helps to increase mothers' level of awareness and their acceptance of new idea and provides better education to other women regarding postnatal care services utilization.

In the present study, the odds of PNC service utilization among women with monthly income greater than 1500 ETB were 2.8 times than those who earn less than 500 ETB. This finding is consistent with a study done in developing countries [18], Rwanda [33], Nigeria [28], Tanzania [34], India [29], Nepal [14] and Addis Ababa, Ethiopia [30].

The possible suggestion for this might be women having better monthly income can afford for all expenses like for transportation.

The analysis also showed that, the odds of PNC service utilization among women with alive birth outcome were 5.7 times than those who gave still birth. This is in line with a study done in Debre Markos town [8]. The possible reason for this similarity may be good birth outcome might have better insight in postnatal care service utilization.

This study also showed that, the odds of PNC service utilization among women with desire of pregnancy were 4 times than those whose pregnancy was unplanned and unsupported. This finding is supported by a study done in three rural districts of Tanzania [35] and California [36].

This study also revealed that the odds of PNC service utilization among women who gave birth at health facility were 3 times than those who delivered at home. This finding is consistent with a study done in three rural districts of Tanzania [35], Rwanda [33], Nigeria [28], Tanzania [34], Nepal [14], Addis Ababa, Ethiopia [30], Hadiya zone, South Ethiopia [22], Debre Markos town [8], Lemo Woreda, Ethiopia [26] and another study done in Jabitena district, Amhara

Table 3 Logistic regression analysis of factors associated with postnatal care utilization of the respondents in Debretabour, Ethiopia, 2017(n = 588)

Variables	Postnatal care utilization		COR(CI)	AOR(CI)	*p*-values
Marital status	Yes	No			
Married	310	211	3.23 (1.50–6.96)	1.27 (0.44–3.68)	
Divorced	13	12	2.38 (0.80–7.04)	2.61 (0.77–8.85)	
Widowed	5	5	2.20 (0.51–9.35)	1.31 (0.24–6.96)	
Single	10	22	1.00	1.00	
Educational status of women					
Unable to read and write	38	64	1.00	1.00	
Can read and write	35	33	1.78 (0.95–3.32)	1.70 (0.88–3.28)	
Primary education	80	78	1.72 (1.03–2.87)	1.47 (0.86–2.53)	
Secondary education and above	185	75	4.15 (2.56–6.73)	3.29 (1.94–5.57)	0.000
Monthly income					
< 500 ETB	9	22	1.00	1.00	
500–1500 ETB	55	66	2.03 (0.86–4.78)	2.18 (0.88–5.41)	
> 1500 ETB	274	162	4.13 (1.85–9.19)	2.85 (1.21–6.68)	0.016
Decision making power on her health					
Self	52	55	1.47 (0.71–3.07)	1.75 (0.64–4.78)	
Both	270	170	2.48 (1.28–4.78)	1.59 (0.69–3.68)	
Husband	16	25	1.00	1.00	
Decision making power on her child health					
Self	38	51	0.88 (0.45–1.73)	0.99 (0.47–2.10)	
Both	274	168	1.94 (1.11–3.38)	1.36 (0.73–2.52)	
Husband	26	31	1.00	1.00	
Parity					
One	122	81	2.07 (1.02–4.18)	1.41 (0.61–3.24)	
Tow-four	200	147	1.87 (0.94–3.68)	1.16 (0.53–2.51)	
Five and above	16	22	1.00	1.00	
Birth outcome of the last pregnancy					
Alive	335	235	7.12 (2.04–24.89)	5.70 (1.53–21.21)	0.009
Still birth	3	15	1.00	1.00	
Nature of the last pregnancy					
Planned and supported	236	160	4.58 (2.10–9.98)	3.94 (1.72–9.01)	0.001
Unplanned but supported	93	62	4.66 (2.06–10.56)	4.40 (1.84–10.52)	0.001
Unplanned and unsupported	9	28	1.00	1.00	
Place of delivery					
Home	7	22	1.00	1.00	
Health facility	331	228	4.56 (1.91–10.85)	3.08 (1.24–7.68)	0.015

region [25].The possible explanation for the similarity between place of delivery and postnatal care services utilization can be evidenced by women who gave birth in health institutions have better opportunity to receive health education related to postnatal care services, get access on benefits and availabilities of PNC services during their stay in health facilities.

Limitation of the study

There could be recall bias since the women were asked for events within the last one year prior to the study. On the other hand the study did not include the rural population which is restricting the scope and relevance. Lastly, since the the design is quantitative it doesn't address cultural issues of the respondents.

Conclusion

This study demonstrated that utilization of postnatal care service is still low.

Educational status of the women, monthly household income, birth outcome of the latest pregnancy, wantedness of the last pregnancy and place of delivery were found to be statistically significant for the current PNC service Utilization.

Abbreviations

EDHS: Ethiopian demographic health survey; MDG: Millennium development goal; MMM: Maternal mortality ratio; PNC: Postnatal care; WHO: World health organization

Acknowledgments

The authors would like to pass their gratitude to Bahirdar University for the approval of ethical clearance. We would like to extend our thanks to Amhara Regional health Bureau, Debretabour health office and respected kebeles for permitting to conduct the study and providing the necessary preliminary information. The authors are also very grateful for data collectors and mothers who participated in this study.

Funding

Bahir Dar University. This study was done by the fund obtained from Bahir Dar University for the design and collection, analysis and interpretation of data. However, the funder has no specific role in the preparation of the manuscript.

Authors' contributions

KGW, AAN and SSG conceived and designed the protocol, performed the data collection, contributed for data analysis, wrote the paper and revised the manuscript. AAT and FYB participate on the editorial and data entry and analysis. All authors read and approved the final paper.

Competing interests

The authors declare that they have no competing interests.

References

1. WHO. Technical Consultation on Postpartum and Postnatal Care: Department of making pregnancy safer; Switzerland; World Health Organization. 2008.
2. WHO, UNFPA, the World Bank. Trends in maternal mortality: 1990 to 2010. World health organization, UNICEF, UNFPA, and the World Bank 2012.
3. Addis Ababa, Maryland, USA: Central Statistical Agency and ICF International; 2012. Central Statistical Agency [Ethiopia] and ICF International: Ethiopia Demographic and Health Survey 2011.
4. Alkema L, Chou D, Hogan D, Zhang S, Moller A-B, Gemmill A, et al. Global, regional, and national levels and trends in maternal mortality between 1990 and 2015, with scenario-based projections to 2030: a systematic analysis by the UN maternal mortality estimation inter-agency group. Lancet. 2016; 387(10017):462–74.
5. Central Statistical Agency [Ethiopia] and ICF International. Ethiopia demographic and health survey 2016 report Addis Ababa, Maryland, USA: central statistical agency and ICF international. Ethiopia demographic and health survey 2016 report Addis Ababa. Rockville, Maryland. In: USA: central statistical agency and ICF international; 2016.
6. FDRE MOH. National reproductive health strategy: 2006–2015. Ministry of health: Department of FH Addis Ababa; 2006.
7. FDRE, MOH. Postnatal Care Blended Learning Module for Health Extension program Ethiopia.
8. Limenih MA, Endale ZM, Dachew BA. Postnatal care service utilization and associated factors among women who gave birth in the last 12 months prior to the study in Debre Markos town, northwestern Ethiopia: a community-based cross-sectional study. International Journal of Reproductive Medicine. 2016;2016.
9. James L, John S, Angelina S. Utilization of maternal postnatal care services among women in selected villages of Bahi District, Tanzania. Curr Res J Soc Sci. 2015;7(4):106–11.
10. Senait B. Assessment of prevalence of postnatal care utilization and associated factors among women who gave birth and attending immunization clinic in selected government health centers in Addis Ababa, Ethiopia, 2015: AAU; 2015.
11. Tesfahun F, Worku W, Mazengiya F, Kifle M. Knowledge, perception and utilization of postnatal care of mothers in Gondar Zuria District, Ethiopia: a cross-sectional study. Matern Child Health J. 2014;18(10):2341–51.
12. Berhe H, Tilahun W, Aregay A, Bruh G, Gebremedhin HGH. Utilization and associated factors of postnatal care in Adwa town, tigray, Ethiopia-a cross sectional study a Peer Reviewed. International Journal for Pharmaceutical and Allied Research. 2012;3(1).
13. Sandeep Kumar Uppadhaya SB, Sivodia SK, et al. Utilization of postnatal care services in rural area of Western Rajasthan, India. National Journal of Community Medicine, July. 2016:7(7).
14. Khanal V, Adhikari M, Karkee R, Gavidia T. Factors associated with the utilization of postnatal care services among the mothers of Nepal: analysis of Nepal demographic and health survey 2011. BMC Womens Health. 2014; 14(1):19.
15. Dhaher E, Mikolajczyk R, Maxwell A, Krämer A. Factors associated with lack of postnatal care among Palestinian women: a cross-sectional study of three clinics in the West Bank. BMC pregnancy and childbirth. 2008;8(1):26.
16. J.Izudi D. Use of early postnatal care among postpartum women in eastern Uganda. Int J Gynecol Obstet. 2015;129:161–4.
17. Yugbare DKS, Goujon A, et al. A review of factors associated with the utilization of health care services and strategies for improving postpartum care in Africa. Afrika Focus. 2015;28(2):83–105.
18. Adhikari C, Yadav RK, Timilshina P, Ojha R, Gaire D, Ghimire A. Proportion and factors affecting for post-natal care utilization in developing countries: a systematic review. Journal of Manmohan Memorial Institute of Health Sciences. 2016;2:14–9.
19. Al. De. Opportunities to improve postpartum care for mothers and infants: design of context -specific packages of postpartum interventions in rural districts in four sub-Saharan African countries. BMC Pregnancy and Childbirth. 2015;15(131):1–11.
20. Regassa N. Antenatal and postnatal care service utilization in southern Ethiopia: a population-based study. African health sciences. 2011;11(3).
21. Birhanu Darega ND, Fikru Tafese and Shimeles Ololo. Institutional delivery and postnatal care services utilizations in Abuna Gindeberet District, west Shewa, Oromiya region, Central Ethiopia: a community-based cross sectional study BMC Pregnancy and Childbirth 2016;16(149).
22. Al ZAe. Magnitude and predictors of postnatal care utilization in Hadiya zone, South Ethiopia. International Journal of Current Research. 2015;7(11): 23176–82.
23. Hordofa M, Almaw S, Berhanu M, Lemiso H. Postnatal Care Service Utilization and Associated Factors Among Women in Dembecha District. Northwest Ethiopia. 2015;3(5):686–92.
24. Tesfaye S, Barry D, Gobezayehu AG, Frew AH, Stover KE, Tessema H, et al. Improving coverage of postnatal care in rural Ethiopia using a community-based, collaborative quality improvement approach. Journal of Midwifery & Women's Health. 2014;59(s1):S55–64.
25. Workineh YG, Hailu DA. Factors affecting utilization of postnatal care service in Jabitena district, Amhara region Ethiopia. Sci J Public Health. 2014;23: 169–76.
26. Tefera B, Ayanos T,Tamiru B. Postnatal care service utilization and associated factors among mothers in Lemo Woreda, Ethiopia Women's Health Care 2016; 5(3).
27. Ith P, Dawson A, Homer C, Whelan A. Practices of skilled birth attendants during labour, birth and the immediate postpartum period in Cambodia. Midwifery. 2013;29(4):300–7.

28. Ibisomi Sa. Determinants of postnatal care non-utilization among women in Nigeria. BMC Res Notes 2016; 9(21).
29. Singh PK, Alagarajan M, Singh L. Determinants of maternity care services utilization among married adolescents in rural India. PLoS One. 2012;7(2).
30. Admassu EA. Factors associated with postnatal care utilization at Entoto Fana health center, Gullele sub-city. Addis Ababa: International Journal of Medical Science and Public Health August; 2015.
31. Dereje Kifle TA, Yalemzewod Assefa Gelaw and Yayehirad Alemu Melsew. Maternal health care service seeking behaviors and associated factors among women in rural Haramaya District, eastern Ethiopia: a triangulated community-based cross-sectional study Reprod Health 2017; 14(6).
32. Alemayeh H, Assefa H, Adama Y. Prevalence and factors associated with post Natal Care utilization in Abi-Adi town, Tigray, Ethiopia: A Cross Sectional Study.
33. Al. Re. Factors associated with postnatal care utilisation in Rwanda: a secondary analysis of 2010 demographic and health survey data BMC Pregnancy and Childbirth 2016; 16(122).
34. James Lwelamira JSaAS. Utilization of maternal postnatal care services among women in selected villages of Bahi District. Tanzania Current Research Journal of Social Sciences. 2015;7(4):106–11.
35. Al. Ke. Factors associated with compliance with the recommended frequency of postnatal care services in three rural districts of Tanzania BMC Pregnancy and Childbirth 2015; 15(341).
36. DiBari JN, Yu SM, Chao SM, Lu MC. Use of postpartum care: predictors and barriers. J Pregnancy. 2014.

15

Physical activity for antenatal and postnatal depression in women attempting to quit smoking

Amanda Daley[1*], Muhammad Riaz[2], Sarah Lewis[3], Paul Aveyard[4], Tim Coleman[5], Isaac Manyonda[6], Robert West[7], Beth Lewis[8], Bess Marcus[9], Adrian Taylor[10], Judith Ibison[11], Andrew Kent[11] and Michael Ussher[12,13]

Abstract

Background: Antenatal depression is associated with harmful consequences for both the mother and child. One intervention that might be effective is participation in regular physical activity although data on this question in pregnant smokers is currently lacking.

Methods: Women were randomised to six-weekly sessions of smoking cessation behavioural-support, or to the same support plus 14 sessions combining treadmill exercise and physical activity consultations.

Results: Among 784 participants (mean gestation 16-weeks), EPDS was significantly higher in the physical activity group versus usual care at end-of-pregnancy (mean group difference (95% confidence intervals (CIs)): 0.95 (0.08 to 1.83). There was no significant difference at six-months postpartum.

Conclusion: A pragmatic intervention to increase physical activity in pregnant smokers did not prevent depression at end-of-pregnancy or at six-months postpartum. More effective physical activity interventions are needed in this population.

Keywords: Pregnancy, Physical activity, Antenatal, Postnatal, Depression

Background

Ten to 20 % of pregnant women become depressed during or after pregnancy [1, 2]. Antenatal depression is associated with harmful consequences for the mother and child, including premature labour, low birth weight, and a compromised mother-child relationship [3–5]. Postnatal depression can adversely affect children's cognitive and emotional development and social behaviour [6]. Antidepressants are effective for treating depression outside of pregnancy [7], but are seldom prescribed during pregnancy due to concerns about potential adverse effects on the fetus or infant [8]. Psychological therapies can be effective [9], but there can be long waiting lists to access treatment and they can be costly. It is important to find alternative effective interventions. One intervention that might be effective is participation in regular physical activity. Thirty minutes of moderate intensity physical activity per day is recommended for mental health benefits during pregnancy [10–13]. However, this guidance is based on studies with non-pregnant individuals and may have limited applicability to pregnant and postnatal populations.

The evidence for using physical activity to prevent or treat depression in pregnancy is mixed: meta-analyses provide evidence for physical activity interventions reducing depression scores both during pregnancy (six trials, $n = 364$) and postnatal (five trials $n = 221$) [14, 15], however, there was significant heterogeneity between trials. Also, the reviewed studies were judged to be of poor to moderate quality. A more recent meta-analysis of antenatal interventions to reduce maternal distress, including depression, did not consider any physical activity trials

* Correspondence: a.daley@lboro.ac.uk
[1]Sport, Exercise and Health Sciences, Loughborough University, Epinal Way, Loughborough, Leicestershire LE11 3TU, UK
Full list of author information is available at the end of the article

as being rigorous enough to be included [16]. Further trials that postdate these systematic reviews showed no benefit of physical activity for preventing antenatal or postnatal depression, [17, 18]. Subsequent trials however have showed a benefit for an exercise intervention for reducing depression during pregnancy and postnatally, although one study did not report exercise adherence [19] and the other failed to show a significant difference in physical activity between the intervention and usual care groups at follow up [20]. There is a need, therefore, for more robust evidence. The recently completed London Exercise and Pregnant Smokers (LEAP) trial investigated whether behavioural support to enhance a woman's physical activity at home, combined with twice-weekly supervised exercise sessions, would increase rates of continuous and biochemically validated smoking abstinence at end of pregnancy [21]. The main rationale for physical activity aiding smoking cessation is the evidence for exercise reducing cigarette cravings and withdrawal symptoms. [22, 23] The LEAP intervention was ineffective at aiding cessation [24].

As a secondary outcome, the present study assessed the effect of the LEAP intervention on antenatal and postnatal depression, in the largest randomised controlled trial (RCT) to date. The outcomes were change in depression from baseline to end-of-pregnancy and six months after birth. In the UK, approximately 12% of pregnant women smoke throughout pregnancy [25] and these women are at heightened risk of depression during pregnancy [26]. We hypothesised that exercise counselling and provision of regular supervised exercise would reduce depression compared with usual care.

Methods

Participants

Pregnant women were recruited via 13 hospital antenatal clinics across the UK. All the hospitals were in localities that included areas of deprivation and social housing. The inclusion criteria for the trial were a desire to stop smoking, wanting help to stop smoking, agreeing to set a date for quitting smoking within one week of the baseline assessment, aged 16-50 years, being between 10 and 24 weeks of gestation, cigarette consumption of five or more daily before pregnancy, currently smoking one or more cigarettes per day, and being able to walk continuously for at least 15 min. Women were not eligible if they had health conditions that had potential to be exacerbated by exercise or advised not to exercise by a medical doctor, unable to provide informed consent or complete the study questionnaires in English, dependence on drugs or alcohol, and currently using or wanting to use nicotine replacement therapy. Written informed consent was obtained from all participants.

Design and interventions

This study reports analysis of depression outcomes from a RCT evaluating the effect of a physical activity intervention on smoking cessation during pregnancy [21]. At the first session, participants were randomly assigned (based on a computer-generated code) to either behavioural cessation support alone (usual care) or to this support plus a physical activity intervention. In the primary analysis, the rates of continuous biochemically validated smoking cessation at end of pregnancy were similar in the physical activity group (7.7%) and usual care group (6.4%) [24].

Intervention

Participants were offered the opportunity to take part in six weekly sessions of 20 min of individual behavioural support for smoking cessation, starting one week before the smoking quit date and ending four weeks later. This intervention seeked to support smoking cessation by reinforcing commitment to abstinence and solving participants' problems about maintaining smoking abstinence. The intervention also aimed to improve the mental health of women.

The physical activity intervention combined supervised exercise sessions with physical activity consultations. All sessions were individual and took place in a private room at the hospital or in a community health centre or children's centre. Fourteen sessions of supervised exercise were offered over eight weeks; twice a week for six weeks, followed by weekly sessions for two weeks. At each session participants were asked to walk at a moderate intensity on a treadmill for up to 30 min. At the first two treadmill sessions, and then on alternate occasions (total of nine consultations), they received the physical activity consultations, which aimed to identify opportunities to incorporate physical activity into women's daily lives and to help them use behavioural strategies to improve adherence to these plans. These 20 min consultations incorporated 19 behaviour change techniques, as previously described in the protocol [21]. Participants were advised to be active for at least 10 bouts, progressing towards 30 min of activity on at least five days a week, with an emphasis on brisk walking. As a motivational tool (not a research measure), participants were given a pedometer (Digi-Walker SW-200; Yamax, Nottingham, UK) and were encouraged to record the number of steps they had achieved each day, with the researcher calculating a 10% increment every two weeks; the overall goal being to work towards accumulating 10,000 steps per day [27]. Participants received £7 for their travel expenses for each session that they attended and were given a DVD on antenatal exercise. On the other occasion the women received behavioural support for smoking sessions (up to six sessions) as for the usual care group.

Measures

One week prior to the quit date, baseline data was collected for demographic variables, smoking characteristics and physical activity behaviours, including the Fagerström Test for Cigarette Dependence score (FTCD, [28, 29]) and self-reported levels of moderate and vigorous intensity physical activity (MVPA) in the previous week using a seven-day physical activity interview [30]. Self-reports of physical activity included all types of activity, irrespective of context (e.g., leisure, occupational). Depression was measured with the Edinburgh Postnatal Depression Scale (EPDS [31], via a face-to-face consultation at baseline and at end of pregnancy and via telephone at six months after the birth. The EPDS is a self-report 10-item scale (each is scored 0-3, range = 0 to 30) designed to assess antenatal and postnatal depression in community samples [32], is widely used and has been validated in many countries [33]. It can be used as a continuous outcome or to classify women as probable cases of antenatal/postnatal depression at a cut-off of 13 or above [34]. Further self-reports of physical activity levels were collected at weeks one, four, and six after the quit date, at end of pregnancy and six months after the birth. In an 11.5% random subsample of participants (the target was 10%) physical activity was objectively measured using an accelerometer (Model GT1M or GT3X; Actigraph, Pensacola, FL, USA). This was worn over the right hip, in the fourth week after the quit date, for seven consecutive days, recording 'dry land' activity during waking hours at one minute epochs.

Analysis & Sample Size

Details of the sample size calculation can be found in previous publications. [21, 24] First, we checked whether those providing EPDS data at the two follow-ups (end-of-pregnancy, six months postnatal) had similar baseline characteristics and physical activity at follow-up as the whole sample. Then we examined whether the baseline characteristics of the physical activity versus usual care group were similar in the sub-samples with EPDS data at the two follow-ups.

For the primary analysis EPDS data was treated as a continuous variable. We used a mixed-effect linear model with EPDS scores at end-of-pregnancy and six months postnatally as dependent variables. To estimate the difference between physical activity and usual care groups at each follow-up adjusting for baseline EPDS and recruitment centre, we fitted a linear mixed effect model including as independent variables the interaction of treatment groups and follow-up times, follow-up times, recruitment centre and the interaction of baseline EPDS score with follow-up times. The model accounts for within-person correlation over time and assumes that data is missing completely at random for the participants with missing EPDS data at follow-ups. In the next step, we further adjusted for the following potential predictors of postnatal depression: marital status, age at leaving full time education (as a proxy for socioeconomic status), body mass index and young age (i.e., age < 20 years). At end-of-pregnancy about half of the women (201/383, 52.5%) provided EPDS data before the birth and half after the birth (182/383, 47.5%); therefore we examined the difference between the mean EPDS scores before and after the birth using t-tests.

As a secondary analysis EPDS was treated as a binary variable. We assessed whether the proportion reaching the EPDS cut-off of ≥ 13 for depression changed at the follow-ups, for physical activity versus usual care, relative to baseline. We used a mixed effect logistic regression model, with the same independent variables as before, to estimate the adjusted odds ratios (OR) of depression for physical activity group versus usual at end-of-pregnancy and 6 month follow-up. This analysis was further adjusted for the same predictors used in the analyses of EPDS as a continuous variable. One recommendation is to use a EPDS cut-off of ≥ 15 antenatally and ≥ 13 postnatally [35], therefore we conducted a further analysis using ≥ 15 for baseline and end-of-pregnancy follow-up before the birth, and ≥ 13 for end-of-pregnancy after the birth. Additionally, in order to explore whether adverse events might have influenced the EPDS outcomes we report these events for the two study groups.

We used multiple imputation analysis to explore the impact of missing data Missing values in the EPDS score at follow-up were replaced by imputed values using chained equations [36] with the predictive mean matching method on the basis of the baseline explanatory variables of EPDS scores at baseline, randomisation groups, body mass index, carbon monoxide level, smoking abstinence at end-of-pregnancy, self-reported minutes of physical activity at baseline, age at leaving full-time education, gestational age (weeks) at baseline, number of cigarettes smoked before pregnancy, number of cigarettes smoked at baseline, FTCD score, marital status, ethnicity, type of physical activity at baseline, parity, partner smoking status, self-efficacy, confidence for physical activity, recruitment centre, perceived positive effects of being physically active. We created twenty imputed datasets and used the same model as above to estimate the treatment effects on EPDS score in these datasets. We combined the imputation-specific estimates using Rubin's rules [37]. All statistical analyses were performed using Stata (version 12).

To explore whether the effect of treatment on depression scores differed according to how physically active the women were at baseline, we tested for an interaction between baseline physical activity (< 150 min/week MVPA versus ≥ 150 min/week MVPA) and the treatment effect for the primary outcome of EPDS score at both follow-ups.

We also explored whether those who adhered better to the physical activity regime had a greater response to treatment by looking at modification of the treatment effect according to whether the individual reported ≥ 150 min/week MVPA at four weeks or six weeks after the quit day in those reporting < 150 min/week MVPA at baseline.

Results

Between April 2009 and November 2012 a total of 789 participants were recruited and randomised. This was 10% of the women recorded as smokers at their first antenatal booking visit (see Fig. 1). Four women were excluded after randomisation; two women in the intervention group were randomised twice in sequential pregnancies and their second enrolment was removed, and two participants in the usual care group were ineligible at their baseline visit and had been randomised erroneously. When using an intention to treat approach it is acceptable to exclude patients' data, without risking bias, when ineligible patients are mistakenly randomised into a trial [38]. One participant was randomised but withdrew consent without giving any reason, before providing any data. A total of 784 women were randomised and included in this study.

EPDS data was provided by all 784 participants at baseline; by 383 (49%) at the end of pregnancy, and by

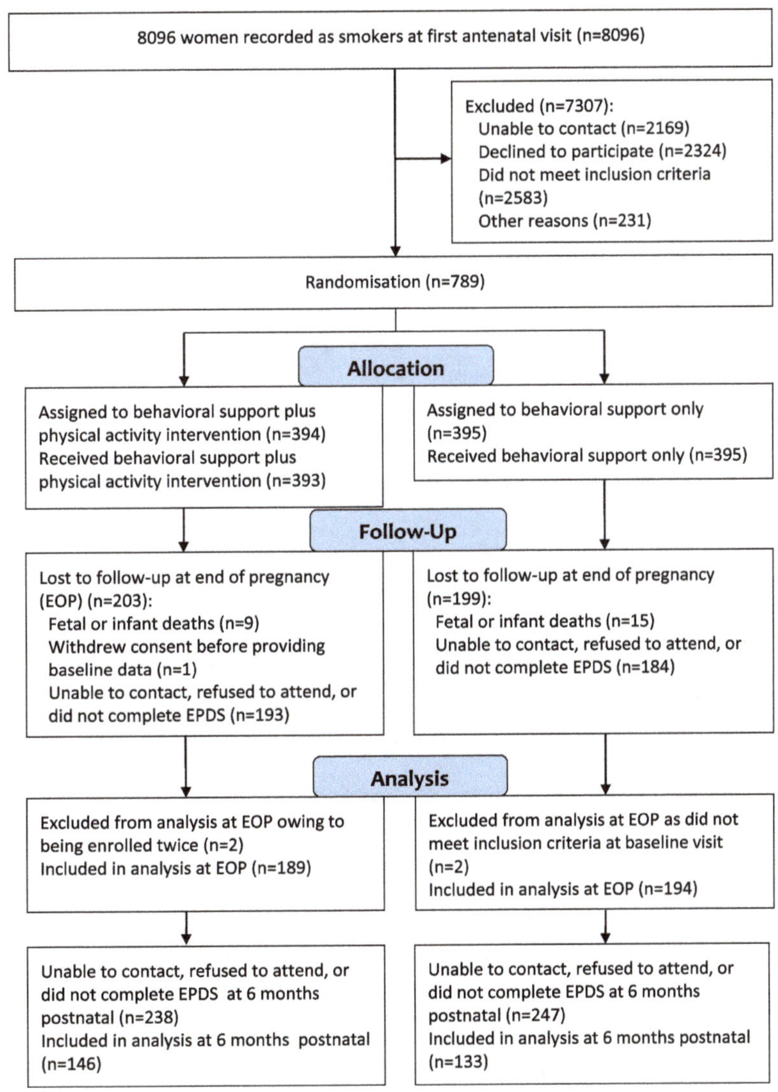

Fig. 1 Numbers of participants who were enrolled in the study and included in the analyses for Edinburgh Postnatal Depression Scale score (EPDS). The participants lost to follow-up included some who had fetal or infant loss and were not assessed for EPDS score

279 (36%) at six-months postnatally (see Fig. 1). The baseline characteristics of those with EPDS data available at end-of-pregnancy and six months were similar to those of recruits as a whole (see Table 1). The baseline characteristics of the trial groups were also very similar and these have been reported elsewhere [24]. In addition, the baseline characteristics and physical activity levels at follow-up were similar for women who did and did not report on their depression.

Participants attended a median (IQR) of four (2-8) treatment sessions in the intervention group and three (2-6) in the usual care group. As reported previously [24], for the physical activity group, compared with the usual care group, the self-reported minutes of MVPA

Table 1 Characteristics for participants in the total trial sample and in the sub-samples providing EPDS data at end-of-pregnancy and 6 months postnatally

	Total sample $n = 784$	End-of-pregnancy $n = 383$	6 months $n = 279$
	Mean (SD)	Mean (SD)	Mean (SD)
Age	27.5 (6.3)	27.7 (6.2)	28.1 (6.2)
Age left full-time education	17.7 (2.9)	17.9 (2.8)	18.0 (2.9)
Weight at booking – kg	68.3 (15.2)	68.8(15.4)	68.9 (15.9)
Body Mass Index kg/m^2	26.1 (5.3)	26.0 (5.2)	26.1 (5.5)
Gestational age – wk	15.6 (3.3)	15.3 (3.2)	15.4 (3.1)
	Median (IQR)	Median (IQR)	Median (IQR)
Fagerström Test of Cigarette Dependence score	4.0 (2.0-5.0)	4.0 (2.0-5.0)	4.0 (2.0-5.0)
EPDS score at baseline	7.0 (3.5-11.0)	8.0 (4.0-12.0)	7.0 (4.0-11.0)
Self-report of weekly MVPA	210.0	210.0	210.0
– mins (at baseline)	(130.0-355.0)	(125.0-330)	(120.0-340.0)
Self-report of weekly MVPA	150.0	150.0	140.0
– mins (at EOP)[a]	(75.0-240.0)	(75.0-240.0)	(70.0-240.0)
Self-report of weekly MVPA	162.5	165.0	155.0
– mins (at 6 months follow up)	(60.0-300.0)	(80.0-310.0)	(60.0-300.0)
Treatment sessions attended[a]	3 (2-6)	6 (3-7)	5(3-7)
	n (%)	n (%)	n (%)
Allocation to physical Activity group	392 (50)	189 (49)	140 (52)
IMD[b] quartiles 3 or 4	555 (74)	259 (71)	191 (72)
Married or living with partner	451 (58)	224 (59)	181 (65)
Caucasian	607 (77)	301 (79)	226 (81)
Professional/managerial occupation	99 (13)	48 (13)	39 (14)
EPDS score at baseline ≥ 13	143 (18)	51 (13)	29 (10)
Thought of harming oneself (EPDS)	20 (3)	11 (3)	7 (3)
Self-report of ≥ 150 mins week MVPA (baseline)	548 (70)	266 (70)	185 (66)
Parity (range = 0 to 5)			
0-1	606 (78)	301 (79)	220 (79)
2-3	155 (20)	75 (20)	54 (19)
≥ 4	21 (3)	7 (2)	5 (2)
Takes alcohol ≥ twice a week	11 (1)	6 (2)	5 (2)
Consumes ≥ 3 alcoholic drinks on a drinking day	17 (10)	7 (8)	6 (10)

EPDS Edinburgh Post-natal Depression Scale, *EOP* End of pregnancy, *IMD* Index of Multiple Deprivation, *MVPA* Moderate and vigorous physical activity. [a]Non-baseline measure [b]*N* = 752 as there were 12 missing postcodes and 20 invalid post codes

were significantly higher by 33% (95% CI: 14, 56%), 28% (7, 52%), and 36% (12, 65%) at one week, four weeks and six weeks, respectively; while among the 11% of participants wearing an accelerometer MVPA levels were very similar for the two study groups.

Primary analysis

EPDS score was significantly higher in the physical activity group versus the usual care group at end-of-pregnancy with both the basic adjustments and in the fully adjusted model (see Table 2). At this time, there was mean increase in EPDS score of 0.4 in the physical activity group and a mean reduction of 0.5 in the usual care group (mean difference between groups (95% CIs) in fully adjusted model: 0.95 (0.08 to 1.83)). At end-of-pregnancy, the EPDS scores did not differ significantly between women who provided data before birth and those who provided after birth. There was no significant difference in EPDS score between the groups at six-months postnatal (fully adjusted mean difference (95% CIs): 0.37(− 0.59 to 1.33)). There was no significant interaction between baseline self-reports of MVPA (< 150 vs ≥ 150 min/week physical activity) and the treatment effect at either time point (at end-of-pregnancy: $p = 0.346$; at 6 months follow up: $p = 0.607$); similar results were found for the fully adjusted model. At end-of-pregnancy, the effect of physical activity was different in those who did and those who did not increase their exercise between baseline and four weeks post quit; for those who did increase, the estimated difference between (95% CI) physical activity versus control was 3.48 (1.46 to 5.51), $p = 0.001$, and for those who did not increase it was 1.14 (− 0.60 to 2.89), $p = 0.199$, but these differences were not significant at 6 months follow-up.

EPDS data as a binary outcome

When treating the EPDS score as a binary variable (i.e., using a cut-off score of ≥13) there was no significant difference between the groups at either follow-up point, although the ORs showed a slightly higher risk of probable depression in the physical activity versus usual care group (fully adjusted OR (95% CIs): 1.11 (0.47 to 2.65; 1. 07 (0.36 to 3.17), for end-of-pregnancy and six months, respectively) (see Table 3). Similar results were produced when using an EPDS cut-off of ≥15 at baseline and end-of-pregnancy (before birth), and ≥ 13 at end-of-pregnancy (after birth).

When we used multiple imputation as an alternative way of dealing with missing data the results were very similar; in particular, the fully adjusted mean difference (95% CIs) in EPDS score between treatment and control groups at end-of-pregnancy was 0.98 (0.10 to 1.85), $p = 0.029$ and at 6 months it was 0.33 (− 0.71 to 1.38), $p = 0.526$.

The rate of at least one adverse event was very similar for the two trial groups (217 (55.5%), 219 (55.7%), in the physical activity and usual care groups, respectively).

Discussion

Main findings

Among pregnant women there was significantly increased depression scores at the end of pregnancy but there was no difference six months after birth. When depression was considered as a binary outcome (those with and without probable depression) there was no evidence of a difference between treatment arms at either follow up. These results emerged despite the physical activity group reporting significantly more minutes of moderate and vigorous physical activity throughout pregnancy.

Our findings are consistent with two trials observing that physical activity did not reduce depression scores/prevalence before or after pregnancy [17, 18], but differ from meta-analyses and recent trials showing benefits for physical activity on both antenatal and postnatal depression [14, 15, 19, 20]. However, there were methodological limitations in these studies and this raises the possibility that the effect of physical activity on depression could have been over-estimated by these trials. This study joins other well conducted trials that have

Table 2 Comparison[a] of depression scores in two trial groups at end-of-pregnancy and six months after birth ($N = 784$[d])

Visit time	EPDS score N, Mean (SD)		β (difference between PA and usual care, basic adjustment[b]) (95% CI)	β (difference between PA and usual care group, fully adjusted[c]) (95% CI)
	Usual care group	Physical activity group		
baseline	393, 7.7 (5.0)	391, 7.6 (5.3)		
End of pregnancy	194, 7.2 (5.0)	189, 8.0 (4.9)	1.06 (0.19, 1.94) $p = 0.017$	0.95 (0.08, 1.83) $p = 0.033$
6 months follow-up	133, 6.6 (4.7)	146, 6.8 (4.8)	0.52 (−0.45, 1.50), $p = 0.293$	0.37 (−0.59, 1.33) $p = 0.450$

EPDS Edinburgh Postnatal Depression Scale, *PA* Physical activity
[a]Results from mixed effect linear model
[b]Adjusted for visit time, baseline EPDS, recruitment centre, the interaction of baseline EPDS and visit time
[c]Adjusted for visit time, baseline EPDS, recruitment centre, the interaction of baseline EPDS and visit time, age at leaving full time education, young age (≤ 20 yrs), BMI, marital status
[d]For the final mixed effect model, $N = 436$

Table 3 Comparison[a] of EPDS score indicating presence or absence of depression in trial groups at end-of-pregnancy and six months after birth ($N = 784$)

Visit time	Depression in each randomisation group		Odds Ratio for PA versus usual care, basic adjustment[b] (95% CI)	Odds Ratio for PA versus usual care, fully adjusted[c] (95% CI) (95% CI)
	Usual care n/N (%)	Physical Activity n/N (%)		
Baseline	75/393 (19)	68/391 (17)	–	–
End of pregnancy	25/194 (12)	26/189 (14)	1.24 (0.52, 2.96) $p = 0.628$	1.11 (0.47, 2.65) $p = 0.808$
6 months follow-up	14/133 (11)	15/146 (10)	1.23 (0.41, 3.70) $p = 0.710$	1.07 (0.36, 3.17) $p = 0.904$

EPDS Edinburgh Postnatal Depression Scale, *PA* Physical activity
[a]Results from mixed effect logistic model for depression (yes = 1, No = 0)
[b]Adjusted for visit time, baseline EPDS scores, the interaction of visit time and baseline EPDS, and recruitment centre
[c]Adjusted for visit time, baseline EPDS scores, the interaction of visit time and baseline EPDS scores, recruitment centre, age at leaving full time education, young age (≤ 20 yrs), BMI, marital status
For the final mixed effect model, $N = 436$

recruited non-pregnant populations which have reported that exercise interventions do not improve depression outcomes [39].

Interpretation in light of other findings

Several explanations are possible for our findings. Women recruited were more active than average, perhaps because active women were attracted to a trial promoting physical activity. This could suggest a ceiling effect where provision of behavioural support to increase activity was ineffective in already active women. We examined whether the effect on depression was greater in women who were inactive at baseline and found no evidence among this subgroup, but there was evidence that depression worsened among women who became active in the intervention group. Taken together, these results suggest that data remain at odds with that from other trials which tend to point towards a benefit from exercise, not an adverse effect, as here.

An alternative explanation is that the difference in the increase in physical activity between the study groups may be less than indicated by the self-reported results and this is supported by the accelerometer results which suggested that physical activity levels were similar in the two groups. Thus, it is possible that the physical activity group did not truly increase their physical activity, as intended. A further explanation relates to the population of interest and the requirements of the intervention. Those in the intervention group were asked to change two health behaviours simultaneously (i.e., smoking and physical activity) while also coping with being pregnant, in addition to dealing with the demands of being asked to attend multiple treatment sessions. These demands might have demoralised some individuals, and they may have found this difficult to achieve, resulting in marginally higher depression scores at the end of pregnancy. It is also possible that treadmill walking/gym based exercise may not be the ideal mode of physical activity and women may well have benefitted more from activity undertaken outside.

Strengths and limitations

The mental health of pregnant smokers is an important clinical question. There has been no other adequately powered trial of pregnant women and exercise, so this study adds new knowledge. This study included a large sample of women ($N = 784$) and the prevalence of probable cases of depression at baseline and follow-up in the usual care group was marginally higher than typical prevalence levels reported in the literature [40], which would be expected among smokers, and this maximises our ability to detect differences due to treatment. Participants were recruited directly from several hospitals in the UK at their antenatal appointment (typically 10-12 weeks of pregnancy) and a large proportion were of non-white ethnicity (23%) and/or living in the two highest IMD deprivation quartiles (74%). This is important as these populations of women can be difficult to recruit and they are the groups at greatest risk of depression, again maximising the ability to detect treatment effects. Attendance at treatment sessions was modest but this was a pragmatic trial of a behavioural intervention that was conducted in a 'real life' NHS setting and women in the intervention group still reported significantly higher physical activity scores than those receiving usual care. Other high quality trials[39] that have had modest to good adherence have also failed to demonstrate an effect for exercise on depression, so our findings may be unrelated to session adherence. We did not include an objective assessment of physical activity behaviour in all women and as previously observed [41], accelerometer validation suggests that participants overestimated their self-reported physical activity.

Less than half the women enrolled provided data on depression at both follow-up points. The relatively low follow-up rates may be because women who have relapsed to smoking are often reluctant to attend further appointments. Loss to follow-up could have introduced bias but women who gave data appeared to have no systematic differences from the whole population. Also, the findings were very similar when using the imputed data. Nonetheless it is unlikely that loss to follow up led to the non-significant effects because we would have to assume that women who failed to be followed up showed a marked improvement in mood while those who remained in the study showed no change or worsening and usually the opposite is the case.

This study reports an outcome from a trial that was powered to detect the effects on the primary outcome of the trial (i.e., smoking abstinence rates) and power calculations were not conducted for the secondary endpoint of EPDS scores. Depression scores did not differ significantly between the groups at six months postnatal follow-up and it is possible that the trial was insufficiently powered to detect this. However, neither the small effect size, nor those indicated as potential effect sizes on the basis of the 95% confidence interval, would be of clinical relevance. Thus, it seems unlikely that lack of power explains the results at six months follow up.

Conclusion

At the end of pregnancy the physical activity group did not report significantly lower depression scores than usual care; in fact the intervention group reported significantly higher depression scores, although the magnitude of this difference was small and unlikely to be clinically relevant [34, 42]. And when treating depression as a binary outcome there were no differences between the two study group. Depression scores did not differ significantly between the groups six months postnatally either. While clinical guidelines recommend that pregnant women exercise for mental health benefits and it is recommended that physical activity be used for treating depression among smokers, the pragmatic facilitated physical activity intervention used in the LEAP trial cannot be recommended as treatment or prevention for antenatal or postnatal depression in pregnant smokers. The lack of a beneficial effect of the intervention on depression scores could be partly explained by the possibility that intervention group did not increase their activity levels sufficiently relative to the usual care group, as reflected in the two groups having similar activity levels among the sub-sample with objectively measured physical activity. This suggests that more effective physical activity interventions may be needed in this population, rather than that physical activity cannot be recommended for moderating depression during pregnancy and postpartum.

Acknowledgements
We thank Dr. Melanie Poudevigne for advice about the assessment of depression.
We thank the following investigators for their contributions: Ory Bolooki (midwife), Janet Brown (midwife), Sarah Cleary (midwife), Caroline Dixon (midwife), Julie Fuller (midwife), Gail Harding (midwife), Maggie Hart (nurse), Tracey Kilbane (research assistant), Rachel Lex (midwife), Zoe Magrath (midwife), Ilia Papachristou (research assistant), Beth Steff (midwife), and Bettina Wanninkhof (midwife). We thank the independent members of the trial steering committee: Jim Thornton (chair), Ann McNeill, Sue Cooper, Kim Watts, and Serena Cox, and we thank Dale Esliger for assistance with analysing and interpreting the accelerometer data.

Funding
This study was funded by the NIHR Health Technology Assessment programme (grant 07.01.14). The funder had no role in the design and conduct of the study; collection, management, analysis, and interpretation of the data; preparation, review, or approval of the manuscript; or decision to submit the manuscript for publication.

Tweetable abstract
Physical activity does not reduce antenatal or postnatal depression in pregnant smokers.

Authors' contributions
MU, TC, SL, PA, IM, RW, BL, BM, and AT conceived the study, wrote the protocol, and obtained funding. MU managed the day to day running of the trial, including all participant follow-up. MR, SL, and MU designed the data analysis. AD, AK and JI advised on the study design and assisted in the design of the analysis for maternal depression. MR conducted all the analyses. All authors had full access to the data, take responsibility for the integrity of the data and the accuracy of the data analysis, contributed to the interpretation of the results, and reviewed and approved the final manuscript. MU, AD and MR drafted the manuscript and MU is the guarantor. The views and opinions expressed in this article are those of the authors and do not necessarily reflect those of the National Institute for Health Research (NIHR) health technology assessment programme, the NIHR, the National Health Service, or the English Department of Health. All authors read and approved the final manuscript.

Competing interests
All authors have completed the ICMJE uniform disclosure form at and declare: no support from any organisation for the submitted work; in the past three years PA has done one day of consultancy for Pfizer concerning general smoking cessation advice and not about particular products and RW has undertaken research and consultancy for companies (Pfizer and GSK) that develop and manufacture smoking cessation drugs; in the past three years TC has been paid for speaking at two educational events that were part or wholly sponsored by a company (Pierre Fabre Laboratories, France) that manufactures nicotine replacement therapy; RW is an unpaid trustee of the stop smoking charity QUIT and an unpaid director of the National Centre for Smoking Cessation and Training; there are no other relationships or activities that could appear to have influenced the submitted work.

Author details
[1]Sport, Exercise and Health Sciences, Loughborough University, Epinal Way, Loughborough, Leicestershire LE11 3TU, UK. [2]Population Health Research Institute, University of Leicester, University Road, Leicester LE1 7RH, UK. [3]Division of Epidemiology and Public Health and UK Centre for Tobacco and Alcohol Studies, University of Nottingham, Nottingham NG5 1PB, UK.

[4]Nuffield Department of Primary Care Health Sciences, Radcliffe Observatory Quarter, University of Oxford, Woodstock Road, Oxford OX2 6GG, UK. [5]Division of Primary Care and UK Centre for Tobacco and Alcohol Studies, University of Nottingham, Nottingham NG5 1PB, UK. [6]Department of Obstetrics and Gynecology, St George's University of London and St George's NHS Trust, Blackshaw Road, London SW17 0QT, UK. [7]Health Behaviour Research Centre, Department of Epidemiology and Public Health, UCL, Gower Street, London WC1E 6BT, UK. [8]School of Kinesiology, University of Minnesota, Minneapolis, MN 55455, USA. [9]Department of Family and Preventive Medicine, University of California, San Diego, CA 92093-0628, USA. [10]Plymouth University Peninsula Schools of Medicine and Dentistry, Plymouth Science Park, Plymouth, Devon PL6 8BX, UK. [11]Institute of Medical and Biomedical Education, St George's University of London, Cranmer Terrace, London SW17 0RE, UK. [12]Population Health Research Institute, St George's University of London, Cranmer Terrace, London SW17 0RE, UK. [13]Institute for Social Marketing, University of Stirling, Stirling, Stirling FK9 4LA, UK.

References

1. Banti S, Mauri M, Oppo A, Borri C, Rambelli C, Ramacciotti D, et al. From the third month of pregnancy to 1 year postpartum. Prevalence, incidence, recurrence, and new onset of depression. Results from the Perinatal Depression–Research & Screening Unit study. Compr Psychiatry. 2011;52:343–51.
2. Bennett HA, Einarson A, Taddio A, Koren G, Einarson TR. Prevalence of depression during pregnancy: systematic review. Obstet Gynecol. 2004;103:698–709.
3. Li D, Liu L, Odouli R. Presence of depressive symptoms during early pregnancy and the risk of preterm delivery: a prospective cohort study. Hum Reprod. 2009;24:46–53.
4. Wisner KL, Sit DK, Hanusa BH, Moses-Kolko EL, Bogen DL, Hunker DF, et al. Major depression and antidepressant treatment: impact on pregnancy and neonatal outcomes. Am J Psychiatry. 2009;166:557–66.
5. Cooper P, Murray L, Wilson A, Romaniuk H. Controlled trial of the short- and long-term effect of psychological treatment of post-partum depression: 1. Impact on maternal mood. Br J Psychiatry. 2003;182:412–9.
6. Murray L. The impact of postnatal depression on infant development. J Child Psychol Psychiatry. 1992;33:543–61.
7. Kendrick T, Chatwin J, Dowrick C, Tylee A, Morriss R, Peveler R, et al. Randomised controlled trial to determine the clinical effectiveness and cost-effectiveness of selective serotonin reuptake inhibitors plus supportive care, versus supportive care alone, for mild to moderate depression with somatic symptoms in primary care: the THREAD (THREshold for AntiDepressant response) study. Health Technol Assess. 2009;13:22.
8. Rai D, Lee BK, Dalman C, Golding J, Lewis G, Magnusson C. Parental depression, maternal antidepressant use during pregnancy, and risk of autism spectrum disorders: population based case-control study. BMJ. 2013;346:f2059.
9. Bower P, Knowles S, Coventry PA, Rowland N. Counselling for mental health and psychosocial problems in primary care. Cochrane Database Syst Rev. 2011;9:CD001025.
10. American College of Obstetrics and Gynecology. American College of Obstetrics and Gynecology committee opinion. Exercise during pregnancy and the postpartum period. Number 267, January 2002. Int J Gynaecol Obstet. 2002;77:79–81.
11. Cooney GM, Dwan K, Greig CA, Lawlor DA, Rimer J, Waugh FR, et al. Exercise for depression. Cochrane Database Syst Rev. 2013;9:CD004366.
12. National Institute for Health and Care Excellence. Antenatal and postnatal mental health. Clinical management and service guidance. *CG45*: National Institute for Health and Care Excellence; 2007. https://www.nice.org.uk/guidance/cg192. Accessed date 12 Oct 2016.
13. Royal College of Obstetricians and Gynaecologists. Recreational exercise and pregnancy: information for you. 2006. https://www.rcog.org.uk/globalassets/documents/patients/patient-information-leaflets/pregnancy/recreational-exercise-and-pregnancy.pdf. Accessed 03 Oct 2016.
14. Daley AJ, Jolly K, MacArthur C. The effectiveness of exercise in the management of postnatal depression: systematic review and meta-analysis. Fam Pract. 2009;26:154–62.
15. Daley AJ, Foster L, Long G, Palmer C, Robinson O, Walmsley H, et al. The effectiveness of exercise for the prevention and treatment of antenatal depression: systematic review with meta-analysis. BJOG. 2015;122:57–62.
16. Fontein-Kuipers YJ, Nieuwenhuijze MJ, Ausems M, Budé L, de Vries R. Antenatal interventions to reduce maternal distress: a systematic review and meta-analysis of randomised trials. BJOG. 2014;121:389–97.
17. Songøygard KM, Stafne SN, Evensen KA, Salvesen KÅ, Vik T, Mørkved S. Does exercise during pregnancy prevent postnatal depression? A randomized controlled trial. Acta Obstet Gynecol Scand. 2012;91:62–7.
18. Lewis BA, Gjerdingen D, Avery M, Sirard J, Guo H, Schuver K, et al. A randomized trial examining a physical activity intervention for the prevention of postpartum depression: the healthy mom trial. Ment Health Phys Activ. 2014;7:42–9.
19. Perales M, Refoyo I, Coteron J, Bacchi M, Barakat R. Exercise during pregnancy attenuates prenatal depression: a randomized controlled trial. Eval Health Prof. 2015;38:59–72.
20. Daley AJ, Blamey RV, Jolly K, Roalfe A, Turner K, Coleman S, et al. A pragmatic randomised controlled trial to evaluate the effectiveness of a facilitated exercise intervention as a treatment for postnatal depression: the PAM-PeRS trial. Psychol Med. 2015;45:2413–25.
21. Ussher M, Aveyard P, Manyonda I, Lewis S, West R, Lewis B, et al. Physical activity as an aid to smoking cessation during pregnancy (LEAP) trial: study protocol for a randomized controlled trial. Trials. 2012;13:186.
22. Haasova M, Warren FC, Ussher M, et al. The acute effects of physical activity on cigarette cravings: systematic review and meta-analysis with individual participant data (IPD). Addiction. 2012;108:26–37.
23. Prapavessis H, De Jesus S, Harper T, Cramp A, Fitzgeorge L, Mottola M, Ussher M, Faulkner G, Selby P. The effects of acute exercise on cravings and withdrawal symptoms in temporary abstinent pregnant smokers. Addict Behav. 2014;39:703–8.
24. Ussher M, Lewis S, Aveyard P, Manyonda I, West R, Lewis B, Marcus B, Riaz M, Taylor A, Daley A, Coleman T. Physical activity for smoking cessation in pregnancy: randomised controlled trial. BMJ. 2015;350:h2145.
25. NHS Information Centre. Infant feeding survey 2010: early results. Leeds: National Health Service Information Centre for Health and Social Care; 2011.
26. Räisänen S, Lehto SM, Nielsen HS, Gissler M, Kramer MR, Heinonen S. Risk factors for and perinatal outcomes of major depression during pregnancy: a population-based analysis during 2002-2010 in Finland. BMJ Open. 2014; 4(11):e004883.
27. Prochaska JJ, Hall SM, Humfleet G, Munoz RF, Reus V, Gorecki J, Hu D. Physical activity as a strategy for maintaining tobacco abstinence: a randomized trial. Prev Med. 2008;47:215–20.
28. Fagerström K. Determinants of tobacco use and renaming the FTND to the Fagerstrom test for cigarette dependence. Nicotine Tob Res. 2012;14:75–8.
29. Heatherton T, Kozlowski L, Frecker T, Fagerström K. The Fagerström test for nicotine dependence: a revision of the Fagerström tolerance questionnaire. Brit J Addict. 1991;86:1119–27.
30. Blair SN, Haskell WL, Ho P, Paffenbarger P, Vranizan KM, Farquhar JW, et al. Assessment of habitual physical activity by seven-day recall in a community survey and controlled experiments. Am J Epidemiol. 1985;122:794–804.
31. Murray D, Cox JL. Screening for depression during pregnancy with the Edinburgh depression scale (EPDS). J Reprod Infant Psyc. 1990;8:99–107.
32. Cox J, Holden J, Sagovsky R. Detection of postnatal depression. Development of the 10-item Edinburgh postnatal depression scale. Brit J Psychiatry. 1987;150:782–6.
33. Gibson J, McKenzie-McHarg K, Shakespeare J, Price J, Gray R. A systematic review of studies validating the Edinburgh postnatal depression scale in antepartum and postpartum women. Acta Psychiatr Scand. 2009;119:350–64.
34. Matthey S. Calculating clinically significant change in postnatal depression studies using the Edinburgh postnatal depression scale. J Affect Disorders. 2004;78:269–72.
35. Matthey S, Henshaw C, Elliott S, Barnett B. Variability in use of cut-off scores and formats on the Edinburgh postnatal depression scale – implications for clinical and research practice. Arch Womens Ment Health. 2006;9:309–15.
36. Azur MJ, Stuart EA, Frangakis C, Leaf PJ. Multiple imputation by chained equations: what is it and how does it work? Int J Methods Psychiatr Res. 2011;20:40–9.
37. Rubin DB. Multiple imputation for nonresponse in surveys. New York: Wiley; 1987.
38. Fergusson D, Aaron SD, Guyatt G, Hébert P. Post-randomisation exclusions: the intention to treat principle and excluding patients from analysis. BMJ. 2002;325:652–4.
39. Chalder M, Wiles NJ, Campbell J, Hollinghurst SP, Haase AM, Taylor AH, et al. Facilitated physical activity as a treatment for depressed adults: randomised controlled trial. BMJ. 2012;344:e2758.

40. Gavin NI, Gaynes BN, Lohr KN, Meltzer-Brody S, Gartlehner G, Swinson T. Perinatal depression: a systematic review of prevalence and incidence. Obstet Gynecol. 2005;106:1071–83.
41. Harrison CL, Thompson RG, Teede HJ, Lombard CB. Measuring physical activity during pregnancy. Int J Behav Nutr Phys Act. 2011;8:19.
42. Affonso DD, De AK, Horowitz JA, Mayberry LJ. An international study exploring levels of postpartum depressive symptomatology. J Psychosom Res. 2000;49:207–16.

16

Identifying and assessing the benefits of interventions for postnatal depression

Binu Gurung[1], Louise J. Jackson[1*], Mark Monahan[1], Ruth Butterworth[2] and Tracy E. Roberts[1]

Abstract

Background: Economic evaluations of interventions for postnatal depression (PND) are essential to ensure optimal healthcare decision-making. Due to the wide-ranging effects of PND on the mother, baby and whole family, there is a need to include outcomes for all those affected and to include health and non-health outcomes for accurate estimates of cost-effectiveness. This study aimed to identify interventions to prevent or treat PND for which an economic evaluation had been conducted and to evaluate the health and non-health outcomes included.

Methods: A systematic review was conducted applying a comprehensive search strategy across eight electronic databases and other sources. Full or partial economic evaluations of interventions involving preventive strategies (including screening), and any treatments for women with or at-risk of PND, conducted in OECD countries were included. We excluded epidemiological studies and those focussing on costs only. The included studies underwent a quality appraisal to inform the analysis.

Results: Seventeen economic evaluations met the inclusion criteria, the majority focused on psychological /psychosocial interventions. The interventions ranged from additional support from health professionals, peer support, to combined screening and treatment strategies. Maternal health outcomes were measured in all studies; however child health outcomes were included in only four of them. Across studies, the maternal health outcomes included were quality-adjusted-life-years gained, improvement in depressive symptoms, PND cases detected or recovered, whereas the child health outcomes included were cognitive functioning, depression, sleep and temperament. Non-health outcomes such as couples' relationships and parent-infant interaction were rarely included. Other methodological issues such as limitations in the time horizon and perspective(s) adopted were identified, that were likely to result in imprecise estimates of benefits.

Conclusions: The exclusion of relevant health and non-health outcomes may mean that only a partial assessment of cost-effectiveness is undertaken, leading to sub-optimal resource allocation decisions. Future research should seek ways to expand the evaluative space of economic evaluations and explore approaches to integrate health and non-health outcomes for all individuals affected by this condition. There is a need to ensure that the time horizon adopted in studies is appropriate to allow true estimation of the long-term benefits and costs of PND interventions.

Keywords: Postpartum depression, Economic analysis, Parental outcomes, Non-health consequences, QALYs, Outcomes for young children

* Correspondence: l.jackson.1@bham.ac.uk
[1]Health Economics Unit, Institute of Applied Health Research, College of Medical and Dental Sciences, University of Birmingham, Edgbaston, Birmingham B15 2TT, UK
Full list of author information is available at the end of the article

Background

Postnatal depression (PND), also called postpartum depression, is a non-psychotic, depressive disorder occurring in women within a year after childbirth [1, 2]. It is a common disorder thought to affect 1 in 10 women within the first postpartum year [2]. The period prevalence of minor or major depressive episodes is estimated to be 19.2% in the first three months following childbirth, with 7.1% of mothers experiencing major depressive episodes [3]. Mothers with PND are likely to experience disturbing emotions and feelings common to depression such as anger, guilt, hopelessness, social withdrawal, and those specific to the perinatal period such as sleep deprivation and bonding difficulty [4, 5].

As well as affecting the mother, PND can also affect others within the family. A meta-analysis of studies documenting depression of fathers in the first postpartum year reported that fathers had a 10% risk of experiencing depression and found the correlation between paternal and maternal depression to be positive and moderate [6]. The experience of PND in the parent or parents can potentially lead to marital problems, the withdrawal of social support between parents can compromise adequate care-giving practices of parents, or parent-baby interactions (e.g. the ability of the mother to respond sensitively to her child), that in turn may negatively affect the cognitive, behavioural and social development of the infant in the short and long-term [7–9].

The economic costs associated with PND are significant [10]. In 2002, Petrou and colleagues reported average additional health and social care costs of £392 (2000 prices; UK pound sterling) in women with PND compared to women without PND over the first 18 months post-partum [11]. Recently, Bauer and colleagues estimated that the societal discounted cost of depression during pregnancy and the postnatal period in the long-term was nearly £74,000 per case (2012/13 prices; UK pound sterling) [12]. Around 70% of the projected costs related to the impacts on children, calculated in terms of pre-term birth, mortality, emotional problems, education and conduct, over a period ranging between birth and overall lifetime.

PND has long been considered a major public health problem [13, 14] and a range of PND interventions have been developed in order to prevent or treat the condition. Compared to evaluations of clinical effectiveness of PND interventions, evaluation of their cost-effectiveness within an economic evaluation (comparative analysis of alternative interventions or programmes in terms of both costs and consequences) has been relatively limited [15–17]. The economic evaluation of a PND intervention is essential to understand the value of the intervention relative to other interventions to allow appropriate allocation of healthcare resources [18]. A key consideration in an economic evaluation of an intervention in health conditions like PND, where the impact could potentially go beyond mothers to children, fathers, and could include non-health aspects such as the child's educational and emotional well-being, is ensuring that all relevant outcomes for all those affected by the intervention are identified and included [19]. Furthermore, it may be necessary to include outcomes that are broader than typical direct health outcomes, as is often the case for public health interventions [20, 21].

Therefore this study was conducted with the aim to systematically review published and unpublished studies of interventions to treat or prevent PND, in which an economic evaluation has been conducted in OECD (Organisation for Economic Cooperation and Development) countries, in order to investigate the outcomes considered and measured. The specific objectives were i) to identify studies of interventions to prevent or treat PND which included an economic evaluation; ii) to ascertain which outcomes were included and how these were measured and valued; and iii) to identify any methodological issues associated with including and measuring outcomes in economic evaluations of PND interventions.

Methods

A systematic review was conducted in adherence with guidance on methods from the Centre for Review and Dissemination [22] and on reporting from Preferred Reporting of Items for Systematic Review and Meta-Analysis (PRISMA) [23].

Search strategy

A comprehensive, systematic search strategy was developed through consultation with an information specialist (Additional file 1). The searches were run from database inception to July 2015 in eight healthcare databases: MEDLINE, MEDLINE in-process and other non-indexed citations, EMBASE, PsychINFO, Cumulative Index to Nursing & Allied Health Literature (CINAHL), National Health Service Economic evaluation database (NHS EED), Health Technology Assessment (HTA) and Web of Science (WOS) core collections. The search was not restricted by the publication date or language. Alongside this process, key journals were hand-searched (these were those which appeared most frequently in results of the searches for relevant papers) and reference lists of all the included studies were screened. Furthermore, key researches in the field and members of the *Birmingham Perinatal and Infant Mental Health Forum* were contacted to identify potential published or unpublished literature.

Inclusion and exclusion criteria

The studies were assessed and selected using the PICOS framework [22] as a guide. The inclusion criteria were: women with or 'at risk' of postnatal depression (i.e. those who are pregnant or have given birth within the 12 months), living in OECD countries, and interventions involving preventive strategies (including screening), and any treatments or other interventions for PND. We restricted our focus to OECD countries, in order to compare economic evaluations concerned with similar health care systems. The comparators included placebo, no intervention and current or standard care. In terms of study design, studies that involved a full or partial economic evaluation or that included economic data were potentially eligible for inclusion.

Broadly speaking, the different forms of economic evaluation can be differentiated by how outcomes are considered (although there are also other key differences, for example, in terms of their theoretical foundations) [10]. A cost-utility analysis (CUA) involves consideration of outcomes in terms of quality-adjusted-life-years (QALYs) which combine measurement of quantity and quality of life [18]. In cost-effectiveness analysis (CEA) outcomes are expressed in natural units (e.g. cases detected) and in cost-benefit analysis (CBA) outcomes are valued in monetary terms. Partial forms of economic evaluation include cost-consequence analysis (CCA) where costs and outcomes are presented in a disaggregated form and cost-minimisation analysis (CMA) that is only recommended in certain circumstances where treatments are proven to have identical outcomes [10].

The following were excluded from the review: epidemiological studies reporting incidence/prevalence; costing studies describing costs only; clinical studies describing and evaluating efficacy or effectiveness only; ongoing or incomplete economic evaluations; discussion papers, letters or commentaries.

Study categorisation

A two-stage process outlined by Roberts and colleagues [24] was used to select and categorise studies based on their eligibility and codes for Stage 1 and 2 are provided in Additional file 2 (and as a Footnote for Fig. 1). Stage 1 involved the initial categorisation of studies into categories A to E based on titles and abstracts according to whether the study involved an economic evaluation or included economic data. One author (BG) carried out the initial coding of the studies and another author (LJ) checked the coding. Studies categorised as potentially relevant to the systematic review were carried forward to Stage 2 and assessed for inclusion based on their full-text. One author (BG) carried out the stage 2 coding from 1 to 7, which was then checked by two authors (LJ and MM) and two authors (BG, LJ) assessed the full-texts of all the studies carried forward to Stage 2.

Data extraction and quality assessment

A data extraction form was used to collect data on the background of the study, details of the outcomes included and any methodological limitations acknowledged by study authors (Additional file 3). The included studies were assessed for quality using an adapted version of Drummond et al.'s checklist [25], which is judged to be suitable for assessing economic evaluations [22]. According to the objectives of the review, the modifications to the checklist included greater focus on outcomes than costs, the addition of a question on the perspective of analysis and the removal of a general question on the study results. The assessment aimed to inform the main analysis rather than to exclude studies based on quality (the full results are available in Additional file 4).

Results

The electronic search of the databases yielded 2360 studies. A further eight studies were identified as potentially relevant to the review from other sources (key researchers in this field and the forum members). After removing 537 duplicates, 1831 records were categorised based on title and abstract (Stage 1). The full-texts of 58 papers were assessed (Stage 2) and 17 studies were identified for synthesis. Figure 1 presents a PRISMA flow diagram of the articles screened, included or excluded in each stage.

Study characteristics

The study characteristics are provided in Table 1. The studies were predominantly from the UK ($n = 13$) with a further four studies conducted in Australia [26], Canada [27], New Zealand [28] and the USA [29].

A variety of interventions were evaluated in the identified studies that conducted an economic evaluation. Nine studies examined interventions concerned with preventive strategies only [26, 27, 29–35], five studies included both screening and treatment [28, 30, 36–38], and the remaining three studies assessed treatment only [39–41]. The most common type of intervention was modified or enhanced support or care in the perinatal period either from a health professional or via peer support [27, 28, 30–35, 41]. Many of the interventions included cognitive behavioural therapy (CBT), either alone [40], or in combination with other therapies such as antidepressants [42], interpersonal therapy [29], listening visits [37, 38] and a range of customised treatments [39]. A pharmacological intervention was delivered as one of the interventions in three studies only [35, 39, 42]. Various screening tools (Edinburgh Postnatal Depression Scale - EPDS, Whooley questions, Beck Depression Inventory, PHQ-9)

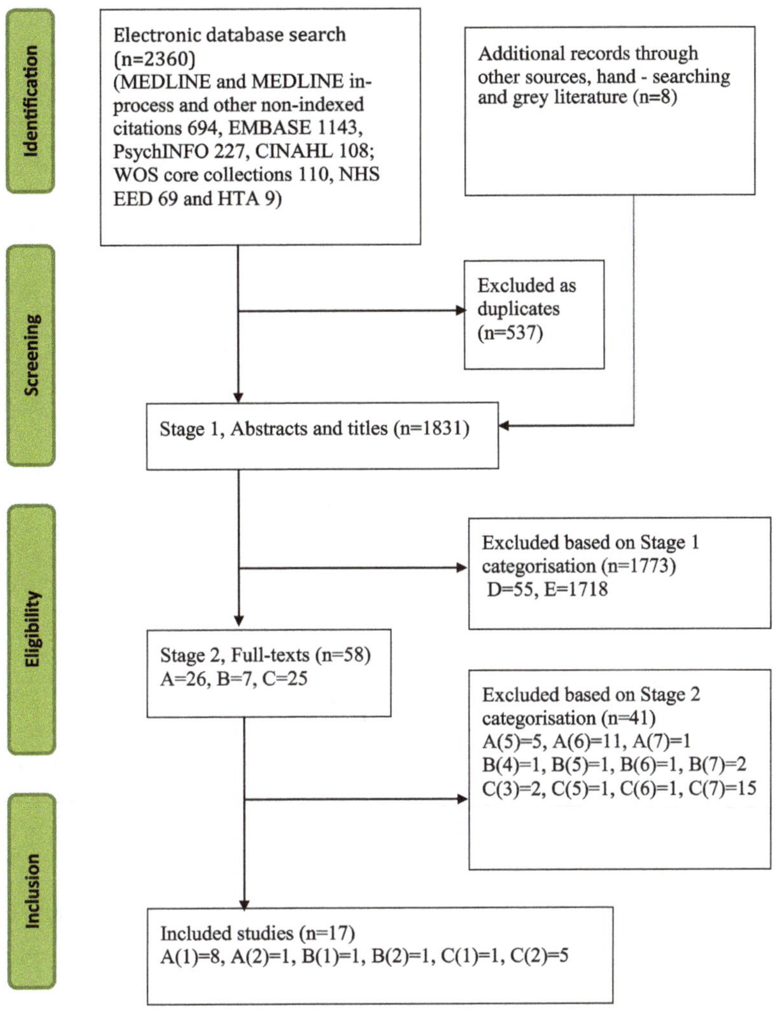

Fig. 1 PRISMA flowchart showing the study selection process.
Notes: Coding- Stage 1) A. The study involves a formal economic evaluation of PND interventions based on primary and/or secondary data (e.g. previously published studies or other sources); B. The study discusses economic aspects of PND interventions and contains relevant primary and/ or secondary data; C. Unclear if the study falls under (A) or (B) but contains useful information; D. The study discusses economic aspects of PND interventions, but is neither (A) nor (B); E. The study is not relevant to the economic evaluation of PND interventions. Stage 2) 1. Full economic evaluation; 2. Partial economic evaluation; 3. Study that measured/valued outcomes of PND interventions but did not consider cost or cost-effectiveness; 4. Other, such as study estimating resource use and/or economic burden of PND and interventions; 5. Secondary study discussing methods or results of economic evaluation; 6. Incomplete economic evaluation of PND interventions (e.g. ongoing studies); 7. Not relevant to the economic evaluation of PND interventions. (See Additional file 2)

were assessed as part of a wider strategy to identify and treat those experiencing PND [28, 36, 38].The comparator adopted was usual, standard or current care/practice/services in nearly all studies. Two studies used 'no intervention' as the comparator [30, 34]. Seven studies did not provide a comprehensive description of their comparators [26, 31, 32, 35, 40–42].

All studies investigating screening considered women in their postnatal period [28, 36–38, 42]. Other preventive strategies focused on pregnant [31, 33] and/or postpartum women [26–28, 30, 33, 35]. For treatment interventions, the targeted population were postpartum women with a PND diagnosis and/or women scoring above the threshold of a screening tool [28, 36, 38–42].

There were some differences in terms of the aims of the interventions evaluated. All but three studies evaluated an intervention that focussed on preventing and/or treating PND alone. These three studies focused on improving other aspects of health and well-being in addition to addressing PND, including women's physical and general health [31, 32], maternal smoking [35] and child injury [35].

There was a greater number of studies that conducted an economic evaluation alongside a Randomised Controlled

Table 1 Study characteristics and aims

Lead author (Year)	Intervention	Comparator	Country	Sample size, N; patient population	Primary aims of economic evaluation	Analytical approach
RCT or cohort-based economic evaluation						
Boath (2003) [39]	PBDU customised treatment (consisting of one or more of the following: individual, couple and family counselling, group therapy, creative therapy, hobbies and activities, stress management, assertiveness training, yoga and relaxation, a group for parents and older children and pharmacotherapy)	RPC	UK	$N = 60$; Women with a baby aged 6 weeks-1 year, with the EPDS score above 12 and with a diagnosis of a major or minor depressive disorder.	Assess the cost-effectiveness of two alternative approaches to the PND treatment.	CEA[a]
Dukhovny (2013) [27]	Telephone-based peer support intervention, access to standard postpartum care	Usual care	Canada	$N = 610$; High-risk women with EPDS score > 9, able to speak English, following a live birth and discharge home	Determine the cost-effectiveness of a peer support intervention to prevent PND.	CEA
Hiscock (2007) [26]	Individual structured maternal and child health consultations, a choice of behavioural interventions, 'controlled crying' or 'camping out'	Usual care	Australia	$N = 328$; Mothers reporting an infant sleep problem in the concurrent 7-month questionnaire	Assess the effectiveness and costs of an intervention targeting infant sleep problems.	CCA
MacArthur (2003) [31]	Redesigned model of community postnatal care (midwifery-led)	Current care	UK	$N = 36$ clusters; All pregnant women registered at the practice antenatally from about 34 weeks gestation.	Develop, implement and test the cost-effectiveness of redesigned postnatal care compared with current care on women's physical and psychological health.	CCA
Morrell (2000) [32]	Community midwifery support worker	Postnatal midwifery care	UK	$N = 471$; All women who delivered a baby at the recruiting hospital living within the study area, were aged 17 or over, and could understand English.	Measure the effect and the total cost per woman of providing postnatal support at home.	CMA
Morrell (2009) [37]	Health visitor trained to identify and deliver CBA or person-centred approach	Health visitor usual care	UK	$N = 418$; Women at risk of PND indicated by EPDS score ≥ 12, registered with participating GP practices, 36 weeks pregnant during recruitment, who had a live baby and were on a collaborating Health Visitor's caseload.	Investigate outcomes for postnatal women attributed to the intervention, and to establish its cost-effectiveness.	CUA[a]
Petrou (2006) [33]	Counselling and support package by trained health visitors	RPC	UK	$N = 151$; Women attending clinics at 26–28 weeks of gestation, identified as at high risk of developing PND	Assess the cost-effectiveness of a preventive counselling and support package for women at high risk of developing PND.	CEA
Price (2015) [29]	Enhanced engagement in home visiting via motivational interviewing and brief intervention (CBT and Interpersonal Therapy)	Usual care	USA	$N = 25$; Pregnant and postpartum women in low-income and ethnic minorities communities meeting risk criteria for major depression	Examine the feasibility of enhanced engagement in routine community care over usual care maternal and child health home visiting.	CCA[a]
Sembi (2016) [41]	Telephone peer support	Standard care	UK	$N = 28$; Women > 16 years when giving birth, experiencing depressive symptom indicated by EPDS threshold ≥10 and/or clinical judgement, and potentially receptive to receiving intervention.	Pilot a telephone peer-support intervention for women experiencing PND.	CCA[a]
Wiggins (2004) [35]	Health visitor support or Community group support	Standard services	UK	$N = 498$; Women living in deprived areas, who gave birth in the specified time period and of any ethnicity.	Measure the impact and cost-effectiveness of two alternative strategies for providing support to mothers in disadvantaged inner city area.	CCA[a]
Model-based economic evaluation						
Battye (2012) [30]	Befriending service (telephone helpline and one-to-one support by trained 'befriender' volunteers)	No intervention	UK	Quantitative study: $N = 39$ Qualitative study: N not provided	Demonstrate value for money of Acacia Family Support's service.	CBA
Bauer (2011) [42]	Universal health visiting (postnatal screening using EPDS and treatment [CBT + antidepressant])	Routine postnatal care	UK	Identification: Hypothetical cohort of women for screening.	Identify and analyse the costs and economic pay-offs of PND interventions.	CUA[a]

Table 1 Study characteristics and aims *(Continued)*

Lead author (Year)	Intervention	Comparator	Country	Sample size, N; patient population	Primary aims of economic evaluation	Analytical approach
				Treatment: Hypothetical cohort of women with moderate to severe PND for the treatment		
Campbell (2008) [28]	Routine screening programme (using PHQ-2) and treatments (antidepressants, psychological therapies or social support) according to severity of PND.	Current practice	New Zealand	N not provided; Mothers who gave birth in any 12 month period, regardless of the number of previous births	Evaluate value for money of implementing a screening programme for PND.	CUA[a], CEA[a]
Hewitt (2009) [36]	Identification 1. EPDS 2. Beck Depression Inventory Treatments 1. Structured psychological therapy 2. Listening visit (Both with preceding additional care)	Current practice	UK	Identification: Hypothetical population of postnatal women (depressed or not) managed in primary care six weeks postnatally Treatment: Hypothetical cohorts of 1000 women with depression in the postnatal period	Identification: Evaluate the cost-effectiveness for a range of feasible identification strategies for PND in primary care. Treatment: Clarify from the NICE guidance whether treatment strategies were cost-effective compared with usual care.	CUA
NCCMH (2014) [38]	Identification 1. EPDS only 2. Whooley questions followed by EPDS 3. Whooley questions followed by PHQ-9 Treatment 1. Facilitated self-help based on CBT principles 2. Listening visits (Both in addition to standard postnatal care)	Standard care	UK	Identification: Hypothetical cohorts of 1000 postnatal women undergoing screening for depression. Treatment: Hypothetical cohorts of 1000 women with sub-threshold/mild to moderate depression	Identification: Assess the relative cost-effectiveness of formal identification methods for PND. Treatment: Assess the cost-effectiveness of different types of psychological and psychosocial, relative to standard postnatal care alone.	CUA[a], CEA[a]
Stevenson (2010) [40]	Group CBT	RPC	UK	Secondary RCT $N = 45$; Women meeting a standardised PND diagnosis or scoring EPDS threshold ≥12.	Evaluate the clinical effectiveness and cost-effectiveness of group CBT compared with currently used packages.	CUA[a]
Taylor (2014) [34]	Social support (e.g. advocacy, befriending)	No intervention	UK	Estimated $N = 100$; Women assessed as vulnerable to PND, either as a self-referral, or referred via the mid-wife/GP.	Determine the benefits and costs of the Perinatal Support Project to prevent PND.	CBA[a]

CBA Cost-Benefit Analysis, *CBA* Cognitive Behavioural Approach, *CBT* Cognitive Behavioural Therapy, *CCA* Cost-Consequence Analysis, *CEA* Cost-Effectiveness Analysis, *CMA* Cost-Minimisation Analysis, *CUA* Cost-Utility Analysis, *EPDS* Edinburgh Postnatal Depression Scale, *NCCMH* National Collaborating Centre for Mental Health, *PBDU* Parent baby day unit, *PHQ* Patient Health Questionnaire, *RCT* Randomised Controlled Trial, *RPC* Routine primary care

[a]Not explicitly stated by authors

Trial (RCT) [26, 27, 31–33, 35, 37, 41] or a cohort study [29, 39] compared to studies that undertook decision modelling [28, 30, 34, 36, 38, 40, 42]. Different approaches to analysis were adopted. CUA was the main approach adopted by six of the 17 studies [28, 36–38, 40, 42]. Of these six studies, two further conducted a CEA [28, 38]. Five of the 17 studies adopted a CCA [26, 29, 31, 35, 41] and three studies conducted a CEA only [27, 33, 39]. Two studies carried out a CBA [30, 34] and only one study conducted a CMA [32].

Health and non-health outcomes

Different types of both health and non-health outcomes were included in the economic evaluations (Tables 2 and 3). All economic evaluations included maternal health outcomes. Thirteen studies included condition-specific outcomes including PND duration [33]; cases recovered or improved [28, 38, 39], cases detected or averted [27, 28]; improvement in PND symptoms [26, 29, 34, 41] or scores from a screening tool [31, 32, 35]. Five studies also used generic outcomes such as well-being [26, 30, 34] and general health [35, 41]. Six studies measured health in terms of QALYs from the maternal perspective [28, 36–38, 40, 42]. However, health outcomes relating to children were considered in only four studies, this was in terms of cognitive functioning [30], sleep [26], temperament [26, 41], and depression [34]. Seven studies acknowledged that outcomes for children and/or partner health were important or likely to be affected but did not include them in their analysis [28, 36–40, 42]. Only three of the seven studies explained their omission; this was typically due to a lack of reliable data [28, 36], or due to missing data [37]. There was no mention of child or partner/family health outcomes in four studies [27, 29, 32, 33].

Similarly, non-health outcomes were explicitly considered by four studies only in relation to PND [29, 30, 34, 41]. Nearly all of these studies included outcomes relating to social or emotional support for PND [29, 30, 41]. Other non-health outcomes included mother's employment and earnings, parent-infant interaction, children's educational attainment and behavioural problems, couples' relationships, satisfaction and efficacy in parenting role, and family functioning. Another four studies explicitly acknowledged the significance of non-health effects, but did not include them [26, 28, 38, 39]. A lack of relevant evidence was the main reason stated for excluding potential non-health effects [30, 34, 38].

Outcome measurement and valuation

Different instruments were used to assess the presence, risk or duration of PND as an outcome in the economic evaluation (Tables 2 and 3). Seven studies employed the Edinburgh Postnatal Depression Scale (EPDS) [26, 27, 31, 32, 35, 38, 41]. However, although the same tool was used, a range of thresholds were used. For example, the thresholds used to define the risk of PND ranged from 9 above [26] to 13 or above [31]. Some defined the EPDS threshold in relation to its level of specificity and sensitivity, by validating it against an existing diagnostic tool [31] or by piloting it on trial participants [32], while others referred to different published sources [26, 27]. Other instruments were also used, with three studies employing the Patient Health Questionnaire [28, 29, 38], two using the Structured Clinical Interview for Depression [27, 33] and one study adopting the Clinical Interview Schedule [39].

In all the economic models that used QALYs, the utility weights were derived from secondary sources (Table 3). Three studies used the same source for utility values [28, 36, 42]. In most cases, the utility values used were based on the health states associated with depressed or general populations rather than women with PND. For other studies involving a monetary valuation of outcomes, some of the valuations of outcomes were based on authors' own estimates, due to a lack of available data [30].

Other methodological considerations

Study perspective

The most common perspective adopted by the economic evaluations was a National Health Service/Personal Social Services (NHS/PSS) or a healthcare perspective only ($n = 10$) [26, 28, 31–33, 36–38, 40, 41]. Three studies adopted a societal perspective only [34, 39, 42]. Two studies took a societal perspective alongside other perspectives such as a public sector perspective [30], a third-party payer perspective, a healthcare perspective and family perspective [27]. In one study [35], a patient perspective was taken alongside a healthcare perspective.

Time horizon and discounting

There were some variations in terms of the time horizon adopted for costs and consequences by the economic evaluations (Table 4). The most common time horizon for outcomes was a year ($n = 9$), followed by six months ($n = 3$), 18 months ($n = 2$), and 12 weeks ($n = 2$). Only two studies adopted time horizons longer than a year, justifying them as necessary due to the short and longer-term impacts of PND [29, 33]. Justifications for adopting a limited time horizon included constraints associated with the trial follow-up period [27, 33], practical limitations and budget constraints [39]. As most studies had the time horizon of a year or less, discounting of benefits was not required. The two studies adopting a longer time period

Table 2 Description of outcomes used in RCT or cohort-based economic evaluations

Study (Year)	Intervention	Outcomes	Outcomes other than maternal and health outcomes	How was the outcome measured and/or valued?	Source	Other outcomes measured in the trial but not used/maybe relevant in the economic evaluation	Outcomes acknowledged but excluded
Boath (2003) [39]	PBDU customised treatment	• PND cases recovered	–	CIS	Cohort study	• Anxiety • Work leisure and family life • Marriage quality and other similar dyads	Child and non-health; reasons for their non-inclusion not provided
Dukhovny (2013) [27]	Telephone-based peer support intervention, access to standard postpartum care	• PND cases averted	–	EPDS (threshold of ≤12 for low risk), SCID	RCT	• Anxiety • Loneliness • Satisfaction with intervention	–
Hiscock (2007) [26]	Individual structured maternal and child health consultations, a choice of behavioural interventions, 'controlled crying' or 'camping out'	• Depression symptoms • Mental and physical health scores • Sleep quality and quantity • Infant's sleep problem (primary outcome) • Infant's temperament	Child	EPDS (threshold > 9 for PND), SF-12, sleep questions, night waking indicator, Global Infant Temperament Scale	RCT	NA	–
MacArthur[a] (2003) [31]	Redesigned model of community postnatal care (midwifery-led)	• PND score	–	EPDS (score of ≥13 indicated risk)	RCT	• Physical and Mental Health • Reported morbidity • 'Good practice' • Women and professionals views about care	Child; reasons for its non-inclusion not discussed
Morrell[a] (2000) [32]	Community midwifery support workers	• PND score	–	EPDS (score of ≥12 indicated risk)	RCT	• General health perception • Functional Social Support • Breastfeeding	–
Morrell (2009) [37]	Health visitor trained to identify and deliver CBA or person-centred approach (listening visits)	• QALY	–	The SF-6D, from a subset of SF-36 questions, was calculated. SF-6D scores estimated using UK tariffs.	RCT	• Proportion of at-risk women (primary) • EPDS score • Physical and mental health • Clinical Outcomes in Routine Evaluation • Anxiety • Perceived stressful impact of having a young child • Couples relationship • Cognitive, social and emotional development of infants • Risk of developing autism	Child, partner/family; these outcomes could not included due to missing data
Petrou (2006) [33]	Counselling and support package by trained health visitors	• Duration of PND experienced	–	SCID-II	RCT	Unclear what other outcomes were measured in the trial	–
Price (2015) [29]	Enhanced engagement in home visiting via motivational interviewing and brief intervention (CBT and Interpersonal Therapy)	• Depressive symptoms • Social support	Non-health	Patient Health Questionnaire-9, Sarason's Social Support Questionnaire-Revised	Cohort study	NA	–
Sembi (2016) [41]	Telephone peer support	• Depressive symptoms • Parent-infant interaction • Anxiety • Emotional support	Child, non-health	EPDS (score of > 9 or 10 indicated mild depression), CARE-Index, Hospital Anxiety and Depression	RCT	NA	–

Table 2 Description of outcomes used in RCT or cohort-based economic evaluations *(Continued)*

Study (Year)	Intervention	Outcomes	Outcomes other than maternal and health outcomes	How was the outcome measured and/or valued?	Source	Other outcomes measured in the trial but not used/maybe relevant in the economic evaluation	Outcomes acknowledged but excluded
		• Parents' satisfaction and efficacy in their parenting role • Optimistic self-beliefs • Couples relationship • Infant temperament • Perceptions of interventions • General health		Scale, Emotional Support Questionnaire, Parenting Sense of Competence scale, Generalised Self-efficacy Questionnaire, Dyadic Adjustment Scale, Infant Temperament Questionnaire and Peer Support Evaluation Inventory, SF-12			
Wiggins[a] (2004) [35]	Health visitor support or Community group support	• PND score	–	EPDS (score $\geq$ 12 indicated high risk)	RCT	• Child injury • Maternal smoking • Social support • Maternal and child health • Infant feeding • Mother-child interaction • Household resources	–

CBA Cognitive Behavioural Approach, *CBT* Cognitive Behavioural Therapy, *CIS* Clinical interview schedule, *EPDS* Edinburgh Postnatal Depression Scale, *PBDU* Parent and baby day unit, *RCT* Randomised Controlled Trial, *SCID* Structured Clinical Interview for Depression, *SF* Short Form, *NA* Not applicable

[a]Study focused on PND and other aspects – other outcomes used in the trial may not necessarily relate to PND

Table 3 Description of outcomes used in model-based economic evaluations

Study (Year)	Intervention	Outcomes	Outcomes other than maternal and health outcomes	How was the outcome measured and/or valued?	Source	Key assumptions	Outcomes acknowledged but excluded
Battye (2012) [30]	Befriending service (telephone helpline and one-to-one support by trained 'befriender' volunteers)	Short-term • Improvements in mental health • Increased awareness of PND and PND support • Increased coping ability Long-term • Reduced infants behavioural problems • Improved infants cognitive functioning • Family functioning improvement Healthcare professionals and volunteers outcomes also measured.	Child, others[a] and non-health	Short Warwick-Edinburgh Mental Wellbeing Scale, qualitative interviews and evaluation form	Questionnaires, qualitative interviews, monitoring data, and published studies	Intervention benefits will sustain in the future with only 20% drop-off.	–
Bauer (2011) [42]	Universal health visiting (postnatal screening using EPDS and treatment [CBT+ antidepressant])	• QALY	–	Utilities for depression states derived from secondary sources.	Bennett et al. [51] and Revicki and Wood [52]	Without treatment, PND will sustain with a short-term resolution. Symptoms of moderate-to-severe PND are comparable to those of moderate-to-severe depression.	Child and non-health; reasons for their non-inclusion not provided
Campbell (2008) [28]	Routine screening programme (using PHQ-2) and treatments (antidepressants, psychological therapies or social support) according to severity of PND.	• PND cases detected • PND cases resolved • QALY	–	PHQ-2, Preference weights for QALYs derived from a secondary source.	Secondary sources, Revicki and Wood [52]	Normal utility six-weeks post-treatment in the treatment responders. Non-responders with mild/moderate depression recover within six months of its onset. PND will sustain in undetected cases and non-responders with severe depression. A linear deterioration or improvement between health states over time.	Child and non-health; child outcomes could not be included due to lack of reliable data
Hewitt (2009) [36]	Identification 1.EPDS 2. Beck Depression Inventory Treatments 1. Structured psychological therapy 2. Listening visit	• QALY	–	Utility weights derived for QALYs from a secondary source.	Effectiveness estimate from a systematic review and meta-analysis, utility values from Revicki and Wood [52]	Non-responders to treatment and usual care would remain depressed until the model endpoint. Women enter the relevant treatment at 6 weeks postnatally.	Child and partner/family; these outcomes could not be included due to lack of reliable data

Table 3 Description of outcomes used in model-based economic evaluations *(Continued)*

Study (Year)	Intervention	Outcomes	Outcomes other than maternal and health outcomes	How was the outcome measured and/or valued?	Source	Key assumptions	Outcomes acknowledged but excluded
	(Both with preceding additional care)					A linear deterioration or improvement between health states over time.	
NCCMH (2014) [38]	Identification 1. EPDS only 2. Whooley questions followed by EPDS 3. Whooley questions followed by PHQ-9 Treatment 1. Facilitated self-help based on CBT principles 2. Listening visits (Both in addition to standard postnatal care)	Identification • QALY Treatment • QALY • PND cases improved and not relapsed	–	EPDS, Whooley question, PHQ-9. Utility weights derived for QALYs from a secondary source.	Effectiveness estimate from meta-analyses, utility values from Sapin and colleagues [53], experts opinion	Identification False negative women could have spontaneous recovery or be identified in the GP follow-up and offered treatment. Only first-line treatments considered and relapse not modelled. Treatment Women who improve remain in the state or relapse until the model endpoint. A linear deterioration or improvement between health states over time.	Child, partner/family and non-health; reasons for excluding non-health outcomes was the lack of relevant evidence
Stevenson (2010) [40]	Group CBT	• QALY	–	Changes in EPDS scores were translated to changes in utility using secondary data.	Data from Morrell et al. [37]	Benefits would sustain over the 6-month period with linear decline afterwards to zero, a year after the treatment.	Child and partner/family; reasons for their non-inclusion not provided
Taylor (2014) [34]	Social support (e.g. advocacy, befriending)	• Increased well-being • Increased chances of employment and higher earnings • Long-term beneficial children outcomes • Reduced use of health and social care services • Increased tax revenues • Volunteers benefits	Child, others[a] and non-health	Hospital Anxiety and Depression Scale, analysis of a cohort study	Experts, a range of secondary sources	Benefits were estimated from an observational study and an RCT of similar service. Benefits for women and society inferred from experts and a range of published studies.	–

CBT Cognitive Behavioural Therapy, *EPDS* Edinburgh Postnatal Depression Scale, *NCCMH* National Collaborating Centre for Mental Health, *PHQ* Patient Health Questionnaire, *QALY* Quality-adjusted-life-year, *RCT* Randomised Controlled Trial

[a]Others include partner/family, volunteers or healthcare professionals

Table 4 Methodological considerations and cost-effectiveness results

Lead author (Year)	Intervention	Perspective (reasons)	Time horizon used in economic evaluation (reasons)	Discounting	Key cost-effectiveness results
RCT or cohort-based economic evaluations					
Boath (2003) [39]	PBDU customised treatment	Societal	6 months (practical considerations, budgetary constraints)	Costs: 6%	"The current treatment of postnatal depression is dominated on the grounds of cost-effectiveness by PBDU treatment. The move from RPC to PBDU would incur an additional cost expended per successfully treated woman of £1945."
Dukhovny (2013) [27]	Telephone-based peer support intervention, access to standard postpartum care	Societal (US and Canadian guidelines) Third-party payer, Healthcare, Family perspective	12 weeks (RCT time horizon)	No**	The intervention was found to be cost-effective. ICER: CAD $10,009 per case of PND averted There is 95% probability that the program would cost less than CAD $20,196 per PND case averted
Hiscock (2007) [26]	Individual structured maternal and child health consultations, a choice of behavioural interventions, 'controlled crying' or 'camping out'	NHS/PSS*	10, 12 months	No	Benefits Infant sleep problems At 10 months, 56% of intervention and 68% of control mothers reported infant sleep problems (OR 0.61, $p = 0.04$); At 12 months, this fell to 39% vs 55% (OR 0.53, $p = 0.007$). EPDS scores Intervention mothers had lower mean EPDS scores than controls at 12 months (5.9 vs 7.2, $p = 0.001$) and higher mental health (SF-12) scores at both 10 months (48.1 vs 45.0, $p = 0.001$) and 12 months (49.7 vs 46.1, $p = 0.001$). Costs Intervention: £96.93 (SD, £249.37) Control: £116.79 (SD, £ 330.31) Mean difference: £19.44 (95% CI £283.70 to £44.81, $p = 0.55$)
MacArthur (2003) [31]	Redesigned model of community postnatal care (midwifery-led)	Healthcare	12 months	No**	"The cost-consequences analysis established that the costs of the intervention and control care were broadly equivalent. The intervention care costing at a maximum £81.90 more per woman to deliver, but possibly representing a saving of £78.30 per woman, depending on assumptions used."
Morrell (2000) [32]	Community midwifery support worker	Healthcare	6 weeks (Valid use of EPDS enabling comparability with other trials)	Costs: 5%	Given that health outcomes were similar for both groups, the economic analysis is limited to a comparison of costs between the intervention and control groups. Mean total cost to the NHS at 6 weeks (primary analysis) Intervention group: £635 (SD, £326) The control group: £456 (SD, £291) Mean difference: £180 (95% CI, £126, £232, $p = 0.001$).
Morrell (2009) [37]	Health visitor trained to identify and deliver CBA or person-centred approach	NHS/PSS (NICE guidelines)	6 months	No**	The intervention dominated the comparator for at-risk women at 6 months (primary analysis). However, a significant difference was not observed in the number of QALYs gained in the intervention groups compared to the control group and there was uncertainty associated with the cost and QALY pairs. The probability of CBT being cost-effective was just over 70%***
Petrou (2006) [33]	Counselling and support package by trained health visitors	Healthcare	18 months (RCT time period)	Outcomes: 1.5% Costs: 6%	The intervention is cost-effective compared to RPC. ICER £43.1 per month of PND avoided. The probability that the intervention is cost-effective exceeds 70% once decision makers express a willingness to invest £1000 to prevent each month of PND.
Price (2015) [29]	Enhanced engagement in home visiting via motivational interviewing	Service providers*	12 weeks	No	Benefits

Table 4 Methodological considerations and cost-effectiveness results *(Continued)*

Lead author (Year)	Intervention	Perspective (reasons)	Time horizon used in economic evaluation (reasons)	Discounting	Key cost-effectiveness results
	and brief intervention (CBT and Interpersonal Therapy)				"A decrease in depressive symptoms associated with the intervention that approached statistical significance ($p = 0.0600$). Significant increase in perceived social support ($t = 3.35$, $p = 0.0027$)." Mean Costs Usual care: $158.30 per participant Enhanced Engagement: $147.50 per participant
Sembi (2016) [41]	Telephone peer support	Healthcare	6 months	No	Benefits (primary outcomes) No significant differences between-subjects and improvement in mother-infant interaction. Costs Mean cost of the combined use of NHS resources For the intervention group: £800.67 (SD, £761.74) For standard care group: £1537.80 (SD, £1936.37). It was not possible to conduct a cost-effectiveness analysis due to the small number of patients.
Wiggins (2004) [35]	Health visitor support or Community group support	Healthcare, Patients	12,18 months	6% (costs)	Benefits There was no clear difference in any of the primary outcomes. Maternal depression: Fewer women in the combined intervention group scored over the depression threshold on the EPDS (−3%) than the control group Mean Costs The Support Health Visitor intervention emerged as a relatively expensive intervention to implement compared with the Community Group Support intervention. Support Health Visitor = £3255 (SD, £2253) Community Group Support: £3231 (SD, £3323) Control group: £2915 (SD, £2349)
Model-based economic evaluations					
Battye (2012) [30]	Befriending service (telephone helpline and one-to-one support by trained 'befriender' volunteers)	Societal, public sector (demonstrate value to society and healthcare)	Outcomes 3, 6 and 30 years Costs 1 year	3.5%	The befriending service was cost-beneficial to both society and the state. Societal perspective For every £1 invested, the estimated SROI: ▪ £3 over the short term ▪ £4 over the medium term ▪ £6.50 over the longer term Public sector perspective For every £1 invested, the estimated SROI: ▪ £0.20 over the short term ▪ £0.20 over the medium term ▪ £1.50 over the longer term
Bauer (2011) [42]	Universal health visiting (postnatal screening using EPDS and treatment [CBT + antidepressant])	Societal*	12 months	No	Health visiting intervention provided a positive net benefit. ICER £4500 per QALY gained Net monetary benefits £640 per mother (at WTP threshold of £20,000). By extrapolation, this amounts to around £300 million for England.
Campbell (2008) [28]	Routine screening programme (using PHQ-2) and treatments	Healthcare	12 months	No**	The proposed routine screening programme appears to be highly cost-effective compared to the current practice from a government perspective. ICERs • NZ $287 per additional case detected

Table 4 Methodological considerations and cost-effectiveness results *(Continued)*

Lead author (Year)	Intervention	Perspective (reasons)	Time horizon used in economic evaluation (reasons)	Discounting	Key cost-effectiveness results
	according to severity of PND.				• NZ $400 per additional case resolved • NZ $3461 per additional QALY gained
Hewitt (2009) [36]	Identification 1.EPDS 2. BDI Treatments 1. Structured psychological therapy 2. Listening visit (Both with preceding additional care)	NHS/PSS	12 months	No**	Identification ICER The identification strategies were not cost-effective compared to the current practice. EPDS at a cut point of 16: 3£41,204 per QALY gained. Other cut points and BDI cut point 10 were either dominated or had ICERs higher than that of EPDS cut point 16. At each of the three WTP thresholds considered (£20,000, £30,000 and £40,000), the strategy with the highest individual probability of being cost-effective was routine case detection. Treatment Structured psychological therapy was a cost effective treatment** but listening home visits was not cost-effective compared to the current practice. ICER Structured psychological therapy: £17,481 per QALY gained Listening home visits: £66,275 per QALY gained There was 50% probability that structured psychological therapy would be cost-effective at a WTP threshold of £20,000 per QALY gained.
NCCMH (2014)[38]	Identification 1. EPDS only 2. Whooley questions followed by EPDS 3. Whooley questions followed by PHQ-9 Treatment 1. Facilitated self-help based on CBT principles 2. Listening visits (Both in addition to standard postnatal care)	NHS/PSS (NICE guidelines)	Identification 12 months Treatment 12 months 7 weeks	No**	Identification The 'Whooley questions' followed by PHQ-9 was estimated to be the most cost-effective identification strategy, however, well above the NICE threshold**. ICER Whooley questions followed by EPDS versus Whooley questions followed by PHQ-9: £45,593 per QALY gained Treatment Facilitated self-help compared with standard care was overall more effective and more costly. ICER Facilitated self-help: £2269 per additional woman improving and not relapsing at the end of the model, or £13,324 per QALY gained. The probability of facilitated self-help being cost effective is 0.59 to 0.72***.
Stevenson (2010) [40]	Group CBT	NHS/PSS (NICE guidelines)	12 months	No**	The group CBT compared with RPC was not found to be cost-effective.*** ICER CBT: £46,462 per QALY gained (95% CI, £37,008 to £60,728).
Taylor (2014) [34]	Social support (e.g. advocacy, befriending)	Societal* (to determine value to society)	12 months-over a lifetime	3.5% (outcomes)	Estimated average direct financial cost of providing support: £2230 per woman. Estimated benefit Using SF-6D: £591–£887 per woman treated Using EQ-5D: £1302–£1954 per woman treated

*Not explicitly stated by authors
**Reasons provided: due to small time horizon
***At a willingness-to-pay threshold of £20,000-£30,000/QALY gained
BDI Beck Depression Inventory, *CAD* Canadian, *CBA* Cognitive Behavioural Approach, *CBT* Cognitive Behavioural Therapy, *EPDS* Edinburgh Postnatal Depression Scale, *EQ-5D* EuroQol-5 dimensions, *ICER* Incremental cost-effectiveness ratio, *NCCMH* National Collaborating Centre for Mental Health, *NHS* National Health Service, *NZ* New Zealand, *OR* Odds ratio, *PBDU* Parent and baby day unit, *PHQ* Patient Health Questionnaire, *PSS* Personal Social Services, *QALY* Quality-adjusted-life-year, *RCT* Randomised Controlled Trial, *RPC* Routine primary care, *SD* Standard deviation, *SF-6D* Short Form- 6 dimensions, *SROI* Social return on investment, *WTP* Willingness-to-pay

discounted the benefits appropriately at the recommended rate [30, 34].

Intermediate outcomes

Some studies used intermediate outcomes such as cases detected or averted [27, 28]. While such outcomes may be meaningful in the context of PND interventions, they can be of more limited general use for commissioners as they do not allow comparison of cost-effectiveness across programme areas [10].

Sensitivity analysis

Almost half of the studies did not explore uncertainty around the estimates of outcomes within a sensitivity analysis. Those studies that performed sensitivity analysis mainly conducted a deterministic sensitivity analysis [28, 30, 32, 39, 40, 42] and a few studies conducted probabilistic sensitivity analysis [27, 38, 40].

Cost-effectiveness of interventions

Of the 11 studies conducting full economic evaluations, 10 reported that the intervention under investigation appeared to be cost-effective (Table 4). Of those 10 studies, three studies found that a combination of PND screening and treatment was cost-effective [28, 37, 42], a further three studies reported that treatments such as psychological therapy, facilitated self-help and customized treatment were more cost-effective than standard care [36, 38, 39], and four studies found positive results for preventive strategies which involved peer support or counselling and other specific support [27, 30, 33, 34]. Group CBT was not found to be cost-effective compared to standard care in one study [40].

Discussion

The systematic review identified 17 studies of interventions to prevent and/or treat PND, in which an economic evaluation was conducted. The majority of the studies focused on psychological or psychosocial interventions and none focused on pharmacological interventions only. Overall, 10 of the 11 full economic evaluations reported that an intervention was cost-effective. These involved a variety of interventions ranging from additional support from health professionals, peer support and combined screening and treatment strategies which were usually compared with standard care. The review identified a number of methodological issues relating to how outcomes were included, measured and valued in the economic evaluations; these related to whose outcomes were included, the inclusion of relevant health and non-health outcomes, study perspective and time horizon.

Guidelines emphasise the need to identify all relevant outcomes in an economic evaluation [25, 43]. However, only four studies considered health outcomes associated with children [26, 30, 34, 41]. This raises concerns since numerous studies have shown the adverse impacts of PND on the child's health and development, and on their interaction with their mothers [20, 44]. The exclusion of children's outcomes from an economic evaluation may mean that an incomplete assessment of cost-effectiveness has been undertaken. For example, an intervention found to be less cost-effective compared to another intervention on the basis of maternal outcomes only, may well be *more* cost-effective when potential benefits to the infant's health are included. However, there could be potential barriers to considering infants' outcomes such as lack of robust data, or an inability to measure outcomes directly for children. A further methodological barrier could be related to concerns about increasing the likelihood of findings of false significance (type I error) due to the inclusion of multiple outcomes in an evaluation. Similarly, health outcomes for the father and wider family are potentially relevant and require consideration [19, 21].

Non-health outcomes are relevant and important in the context of PND [18]. However, presently, there is no accepted method to determine which non-health effects are important and how they should be incorporated in an economic analysis [43]. A range of potential approaches for public health interventions have been outlined that allow for the inclusion of health and non-health outcomes (e.g. cost-consequence analysis, cost-benefit analysis etc.) [21]. The focus of most of the studies was exclusively on health, with only four studies measuring some kind of non-health outcomes. Several authors deemed non-health outcomes to be important but did not include them in their evaluation due to challenges such as a lack of reliable and quantifiable data, missing data, and more than one primary outcome being included in the trial.

Some methodological issues were evident relating to the measurement and valuation of outcomes. A detailed analysis of the properties and limitations of the existing instruments used to capture outcomes is essential to inform appropriate ways to measure those outcomes. For example, the frequently used EPDS tool had various cut-off thresholds, indicating differing approaches to using this tool. Many authors of the included studies also mentioned the lack of reliable data on utilities. For example, Stevenson et al. [40] used regression techniques to estimate utilities (based on data from a different trial) but acknowledged that this introduced further uncertainty in the analysis. Other authors used utility weights based on the health states associated with general depression and not PND. Although PND and general depression share some similar symptoms they differ in certain characteristics such as the experience of childbirth and sleep deprivation [44]. If utility estimates do not directly relate to PND, there is a possibility that the utilities may overestimate or underestimate the intervention effects.

A societal perspective is generally considered the most appropriate perspective for PND interventions due to the wide range of impacts associated with the condition [21, 45, 46]. This is in keeping with guidance relating to the economic evaluation of public health interventions, where a perspective broader than the healthcare perspective may be necessary [21]. This would enable outcomes beyond health to be considered, such as those relating to education, housing, crime etc. However, the results of this review demonstrated that only five studies adopted a societal perspective.

Another recurrent issue observed was the limited time length adopted by most of the studies. The time horizon was no more than 18 months in the trial-based economic evaluations. It can be argued that important differences between the interventions may not be captured using short time-horizons. For example, a prospective longitudinal study showed that the children, who were adversely affected in their infancy due to their mother's PND at 3 months postpartum, experienced more problems with intellectual and academic performance at 11 years of age compared to the children of healthy mothers [20] and those problems could have potential economic consequences such as additional school support costs and productivity losses from leaving school without qualifications [10]. Thus, studies adopting a longer time horizon are needed to be able to capture the long-term effects of PND.

This review has several strengths. Systematic and rigorous processes were adopted to identify and assess studies. A comprehensive search strategy was implemented which also included searches for unpublished reports. Both prevention and treatment strategies were included, providing a holistic overview of several methodological issues concerning outcome identification and measurement for the economic evaluation of PND interventions. Using established criteria [25] a quality appraisal process was undertaken analysing all key elements relating to outcomes.

Nonetheless, the review is subject to some limitations. Firstly, potential studies may have been missed by the search strategy either due to inadequate classifications of economic terms in the databases or due to the different ways interventions to improve mental health in the postpartum period can be coded depending on the type or the focus of intervention (e.g. on the mother, the infant etc.) [47]. Secondly, since we could not find detailed guidelines focussed on economic evaluations of PND interventions, our analysis of the quality of the studies was based on generic guidance. Lastly, an in-depth analysis of evidence on the clinical and cost-effectiveness of the interventions was beyond the review's scope.

This is the first systematic review to examine the approaches taken and types of outcomes used in economic evaluations of PND interventions (for prevention and treatment). A systematic review undertaken by the National Collaborating Centre for Mental Health [38] was concerned with accumulating evidence on the cost-effectiveness of interventions to prevent or treat mental health problems in pregnancy and the postnatal period. More recently a systematic review [16] was conducted to inform parameters for a model-based economic evaluation of antenatal and postnatal interventions for pregnant and postnatal women to prevent PND. While these studies attempted to identify economic evaluations of PND interventions, they did not explore the methodological issues associated with the approaches taken and outcomes adopted in the studies.

The findings of this review highlight several implications for future research. Future economic evaluations should identify and consider the full range of potential outcomes that are relevant in the context of PND: health and non-health outcomes, maternal, family and child outcomes. The development of new methods and refinement of existing approaches that can incorporate both health and non-health benefits of intervention are essential for a complete evaluation of the cost-effectiveness of PND interventions. The list of outcomes generated from this review, as a preliminary framework, could be refined further through engagement with key stakeholders including mothers, family members, clinicians and healthcare commissioners to reach consensus on what outcomes are important for use in economic evaluations of PND interventions and in wider evaluations of interventions and services. Given the wide range of impacts associated with PND, in order to allow a full assessment of costs and consequences, a societal perspective should be considered. However, key challenges remain around the monetary valuation of outcomes to enable analyses adopting a societal perspective to be carried out more robustly. Research addressing this issue could explore methods that have been used before in relation to general depression [48, 49]. Similarly, if QALYs are used as outcome, there is an urgent need to address the paucity of estimates of health state utility values relevant to PND. The limited time period inherent in trial-based economic evaluations could be overcome by exploiting modelling techniques that extrapolate outcomes and costs over an extended timeframe [50] and the most appropriate time horizons could be further explored in consultation with decision-makers. In all types of economic evaluation, robust sensitivity analyses will need to be undertaken to explore the implications associated with uncertainty around outcome estimates.

Conclusion

This systematic review has demonstrated that very few economic evaluations included and identified all outcomes relevant to PND interventions. For example, outcomes for the child were not included in most studies, and only a minority included non-health outcomes. Thus, the review paves the way for further work to explore new approaches and methods that enable inclusion of relevant health and non-health outcomes. In addition, the time horizons adopted in the studies did not allow long-term outcomes for the child to be addressed, which have been shown to be important for PND. The review also shows that a broader perspective can facilitate the assessment of the overall impact of interventions in this area. To achieve optimal policy decisions for interventions to prevent and treat PND, addressing these methodological issues is essential.

Additional files

Additional file 1: A search strategy carried out in Ovid MEDLINE (from 1946 to July Week 1 2015).

Additional file 2: Categorisation Criteria (details of the two-stage process used for study screening and selection).

Additional file 3: Description of key methodological issues relating to outcomes (limitations as acknowledged by the authors of the included studies).

Additional file 4: Results of study assessment using Drummond's checklist (adapted).

Abbreviations

CBA: Cost-benefit analysis; CCA: Cost-consequence analysis; CEA: Cost-effectiveness analysis; CINAHL: Cumulative Index to Nursing & Allied Health Literature; CMA: Cost-minimisation analysis; CUA: Cost-utility analysis; EPDS: Edinburgh postnatal depression scale; HTA: Health Technology Assessment; NHS EED: National Health Service Economic evaluation database; NHS: National Health Service; NICE: National Institute of Health and Care Excellence; OECD: Organisation for Economic Co-operation and Development; PND: Postnatal depression; QALY: Quality-adjusted-life-year; RCT: Randomised controlled trial

Acknowledgements

This systematic review was undertaken at the Health Economics Unit at the University of Birmingham as part of Binu Gurung's MSc dissertation. We are grateful to Jane Barlow (University of Warwick), Annette Bauer (The London School of Economics), Sukhdev Sembi (University of Warwick) and the members of *'Birmingham Perinatal Maternal and Infant Mental Health Forum'* for providing us access to relevant unpublished studies and data. We also thank Susan Bayliss (University of Birmingham) for her support in refining the search strategy.

Authors' contributions

LJ conceived and coordinated the study. BG assessed the title, abstract and full texts, performed the data extraction, analysis and drafted the manuscript with advice from LJ, MM, RB and TR. LJ checked the coding in the two-stage process and assessed the full-texts. All authors read and approved the final manuscript.

(The manuscript does not report on or involve the use of any animal or human data or tissue, as it is a systematic review)

Competing interests

The authors declare that they have no competing interests.

Author details

[1]Health Economics Unit, Institute of Applied Health Research, College of Medical and Dental Sciences, University of Birmingham, Edgbaston, Birmingham B15 2TT, UK. [2]Cheshire and Mersey Specialist Perinatal Mental Health Service, Thorn Road Clinic, Thorn Road, Runcorn WA7 5HQ, UK.

References

1. American Psychiatric Association. Diagnostic and statistical manual of mental disorders: DSM-5. 5th ed. Arlington: American Psychiatric Association; 2013.
2. Cox J, Holden J, Henshaw C. Perinatal mental health: the Edinburgh postnatal depression scale (EPDS) manual. 2nd ed. The Royal College of Psychiatrists: UK; 2014.
3. Gavin NI, Gaynes BN, Lohr KN, Meltzer-Brody S, Gartlehner G, Swinson T. Perinatal depression: a systematic review of prevalence and incidence. Obstet Gynecol. 2005;106(5):1071.
4. Beck CT. Postpartum depression: a metasynthesis. Qual Health Res. 2002; 12(4):453.
5. National Health Service. Postnatal depression: symptoms. 2015. http://www.nhs.uk/Conditions/Postnataldepression/Pages/Symptoms.aspx. Accessed 15 July 2015.
6. Paulson JF, Bazemore SD. Prenatal and postpartum depression in fathers and its association with maternal depression: a meta-analysis. JAMA. 2010; 303(19):1961–9.
7. Hay DF, Asten P, Mills A, Kumar R, Pawlby S, Sharp D. Intellectual problems shown by 11-year-old children whose mothers had postnatal depression. J Child Psychol Psychiatry. 2001;42(7):871–89.
8. Murray L, Cooper P. Effects of postnatal depression on infant development. Arch Dis Child. 1997;77(2):99–101.
9. Letourneau NL, Dennis C, Benzies K, Duffett-Leger L, Stewart M, Tryphonopoulos PD, Este D, Watson W. Postpartum depression is a family affair: addressing the impact on mothers, fathers, and children. Issues Ment Health Nurs. 2012;33(7):445–57.
10. Bauer A, Pawlby S, Plant D, King D, Pariante C, Knapp M. Perinatal depression and child development: exploring the economic consequences from a South London cohort. Psychol Med. 2014;45:51–61.
11. Petrou S. Economic costs of post-natal depression in a high-risk British cohort. Br J Psychiatry. 2002;181(6):505–12.
12. Bauer A, Parsonage M, Knapp M, Lemmi V, Adelaja B. The costs of perinatal mental health problems. Centre for Mental Health and London School of Economics. 2014. http://eprints.lse.ac.uk/59885/1/__lse.ac.uk_storage_LIBRARY_Secondary_libfile_shared_repository_Content_Bauer%2C%20M_Bauer_Costs_perinatal_%20mental_2014_Bauer_Costs_perinat. Accessed 17 June 2015.
13. Robertson E, Celasun N, Stewart DE. Risk factors for postpartum depression. In Stewart DE, Robertson E, Dennis CL, Grace SL, Wallington T. Postpartum depression: Literature review of risk factors and interventions. 2003. http://www.who.int/mental_health/prevention/suicide/mmh&chd_chapter_1.pdf. (Accessed 4 Mar 2016).
14. Community Practitioners' and Health Visitors' Association conference proceedings. Postnatal depression and maternal mental health: a public health priority. London: Community practitioners' and Health Visitors' Association; 2001.
15. Dennis C, Dowswell T. Psychosocial and Psychological interventions for preventing postpartum depression. Cochrane Database Syst Rev. 2013;2: CD001134.
16. Morrell CJ, Sutcliffe P, Booth A, Stevens J, Scope A, Stevenson M, Harvey R, Bessey A, Cantrell A, Dennis C-L, Ren S, Ragonesi M, Barkham M, Churchill D, Henshaw C, Newstead J, Slade P, Spiby H, Stewart-Brown S. A systematic review, evidence synthesis and meta-analysis of quantitative and qualitative

studies evaluating the clinical effectiveness, the cost-effectiveness, safety and acceptability of interventions to prevent postnatal depression. Health Technol Assess. 2016;20(37):1–414.
17. Sockol LE, Epperson CN, Barber JP. A meta-analysis of treatments for perinatal depression. Clin Psychol Rev. 2011;31(5):839–49.
18. Brazier J, Ratcliffe J, Tsuchiya A, Salomon J. Measuring and Valuing health benefits for economic evaluation. UK: Oxford University Press; 2007.
19. Drummond MF, Sculpher MJ, Torrance GW, O'Brien BJ, Stoddart GL. Methods for the economic evaluation of health care programmes. 3rd ed. Oxford: Oxford University Press; 2005.
20. Lorgelly PK, Lawson KD, Fenwick EAL, Briggs AH. Outcome measurement in economic evaluations of public health interventions: a role for the capability approach? Int J Environ Res Public Health. 2010;7(5):2274–89.
21. National Institute for Health and Care Excellence. Method for the Development of NICE Public Health Guidance. 3rd ed. National Institute for Health and Care Excellence. 2012. https://www.nice.org.uk/process/pmg4/chapter/introduction. Accessed 17 June 2015.
22. Centre for Reviews and Dissemination. CRD's guidance for undertaking reviews in health care. UK: York, Centre for Reviews and Dissemination; 2009.
23. Moher D, Liberati A, Tetzlaff J, Altman DG. Preferred reporting items for systematic reviews and meta-analyses: the PRISMA statement. Ann Intern Med. 2009;151(4):264–9.
24. Roberts T, Henderson J, Mugford M, Bricker L, Neilson J, Garcia J. Antenatal ultrasound screening for fetal abnormalities: a systematic review of studies of cost and cost effectiveness. BJOG Int J Obstet Gynaecol. 2002;109(1):44–56.
25. Drummond MF, Jefferson TO. Guidelines for authors and peer reviewers of economic submissions to the BMJ. BMJ. 1996;313(7052):275–83.
26. Hiscock H, Bayer J, Gold L, Hampton A, Ukoumunne OC, Wake M. Improving infant sleep and maternal mental health: a cluster randomised trial. Arch Dis Child. 2007;92(11):952–8.
27. Dukhovny D, Dennis CL, Hodnett E, Weston J, Stewart DE, Mao W, Zupancic JA. Prospective economic evaluation of a peer support intervention for prevention of postpartum depression among high-risk women in Ontario, Canada. Am J Perinatol. 2013;30(8):631–42.
28. Campbell S, Norris S, Standfield L, Suebwongpat A. Screening for postnatal depression within the well child Tamariki Ora framework. Christchurch: Health Services Assessment Collaboration (HSAC; 2008.
29. Price SK, Gray LA, Thacker LR. Enhanced engagement: an intervention pilot for mental health promotion among low-income women in a community home visiting program. Best Pract Ment Health. 2015;11(1):69–82.
30. Battye F, Salisbury D, O'Brien D. An economic analysis of Acacia Family Support's befriending service. GHS Consulting Ltd: Birmingham; 2012.
31. MacArthur C, Winter HR, Bick DE, Lilford RJ, Lancashire RJ, Knowles H, Braunholtz DA, Henderson C, Belfield C, Gee H. Redesigning postnatal care: a randomised controlled trial of protocol-based midwifery-led care focused on individual women's physical and psychological health needs. Health Technol Assess. 2003;7(37):iii.
32. Morrell CJ, Spiby H, Stewart P, Walters S, Morgan A. Costs and benefits of community postnatal support workers: a randomised controlled trial. Health Technol Assess. 2000;4(6):1.
33. Petrou S, Cooper P, Murray L, Davidson LL. Cost- effectiveness of a preventive counseling and support package for postnatal depression. Int J Technol Assess Health Care. 2006;22(4):443–53.
34. Taylor R, Lee A, Simmons D. The benefits of family action: an economic assessment of the potential benefits from family action interventions for women at risk of perinatal depression. Pro Bono Economics: UK; 2014.
35. Wiggins M, Oakley A, Roberts I, Turner H, Rajan L, Austerberry H, Mujica R, Mugford M. The social support and family health study: a randomised controlled trial and economic evaluation of two alternative forms of postnatal support for mothers living in disadvantaged inner-city areas. Health Technol Assess. 2004;8(32):iii.
36. Hewitt C, Gilbody S, Brealey S, Paulden M, Palmer S, Mann R, Green J, Morrell J, Barkham M, Light K, Richards D. Methods to identify postnatal depression in primary care: an integrated evidence synthesis and value of information analysis. Health Technol Assess. 2009;13(36):1–145. 147-230
37. Morrell C, Warner R, Slade P, Dixon S, Walters S, Paley G, Brugha T. Psychological interventions for postnatal depression: cluster randomised trial and economic evaluation. The PoNDER trial. Health Technol Assess. 2009;13(30):1–176.
38. National Collaborating Centre for Mental Health: Case identification and assessment, psychological and psychosocial interventions for the prevention or treatment of mental health problems. In Antenatal and postnatal mental health: the NICE guideline on clinical management and service guidance (update). Edited by Anonymous UK: British Psychological Society and The Royal College of Psychiatrists; 2014:81–647.
39. Boath E, Major K, Cox J. When the cradle falls II: the cost- effectiveness of treating postnatal depression in a psychiatric day hospital compared with routine primary care. J Affect Disord. 2003;74(2):159–66.
40. Stevenson MD, Scope A, Sutcliffe PA, Booth A, Slade P, Parry G, Saxon D, Kalthenthaler E. Group cognitive behavioural therapy for postnatal depression: a systematic review of clinical effectiveness, cost-effectiveness and value of information analyses. Health Technol Assess. 2010;14(44):1.
41. Sembi S, Barlow J, McKenzie-McHarg K, Longo R. Mums4Mums: pilot RCT of the clinical and cost-effectiveness of telephone peer support for postnatal depression (submitted for publication). 2016.
42. Bauer A, Knapp M, McDaid D. Health visiting and reducing post-natal depression. In: Knapp M, McDaid DM, Parsonage M, editors. Mental health promotion and mental illness prevention: the economic case. London: Department of Health; 2011. p. 4–5.
43. Drummond MF, Sculpher MJ, Claxton K, Stoddart GL, Torrance GW. Methods for the economic evaluation of health care programmes. 4th ed. Oxford: Oxford University Press; 2015.
44. Tsivos Z, Calam R, Sanders MR, Wittkowski A. Interventions for postnatal depression assessing the mother–infant relationship and child developmental outcomes: a systematic review. Int J Womens Health. 2015;7:429–47.
45. O'Donnell O, Maynard A, Wright K. Evaluating mental health care: the role of economics / by Owen O'Donnell, Alan Maynard, Ken Wright. York: Centre for Health Economics, University of York; 1988.
46. Petrou S, Morrell CJ, Knapp M. An overview of health economics aspects of perinatal depression. In: Milgrom J, Gemmill AW, editors. Identifying perinatal depression and anxiety: evidence-based practice in screening, psychosocial assessment and management. UK: John Wiley & Sons; 2015. p. 228–38.
47. Sassi F, Archard L, Mcdaid D. Searching literature databases for health care economic evaluations: how systematic can we afford to be? Med Care. 2002;40(5):387–94.
48. Unützer J, Katon WJ, Russo J, Simon G, von Korff M, Lin E, Walker E, Ludman E, Bush T. Willingness to pay for depression reatment in primary care. Psychiatr Serv. 2003;54:340–5.
49. Van DP, Shiell A, Au F, Jonhston D, Tough S. Eliciting individual preferences for health care: a case study of perinatal care. Health Expect. 2010;13(1):4–12.
50. Gray AM, Clarke PM, Wolstenholme JL, Wordsworth S. Applied methods of cost-effectiveness analysis in health care. Oxford: Oxford University Press; 2011.
51. Bennett KJ, Torrance GW, Boyle MH, Guscott R. Cost-utility analysis in depression: the McSad utility measure for depression health states. Psychiatr Serv. 2000; 2000(5):1171–6.
52. Revicki DA, Wood M. Patient-assigned health state utilities for depression-related outcomes: differences by depression severity and antidepressant medications. J Affect Disord. 1998;48:25–36.
53. Sapin C, Fantino B, Nowicki ML, Kind P. Usefulness of EQ-5D in assessing health status in primary care patients with major depressive disorder. Health Qual Life Outcomes. 2004;2:20.

17

Self-medication among pregnant women attending antenatal clinic at Makongoro health centre in Mwanza, Tanzania: a challenge to health systems

Karol J. Marwa[1*], Agnes Njalika[3], Deodatus Ruganuza[2], Deogratias Katabalo[3] and Erasmus Kamugisha[4]

Abstract

Background: Self-medication is a universal challenge that requires attention because of the potential threat not only to the pregnant women but also to unborn child. Data on self-medication practice and predictors among pregnant women is lacking in Tanzania. Information on the effects of this practice to the pregnant woman and the foetus globally is also scanty.

Methods: This was a cross sectional study which was conducted using face to face interview with 372 pregnant women at Makongoro health centre. Semi-structured questionnaires were used. Data were analysed using STATA 13 (Statistical Corporation, College Station, Texas, US).

Results: A total of 372 pregnant women participated in the study. The prevalence of self-medication among pregnant women was 172 (46.24%). There was a significant statistical association between self-medication and occupation (P value =0.01), gestation age ($P < 0.01$) and education ($P < 0.01$). Age, marital status and gravidity were not associated with self-medication ($P = 0.809$, $P = 0.243$ and $P = 0.922$) respectively. When bivariate logistic regression was performed, occupation and education were the only determining factors for self-medication. Pregnant women who were unemployed, doing business and house wife were most likely to practice self-medication than employed pregnant women ($P = 0.03$; OR = 2.33; 95% CI, 1.06–5.31, $P = 0.01$; OR = 2.31; CI 1.21–4.41, $P = <0.01$, OR = 2.73, 95% CI 0.52–2.43) respectively. Pregnant women with no formal education, incomplete primary education, primary education and secondary education were most likely to practice self-medication than pregnant women with college or university education ($P < 0.01$, OR = 6.37 95% CI 2.37–19.03, $P < 0.01$, OR = 6.58, 95% CI 2.36–18.25, $P < 0.01$, OR = 3.78, 95% CI 1.89–7.56, $P < 0.01$, OR = 2.59 95% CI = 1.30–5.17). The leading illness/ symptoms which led to self-medication among pregnant women attending clinic were malaria 56 (32.56%, morning sickness 44 (25.55%) and headache 33(19.19%). Drugs commonly used in self-medication among pregnant women were ant malarial 42 (24.42%), antiemetics 59 (34.30%) and analgesics 33 (19.19%).

Conclusion: Prevalence of self-medication among pregnant women is high in Tanzania. This is a threat to the safety of the developing foetus and the pregnant woman. Therefore there is a need of interventions to minimize the practice among pregnant women.

Keywords: Self-medication, Pregnancy, Predictors, Antenatal clinic and Tanzania

* Correspondence: carol_maro@yahoo.com
[1]Department of Pharmacology, Catholic University of Health and Allied Sciences, Mwanza, Tanzania
Full list of author information is available at the end of the article

Background

Self-medication is defined as self-administration of medication not prescribed by or in a manner not directed by a physician [1] and is regarded as part of self-care among patients assuming the responsibility of the medical personnel to treat or prevent illnesses by using non-prescription or prescription only medicines (POMs) [2]. Self-medication may extend to prescription and herbal drugs and may be propagated by counselling or advice offered from health care professionals [2–4]. Self-medication carries serious risk of drug interactions, polypharmacy, misdiagnosis, excessive drug dosage use, prolonged drug use, incorrect drug choice, rare but severe adverse events, dependence or abuse and increased antimicrobial resistance [2, 5–8].

Self-medication is common in African countries including Tanzania [9–14]. Many studies have addressed the use drugs after prescriptions/directions from physicians; however data on self-medication during pregnancy is scanty.

Herbal drugs are commonly used in self-medication in developing countries [13–15]. The wide use of herbal drugs in pregnancy is also observed in developed countries [15] Norway being an example (36%) [16]. Studies have shown that herbal drugs are also not safe during pregnancy unlike what most people think [17] though information on effects to the foetus is limited [15].

The main reason for self-medication as reported from different countries include; the feeling that the condition /disease is mild thus not requiring doctor's consultation, previous good experience of treating similar illness, prompted by a pharmacist, feeling of independence to take care of him/herself and non-availability of doctors [4, 14, 18–20]. Advertisement by pharmaceutical companies or their agencies on drugs has also been established as a promoting factor for self-medication [21].

Despite the fact that the use of prescription and non-prescription drugs is common among pregnant women [22, 23], most drugs used in clinical practice have limited information on the safety in pregnancy, hence not recommended for use in pregnant women [24, 25]. This is due to the fact that pregnant women are excluded from clinical trials owing to the fear of harming the mother or the developing foetus [26, 27]. The only available information on drug effects during pregnancy are derived from pre-clinical studies which involve animals and cannot be directly extrapolated to human beings including pregnant women [25, 27, 28], however such studies give us insight on the possibility of toxic effects to the foetus and the pregnant woman [27, 29].

Drug use cannot be avoided in pregnancy in acute illnesses which can harm the mother or foetus if left untreated [24]. In such situation drug use in these patients is based on risk-benefit ratio assessment whereby the potential benefits to the mother must outweigh the risks to the foetus [27]. Drugs effects in pregnancy can be detected in post marketing surveillance studies when a drug is introduced to a large population, nevertheless there is limited information on drug risk to the foetus and pregnant woman, consequently health professionals are deprived of this important information during prescribing and dispensing [27, 30].

There is Food and Drug Authority (FDA) classification placing drugs in categories in relation to safety in pregnancy from class A (the safest) to class X (the teratogenic group) [27]. Unfortunately only few drugs (40%) are listed in this classification [27] indicating that only a safety of few drugs can be predicted during pregnancy considering facts that self-medication is a common practice among pregnant women [31, 32] and presence of a large number of counterfeit drugs in developing countries and the world at large [33–35]. The illicit trade on counterfeit drugs makes self-medication dangerous to the pregnant women and the foetus in developing countries like Tanzania.

There has been expansion of primary health care facilities which include health centres and dispensaries over the past decades [36] in Tanzania. However lack and absenteeism of trained staff, unreliable drug and medical equipment supply chains, resource constrains and sometimes health system failure [37–39] affect delivery of antenatal care services to pregnant women in Tanzania thus driving this group to self-medication and alternative medicine seeking.

It is important to evaluate self-medication among pregnant women considering the above barriers in provision of antenatal care services to this population in Tanzania and a high prevalence of congenital anomalies among infants (29%) reported during birth in Mwanza, Tanzania with central nervous system as the most affected organ system [40]. Close monitoring of drug use during pregnancy is of paramount importance towards protecting the pregnant woman and the unborn foetus.

Therefore in this study we estimated the prevalence of self-medication and evaluated predictors of self-medication among pregnant women at Makongoro antenatal clinic in Mwanza, Tanzania.

Methods

Study area and subjects

This was a cross sectional study conducted at Makongoro antenatal clinic which is the largest antenatal clinic in Mwanza city in North West, Tanzania. The city has approximately half a million inhabitants, and is located on the southern shores of Lake Victoria [41]. Approximately more than 50 pregnant women attend at Makongoro clinic in a day. About 17,431 pregnant women seek health services at this clinic per year [42]. There are no admissions at the clinic, patients are referred to the nearby by Sekou-toure regional hospital. The clinic was chosen because it gives a representation of the entire population of the city and is located in the city centre.

Sampling procedure

A prevalence of self-medication of 36% among pregnant women on the basis of previous data was used to calculate a sample size of 372 respondents using the Kish Leslie (1965) formula. A systematic sampling method was employed where by numbers were assigned on the daily patient register from 1 to 10; then all 1st, 3rd and 7th numbers were picked randomly. Pregnant women who were represented by these numbers were included in the study regardless of their gestation age until when the sample size was reached. The picked women were interviewed on the same date of their visit to the clinic.

Data collection

A questionnaire was developed in English and translated into the local language (Swahili) and then administered through face to face interviews after consent from the respondents. Pre-testing of the questionnaire was done at the same clinic two weeks before to assess practicability and respondent's understanding of the questionnaire. The questionnaire captured the information on the socio-demographic characteristics, self-medication and predictors for the practice. Antenatal care follow up cards were also reviewed to document socio-demographic characteristics and substantiate some of the information given during the interview. The questionnaire instrument can be found in Additional file 1.

Statistical analysis

Data were analysed using STATA 13 (Statistical Corporation, College Station, TX, US). Chi-square and Fischer's exact tests were performed for determining association between categorical variables where appropriate. Demographic and socio-economic variables were assessed using logistic regression. The potential associations were first assessed at a bivariate level; then, factor with a *P*-value <0.2 were entered into the multivariate model. Age group term was entered as a priori into the multivariate model. Stepwise backward logistic regression was used to determine whether these variables were independent factors for self-medication during pregnancy; odds ratios (OR) and 95% confidence intervals (95% CI) were reported as a measure of effect. *P* value of ≤0.05 was considered as statistically significant.

Results

Demographic characteristics

Three hundred and seventy two (372) out of 376 pregnant women gave a consent to participate in the study, of whom 221(59.1%) and 139 (33.4%) were aged 18–27 and 28–37 years respectively while only 12(3.2%) were ≥38 years. Majority 254 (68.3%) of participants were married while 95(25.6%) were unmarried. One hundred and four (28.0%) were business women while 70 (18.8%) were employed, 41(11%) unemployed and 157(42.1%) were house wives. Twenty (5.4%) had never attended any formal education, 38 (10.2%) did not complete primary education, 122(32.8%) had primary school education, 130(35.0%) had secondary education and 62(16.6%) were college/university graduates. All pregnant women (372) who consented completed the interview successfully. This could be due to the design of the interview which was short and pregnant women were interviewed just before seeing the doctor early in the morning whereby they were not tired and were still on the wait list.

Self-medication

Self-medication during pregnancy was practiced by 172 (46.24%) pregnant women. Self-medication was 59 (57.84%) during first trimester (<12 weeks), 87 (49.43%) during second trimester (13–24 weeks) and 26 (27.66%) during third trimester (Table 1).

There was a significant statistical association between self-medication and occupation (*P* value =0.01), gestation age ($P < 0.01$) and education (P < 0.01). Nevertheless age, marital status and gravidity were not associated with self-medication ($P = 0.809$, $P = 0.243$ and $P = 0.922$) respectively (Table 1).

When bivariate logistic regression was performed, only occupation and education were the determining factors for self-medication (Table 2). Pregnant women who were unemployed 20 (48.78%), doing business 50(48.08%) and house wives 82 (52.23%) were most likely to self-medicate than employed pregnant women 20 (28.57%) ($P = 0.03$; OR = 2.33; 95% CI, 1.06–5.31, $P = 0.01$; OR = 2.31; CI 1.21–4.41, P = <0.01, OR = 2.73, 95% CI 0.52–2.43) respectively. Pregnant women with non-formal education 13 (65.00%), incomplete primary education 25 (65.79%), primary education 64 (52.46%) and secondary education 56 (43.08%) were most likely to practice self-medication than pregnant women with college or university education 14(22.58%) ($P < 0.01$, OR = 6.37 95% CI 2.37–19.03, $P < 0.01$, OR = 6.58, 95% CI 2.36–18.25, $P < 0.01$, OR = 3.78, 95% CI 1.89–7.56, $P < 0.01$, OR = 2.59 95% CI = 1.30–5.17).

Conversely when multivariate logistic regression was performed, education was the only factor established to be associated with self-medication (Table 2).

Table 1 Prevalence and factors associated with self-medication among pregnant women attending at Makongoro clinic

Variable	Yes	No	Chi square	*P* value
Age				
18–27	104 (47.06%)	117 (52.94%)	0.9694	0.809
28–37	63 (45.32%)	76 (54.68%)		
38–47	5 (45.45%)	6 (54.55%)		
> 47	0 (0.00%)	1 (100%)		
Marital Status				
Not Married	47 (49.47%)	48 (50.53%)	5.47	0.243
Married	111 (43.70%)	143 (56.30%)		
Separated	6 (50.00%)	6 (50.00%)		
Divorced	5 (62.50%)	3 (37.50%)		
Widowed	3 (100.00%)	0 (0.00%)		
Occupation				
Employed	20 (28.57%)	50 (71.43%)	11.3	0.01
Business	50 (48.08%)	54 (51.92%)		
Unemployed	20 (48.78%)	21 (51.22%)		
House wife	82 (52.23%)	75 (47.77%)		
Education				
No formal education	13 (65.00%)	7 (35.00%)	25.06	<0.01
Incomplete Primary school	25 (65.79%)	13 (34.21%)		
Primary School	64 (52.46%)	58 (47.54%)		
Secondary School	56 (43.08%)	74 (56.92%)		
College or University Level	14 (22.58%)	48 (77.42%)		
Gestation Age				
First Trimester (<12 weeks)	59 (57.84%)	43 (42.16%)	19.3	<0.01
Second Trimester (13–24 weeks)	87 (49.43%)	89 (50.57%)		
Third Trimester (>25 weeks)	26 (27.66%)	68 (72.34%)		
Gravidity				
1	55 (45.83%)	65 (54.17%)	1.9786	0.922
2	51 (43.97%)	65 (56.03%)		
3	41 (46.59%)	47 (53.41%)E		
4	15 (50.00%)	15 (50.00%)		
5	5 (50.00%)	5 (50.00%)		
6	4 (57.14%)	6 (42.86%)		
7	1 (100.0%)	0 (0.00%)		

The leading illness/symptoms which necessitates self-medication among pregnant women attending clinic were malaria 56 (32.56%, morning sickness 44 (25.55%) and headache 33(19.19%) (Table 3).

Drugs commonly used in self-medication among pregnant women were ant malaria 42(24.42%), antiemetic 59 (34.30%) and analgesics 33 (19.19%) (Table 4).

The overall use of traditional herbs among pregnant women was 94(25.3%). The use of traditional herbs among pregnant women who self-medicated with modern drugs was significantly higher 57(33.2%) than among pregnant women who did not self-medicate with modern drugs 37(18.5%) (*P*-value 0.001) as shown in Table 5.

Discussion

The present study was carried out to establish prevalence and predictors of self-medication among pregnant women attending antenatal clinic in Mwanza, Tanzania. Prevalence of self-medication during pregnancy 172 (46.24%) was high. These findings are comparable to other developing countries particularly South Africa [31] and lower than Ethiopia(20.4%) [32].

Table 2 Predictors for self-medication among pregnant women attending clinic

Variable	N	*n* (%)	Odd Ratio	95% CI	*P* Value	adjusted Odd Ratio	95% CI	*P* Value
Age								
18–27	221	104 (47.06%)	1			1		
28–37	139	63 (45.32%)	0.93	0.6–142	0.74	1.04	0.66–1.64	0.88
38–47	11	5 (45.45%)	0.93	0.27–3.16	0.91	0.88	0.24–3.13	0.84
> 47	1	0 (0.00%)	1			1		
Occupation								
Employed	70	20 (28.57%)	1			1		
Business	104	50(48.08%)	2.31	1.21–4.41	0.01	1.38	0.67–2.83	0.38
Unemployed	41	20 (48.78%)	2.33	1.06–5.31	0.03	1.57	0.6–3.79	0.32
House wife	157	82 (52.23%)	2.73	1.49–5.00	<0.01	1.12	0.52–2.42	0.78
Education								
College or University	62	14 (22.58%)	1			1		
No formal education	20	13 (65.00%)	6.37	2.37–19.03	<0.01	7.52	2.15–26.28	0.02
Incomplete Primary	38	25 (65.79%)	6.59	2.69–16.15	<0.01	6.56	2.36–18.35	0.04
Primary School	122	64 (52.46%)	3.78	1.89–7.56	<0.01	3.64	1.59–8.32	0.02
Secondary School	130	56 (43.08%)	2.59	1.3–5.19	<0.01	2.50	1.2–5.22	0.01

This study has identified level of education as a strong predictor of self-medication among pregnant women (Tables 1 and 2). Pregnant women with non-formal education, incomplete primary education, primary education and secondary education were most likely to practice self-medication than pregnant women with college or university education. These findings are similar to those documented in developing countries like Sudan, Sri-Lanka, Mexico, Ghana and Nigeria [5, 20, 43–45] but different to developed European countries where higher levels of education is associated with self-medication [10, 18, 46]. The educated patients in developing countries may have a high income as most are employed therefore can afford health care service hence would not prefer self-medication. Low income is a predictor of self-medication in poor/developing countries [14, 45, 47] while high education level is associated with promptness in seeking care from health care providers [48] and attendance to clinic [49].

Conversely in developed countries people with high level of education opt for self-medication because there are internet pharmacies and these patients can easily understand drug leaflets hence they believe they can treat mild illnesses without consulting a doctor whereas the illiterate patients may not understand the drug leaflets and information on internet on drugs therefore

Table 3 Common cause and illness/symptoms that necessitates self-medication among pregnant women

No.	Illness	Self-Medication
1	Malaria	56 (32.56%)
2	Urinary Tract Infection	16 (9.3%)
3	Morning Sickness	44 (25.55%)
4	Heartburn	4 (2.34%)
5	Headache	33 (19.19%)
6	Asthma	3 (1.74%)
7	Epilepsy	2 (1.16%)
8	Hypertension	2 (1.6%)
9	Cough & Cold	9 (5.25%)
10	Diarrhoea	1 (1.58%)
11	Helminth's	1 (1.58%)
12	None	0 (0%)
13	Fungal Infection	1 (0.58%)
	TOTAL	172 (100%)

Table 4 Drugs commonly used in self-medication among pregnant women

No.	Illness	Self-Medication
1	Antimalarial	42 (24.42%)
2	Antibiotics	17 (9.58%)
3	Antiemetic	59 (34.30%)
4	Analgesics	33 (19.19%)
5	Antiasthma	3 (1.74%)
6	Antiepileptic	2 (1.16%)
7	Antihypertensive	2 (1.16%)
8	Cough & Cold Remedies	9 (5.23%)
9	Heartburn	3 (1.74%)
10	Antihelmintics	2 (1.16%)
	Total	172 (100%)

Table 5 Self-medication with modern drugs and herbal drugs use among pregnant women

Self-medication	Herbal drugs use		Total	Chi2	*P*-value
	Yes	No			
Yes	57 (33.1%)	115 (66.9%)	172 (100%)	10.49	0.001
No	37 (18.5%)	163 (81.5%)	200 (100%)		
Total	94 (25.3%)	278 (74.7%)	372 (100%)		

relying on health care services which are reliable and affordable.

Occupation was also strong predictor for self-medication among pregnant women attending antenatal clinic (Table 1). Pregnant women who were unemployed, doing business and house wives were most likely to self-medicate than employed pregnant women. As shown above, high level of education was not associated with self-medication. Employment is associated with level of education. The recorded low level of self-medication among employed pregnant women could be attributed to their high level of education too which is the opposite with regards to unemployed or house wives. These findings are consistent with data from other developing countries like India [50].

Self-medication was highest during first trimester and decreased as gestation age increased where by less pregnant women self-medicated in the third trimester of pregnancy (Table 1). This finding is an alarmingly threat because drug exposure in this period is likely to cause congenital malformations [51, 52] considering high prevalence of congenital malformations reported during birth in our study area [40]. The higher self-medication practice in the first trimester may be attributed to the occurrence of many symptoms, discomforts and illness such as nausea or vomiting, headache, dizziness and fevers in the first trimester than other trimesters during pregnancy. However, when Multivariate logistic regression was performed, gestation did not emerge as a strong predictor for self-medication in pregnancy (Table 2).

Age was not observed as a predictor of self-medication similar to documentations in Nigeria [20] and different to findings in Portugal [53].

Self-medication with herbal drugs was substantially high (25.3%) among pregnant women. Surprisingly even those who did not self-medicate with modern drugs were also using herbal drugs though to a lesser extent than those who self-medicated with modern drugs as shown in Table 5. This is not surprising because self-medication with traditional herbal drugs is part of culture in Africa due to its availability, affordability and easy access [54]. Findings from this study are similar to other African countries particularly South Africa, where self-medication with herbal drugs during pregnancy is common [31]. The wide use of herbal drugs in pregnancy is also observed in developed countries Norway being an example (36%) [16, 55]. The high use of herbal drugs in developed and developing countries may be due to promotions and beliefs that herbs are natural and safe which attract pregnant women who are in most cases concerned about the health of their unborn children [55].

The prominent illness/symptoms which necessitate self-medication among pregnant women attending clinic were malaria, morning sickness and headache (Table 3). Malaria being among the leading illnesses among pregnant women is not surprising because women in malaria endemic areas like Mwanza are at a higher risk of being infected with malaria which is often associated with headache. Motion sickness is a common symptom experienced in pregnancy especially in the first trimester matching with the findings from the present study that most pregnant women self-medicate when they have nausea/vomiting.

Drugs commonly used in self-medication among pregnant women were antimalarial, antiemetics and analgesics. The use of drugs matches with prominent symptoms/illnesses compelling self-medication among pregnant women as discussed above. Self-medication with antimalaria drugs is already known to be a common practice among communities in malaria endemic countries like Tanzania. This is similar to the observed findings among pregnant women in this study [56–58]. Though malaria is endemic in Tanzania drug use is restricted for safety purposes in the first trimester (Artemisinin based combination therapies (ACTs) due to teratogenicity potential and third trimester (Quinine and its derivatives) due to ability to induce abortion and increased risk of hypoglycaemia as per WHO recommendation [59].

The antimalarial drugs mostly used in self-medication were Sulphadoxine-Pyrimethamine (54%) known as SP and Artemether-Lumefantrine (40%) known as ALU. The higher use of Sulphadoxine-Pyrimethamine (SP) which is used as drug of choice in Intermittent Preventive Therapy (IPT) among pregnant women and provided as DOT may be attributed to perception that the drug is used in treatment of malaria in pregnancy which is misleading since the drug is reserved for prevention of malaria infection only among pregnant women. Artemether-Lumefantrine is a first line drug for treatment of uncomplicated malaria in Tanzania but contra-indicated in the first trimester of pregnancy [59] thus rising a concern on the safety of the unborn child resulting from self-medication.

Study limitations

The current study did not evaluate the impact of self-medication to the pregnant women and infants during birth among those who practiced self-medication. Another limitation was that respondents were not asked if they reported their drug use to the nurses and doctors at the clinic. This information could help doctors in decision making during prescribing thus considering issues like drug interactions and overdose (repetition in using the same drug). It should also be borne in mind that the completeness of reporting of the past self-medication is prone to recall bias and the position for the first sample was chosen arbitrarily. Sensitivity analysis restricted to women on third trimester who have a full overview of the pregnancy was not done. Women in early pregnancy might have not have the chance yet to use medications consequently affecting the reported results on drugs commonly used in pregnancy.

This study has addressed a gap in knowledge on self-medication during pregnancy in the area. Findings from the present study is expected to raise awareness among health care providers especially clinicians and the ministry of health thus calling for appropriate intervention(s) to prevent unnecessary drug use and control self-medication among pregnant women .

Conclusion

Prevalence of self-medication with modern drugs and herbal drugs among pregnant women in Tanzania is alarmingly high. The practice is common among illiterate, unemployed and during first trimester of pregnancy.

Abbreviations

ACTs: Artemisinin based combination therapies; ALU: Artemether-Lumefantrine; DOT: Directly Observed Therapy; FDA: Food and Drug Authority; IPT: Intermittent Preventive Therapy; POMs: Prescription Only Medicines; SP: Sulphadoxine-Pyrimethamine; WHO: World Health Organization

Acknowledgements

We sincerely thank pregnant women who participated in the study, nurses at Makongoro antenatal clinic for their valuable support with records retrieving and logistic issues, the Catholic University of Health and Allied Sciences and Regional Medical Officer for granting us a permission to conduct the study.

Funding

Not applicable.

Authors' contributions

KJ participated in proposal development, data collection, data analysis, manuscript drafting and submitting. AN participated in proposal development, data collection and data analysis. DR, DK and EK participated in proposal development, data analysis and manuscript revising and approval for publication. All authors have read and approved the final version of this manuscript.

Competing interests

All authors declare to have no competing interests.

Author details

[1]Department of Pharmacology, Catholic University of Health and Allied Sciences, Mwanza, Tanzania. [2]Department of Parasitology, Catholic University of Health and Allied Sciences, Mwanza, Tanzania. [3]School of Pharmacy, Catholic University of Health and Allied Sciences, Mwanza, Tanzania. [4]Department of Biochemistry, Catholic University of Health and Allied Sciences, Mwanza, Tanzania.

References

1. Guarlink D. Webster's new world dictionary. New Delhi, Bombay: Oxford, MBH Publishing Co; 1998.
2. Hughes CM, McElnay JC, Fleming GF. Benefits and risks of self medication. Drug Saf. 2001;24(14):1027–37.
3. Kamat VR, Nichter M. Pharmacies, self-medication and pharmaceutical marketing in Bombay, India. Soc Sci Med. 1998;47(6):779–94.
4. Haider S, Thaver IH. Self medication or self care: implication for primary health care strategies. Self. 1995;
5. Awad A, Eltayeb I, Matowe L, Thalib L. Self-medication with antibiotics and antimalarials in the community of Khartoum state, Sudan. J Pharm Pharm Sci. 2005;8(2):326–31.
6. Hardon A, Van der Geest S. Hazards of self-medication. World Health Forum: 1987. 1987:469–71.
7. Pfeiffer K, Some F, Müller O, Sie A, Kouyate B, Haefeli W, Zoungrana A, Gustafsson L, Tomson G, Sauerborn R. Clinical diagnosis of malaria and the risk of chloroquine self-medication in rural health centres in Burkina Faso. Tropical Med Int Health. 2008;13(3):418–26.
8. Organization WH: Guidelines for the regulatory assessment of medicinal products for use in self-medication. 2000.
9. Basco LK. Molecular epidemiology of malaria in Cameroon. XIX. Quality of antimalarial drugs used for self-medication. Am J Trop Med Hyg. 2004;70(3): 245–50.
10. Grigoryan L, Haaijer-Ruskamp FM, Burgerhof JG, Mechtler R, Deschepper R, Tambic-Andrasevic A, Andrajati R, Monnet DL, Cunney R, Di Matteo A. Self-medication with antimicrobial drugs in Europe. Emerg Infect Dis. 2006;12(3):452.
11. Mangesho P, Shayo E, Makunde W, Keto G, Mandara C, Kamugisha M, Kilale A, Ishengoma D. Commnity knowledge, attitudes and practices towards tberculosis and its treatment inMpwapwa district, central Tanzania. Tanzania Journal of Health Research. 2007;9(1):38–43.
12. Nsimba S, Rimoy G. Self-medication with chloroquine in a rural district of Tanzania: a therapeutic challenge for any future malaria treatment policy change in the country. J Clin Pharm Ther. 2005;30(6):515–9.
13. Awad AI, Eltayeb IB, Capps PA. Self-medication practices in Khartoum state, Sudan. Eur J Clin Pharmacol. 2006;62(4):317–24.
14. Shankar P, Partha P, Shenoy N. Self-medication and non-doctor prescription practices in Pokhara valley, western Nepal: a questionnaire-based study. BMC Fam Pract. 2002;3(1):17.
15. Moussally K, Bérard A. Exposure to specific herbal products during pregnancy and the risk of low birth weight. Altern Ther Health Med. 2011;18(2):36–43.
16. Nordeng H, Havnen GC. Use of herbal drugs in pregnancy: a survey among 400 Norwegian women. Pharmacoepidemiol Drug Saf. 2004;13(6):371–80.
17. Mitri F, Hofmeyr G, Van Gelderen C: Meconium during labour–self-medication and other associations. South African medical journal=Suid-Afrikaanse tydskrif vir geneeskunde 1987, 71(7):431–433.
18. Garofalo L, Di Giuseppe G, Angelillo IF. Self-medication practices among parents in Italy. Biomed Res Int. 2015;2015

19. Suleman S, Ketsela A, Mekonnen Z. Assessment of self-medication practices in Assendabo town, Jimma zone, southwestern Ethiopia. Res Soc Adm Pharm. 2009;5(1):76–81.
20. Afolabi A. Factors influencing the pattern of self-medication in an adult Nigerian population. Annals of African medicine. 2009;7(3):120–7.
21. TYK BIDUKI. The effects of advertisement on self-medication: case study of Ejura-Sekyedumase municipality. Department of Economics, Kwame Nkrumah university of Sci Technol. 2013;
22. Rubin JD, Ferencz C, Loffredo C. Group T-WIS: use of prescription and non-prescription drugs in pregnancy. J Clin Epidemiol. 1993;46(6):581–9.
23. Lacroix I, Damase-Michel C, Lapeyre-Mestre M, Montastruc J. Prescription of drugs during pregnancy in France. Lancet. 2000;356(9243):1735–6.
24. Dellicour S, ter Kuile FO, Stergachis A. Pregnancy exposure registries for assessing antimalarial drug safety in pregnancy in malaria-endemic countries. PLoS Med. 2008;5(9):e187.
25. Ward SA, Sevene EJ, Hastings IM, Nosten F, McGready R. Antimalarial drugs and pregnancy: safety, pharmacokinetics, and pharmacovigilance. Lancet Infect Dis. 2007;7(2):136–44.
26. Mitchell AA. Special considerations in studies of drug-induced birth defects. In: Pharmacoepidemiology. Third ed; 2002. p. 749–63.
27. Wood AJ, Koren G, Pastuszak A, Ito S. Drugs in pregnancy. N Engl J Med. 1998;338(16):1128–37.
28. Czeizel AE, Gidai J, Petik D, Timmermann G, Puhó E. Self-poisoning during pregnancy as a model for teratogenic risk estimation of drugs. Toxicol Ind Health. 2008;24(1–2):11–28.
29. Fantel AG, Shepard TH, Newell-Morris LL, Moffett BC. Teratogenic effects of retinoic acid in pigtail monkeys (Macaca Nemestrina) I. General features. Teratology. 1977;15(1):65–71.
30. Lacroix I, Hurault C, Sarramon M, Guitard C, Berrebi A, Grau M, Albouy-Cossard C, Bourrel R, Elefant E, Montastruc J. Prescription of drugs during pregnancy: a study using EFEMERIS, the new French database. Eur J Clin Pharmacol. 2009;65(8):839–46.
31. Abrahams N, Jewkes R, Mvo Z. Indigenous healing practices and self-medication amongst pregnant women in cape town, South Africa. Afr J Reprod Health. 2002:79–86.
32. Kebede B, Gedif T, Getachew A. Assessment of drug use among pregnant women in Addis Ababa, Ethiopia. Pharmacoepidemiol Drug Saf. 2009;18(6):462–8.
33. Cockburn R, Newton PN, Agyarko EK, Akunyili D, White NJ. The global threat of counterfeit drugs: why industry and governments must communicate the dangers. PLoS Med. 2005;2(4):302.
34. Petersen E. Antimalaria drug resistance: the mono–combi–counterfeit triangle. Expert Rev Anti-Infect Ther. 2009;7(9):1039–42.
35. Glass BD. Counterfeit drugs and medical devices in developing countries. Research and Reports in Tropical Medicine. 2014;2014:11–22.
36. Kanté AM, Exavery A, Phillips JF, Jackson EF. Why women bypass front-line health facility services in pursuit of obstetric care provided elsewhere: a case study in three rural districts of Tanzania. Tropical Med Int Health. 2016;21(4):504–14.
37. Kahabuka C, Moland KM, Kvåle G, Hinderaker SG. Unfulfilled expectations to services offered at primary health care facilities: experiences of caretakers of underfive children in rural Tanzania. BMC Health Serv Res. 2012;12(1):158.
38. Gross K, Schellenberg JA, Kessy F, Pfeiffer C, Obrist B: Antenatal care in practice: an exploratory study in antenatal care clinics in the Kilombero Valley, south-eastern Tanzania. BMC pregnancy and childbirth 2011, 11(1):1.
39. Manzi F, Schellenberg JA, Hutton G, Wyss K, Mbuya C, Shirima K, Mshinda H, Tanner M, Schellenberg D. Human resources for health care delivery in Tanzania: a multifaceted problem. Hum Resour Health. 2012;10(1):1.
40. Mashuda F, Zuechner A, Chalya PL, Kidenya BR, Manyama M. Pattern and factors associated with congenital anomalies among young infants admitted at Bugando medical centre, Mwanza, Tanzania. BMC research notes. 2014;7(1):1.
41. Faurholt-Jepsen D, Range N, PrayGod G, Jeremiah K, Faurholt-Jepsen M, Aabye MG, Changalucha J, Christensen DL, Pipper CB, Krarup H. Diabetes is a risk factor for pulmonary tuberculosis: a case-control study from Mwanza, Tanzania. PLoS One. 2011;6(8):e24215.
42. Msaki BP, Mshana SE, Hokororo A, Mazigo HD, Morona D. Prevalence and predictors of urinary tract infection and severe malaria among febrile children attending Makongoro health centre in Mwanza city, north-western Tanzania. Archives of Public Health. 2012;70(1):1.
43. Abosede O. Self-medication: an important aspect of primary health care. Soc Sci Med. 1984;19(7):699–703.
44. Balbuena FR, Aranda AB, Figueras A. Self-medication in older urban mexicans. Drugs Aging. 2009;26(1):51–60.
45. Biritwum R, Welbeck J, Barnish G. Incidence and management of malaria in two communities of different socio–economic level, in Accra, Ghana. Ann Trop Med Parasitol. 2000;94(8):771–8.
46. Figueiras A, Caamano F, Gestal-Otero JJ. Sociodemographic factors related to self-medication in Spain. Eur J Epidemiol. 2000;16(1):19–26.
47. Keche Y: Self Medication Use in Urban Population of Pune, Maharashtra, India. Drugs, 125:48.45.
48. Tarimo DS, Lwihula GK, Minjas JN, Bygbjerg I. Mothers' perceptions and knowledge on childhood malaria in the holendemic Kibaha district, Tanzania: implications for malaria control and the IMCI strategy. Tropical Med Int Health. 2000;5(3):179–84.
49. Slutsker L, Chitsulo L, Macheso A, Steketee R. Treatment of malaria fever episodes among children in Malawi: results of a KAP survey. Tropical medicine and parasitology: official organ of Deutsche Tropenmedizinische Gesellschaft and of Deutsche Gesellschaft fur Technische Zusammenarbeit (GTZ). 1994;45(1):61–4.
50. Deshpande S, Tiwari R. Self medication-a growing concern. Indian J Med Sci. 1997;51(3):93.
51. Bérard A, Ramos E, Rey E, Blais L, St-André M, Oraichi D. First trimester exposure to paroxetine and risk of cardiac malformations in infants: the importance of dosage. Birth Defects Research Part B: Developmental and Reprod Toxicol. 2007;80(1):18–27.
52. Gidai J, Acs N, Bánhidy F, Czeizel A. A study of the teratogenic and fetotoxic effects of large doses of chlordiazepoxide used for self-poisoning by 35 pregnant women. Toxicol Ind Health. 2008;24(1–2):41–51.
53. de Melo MN, Madureira B, Ferreira APN, Mendes Z, da Costa Miranda A, Martins AP. Prevalence of self-medication in rural areas of Portugal. Pharm World Sci. 2006;28(1):19–25.
54. Kasilo OM, Soumbey-Alley E, Wambebe C, Chatora R. Regional overview: African region. WHO Global Atlas of Traditional, Complementary and Alternative Medicine. 2005:3–12.
55. Nordeng H, Havnen GC. Impact of socio-demographic factors, knowledge and attitude on the use of herbal drugs in pregnancy. Acta Obstet Gynecol Scand. 2005;84(1):26–33.
56. Thomas F, Erhart A, D'Alessandro U. Can amodiaquine be used safely during pregnancy? Lancet Infect Dis. 2004;4(4):235–9.
57. Ndyomugyenyi R, Neema S, Magnussen P. The use of formal and informal services for antenatal care and malaria treatment in rural Uganda. Health Policy Plan. 1998;13(1):94–102.
58. McCombie S. Self-treatment for malaria: the evidence and methodological issues. Health Policy Plan. 2002;17(4):333–44.
59. Organization WH: Guidelines for the treatment of malaria: World Health Organization; 2015.

18

Antepartum urinary tract infection and postpartum depression in Taiwan

Jui-Ming Liu[1,2,3†], Feng-Hsiang Chiu[4,5†], Yueh-Ping Liu[6], Shu-Pin Chen[7], Hsun-Hao Chan[8], Jing-Jung Yang[9,10], Fung-Wei Chang[11*] and Ren-Jun Hsu[3,12,13*]

Abstract

Background: Urinary tract infections (UTIs) are among the most common bacterial infections in pregnant women due to anatomic and physiologic changes in the female urinary tract during pregnancy, and antepartum UTIs can cause adverse pregnancy outcomes that may induce mental stress. There have only been a few studies, however, investigating antepartum UTIs and mental stress. As such, the present study was conducted in order to investigate the association between antepartum UTIs and postpartum depression (PPD).

Methods: We used data from the 2000–2013 National Health Insurance Research Database (NHIRD) of Taiwan. Data regarding a total of 55,087 singleton pregnancies was utilized, including data regarding 406 women who were newly diagnosed with PPD in the first 6 months postpartum. The associations between PPD and antepartum UTIs or other risk factors were examined by multiple logistic regression analysis.

Results: The logistic regression analysis results indicated that PPD was associated with antepartum UTIs (adjusted odds ratio [aOR] 1.27; 95% confidence interval [CI] (1.07–1.65). Furthermore, the risk of PPD was higher in women with an upper antepartum UTI (aOR 2.97 (1.31, 6.77) than in those with a lower antepartum UTI (aOR 1.21 (1.02, 1.58)).

Conclusions: Antepartum UTIs, particularly upper antepartum UTIs, are significantly associated with PPD. This information may encourage physicians to pay greater attention to the mental health of women who have suffered upper UTIs during their pregnancies.

Keywords: Urinary tract infection, National health insurance research database, Postpartum depression, Female

Background

Previous epidemiological studies have reported that postpartum depression (PPD) occurs in approximately 10–15% of women after delivery [1–3]. PPD is defined in the fifth edition of the Diagnostic and Statistical Manual of Mental Disorders (DSM-V) [4] as a major depressive episode occurring during pregnancy or in the 4 weeks following delivery. However, PPD usually occurs in the first 6 months after delivery [5, 6]. A recent study of postnatal women in the UK and Taiwan showed that 19% of Taiwanese women and 18% of British women reported experiencing PPD [7].

During pregnancy, women experience substantial physiological and psychological changes. These changes may lead postpartum depressive mood. Previous studies have highlighted numerous risk factors associated with PPD including physical, psychological, obstetric, pediatric, socio-demographic, and cultural factors [8, 9].

Pregnancy also causes anatomic and physiologic changes to the female urinary tract. Urinary tract infections (UTIs) are among the most common bacterial infections during pregnancy [10], with approximately 2–10% of pregnant women experiencing a UTI [11]. Antepartum UTIs are associated with some adverse pregnancy outcomes [12] and are also one of the major causes of antepartum admissions [13].

* Correspondence: doc30666@gmail.com; hsurnai@gmail.com
†Equal contributors
[11]Superintendent, Tri-Service General Hospital Penghu Branch, National Defence Medical Center, Penghu Branch, Taiwan
[3]Graduate Institute of Life Sciences, National Defense Medical Center, Taipei, Taiwan
Full list of author information is available at the end of the article

To the best of our knowledge, however, there have been very few reports on the relationship, if any, between antepartum UTIs and PPD. As such, the present population-based study sought to (1) determine whether there is a relationship between antepartum UTIs and PPD and (2) determine whether different locations of antepartum UTIs (that is, in the upper or lower urinary tract) result in different effects on the mental health of pregnant women.

Methods

Data source and collection

We used the National Health Insurance Research Database (NHIRD) for this population-based study. The NHIRD is a database collected by the National Health Insurance (NHI) program of Taiwan, which is a unique health insurance system covering almost all the citizens of Taiwan. The NHI program was begun in 1995 and provided coverage for 99.9% of the 23 million people in Taiwan as of 2013 [14]. The NHIRD is a large-scale database that contains outpatient and inpatient medical information about the patients included in the database, including information on their medication use, surgical procedures, intervention procedures, and clinical prescriptions [15, 16]. At present, there are more than 2000 published studies that have utilized data included in this database [17]. The present retrospective population-based study used a sub-dataset of the NHIRD called the Longitudinal Health Insurance Database 2000 (LHID 2000) that included data from January 2000 to December 2013. The LHID 2000 contains 1 million people who were randomly selected from the total of 23 million residents included in the NHIRD in 2000 [18, 19]. The disease diagnoses of the people included in the database were made according to the International Classification of Diseases, 9th revision, Clinical Modification (ICD-9-CM).

Study population

The study population was selected from the LHID 2000 covering the period from January 2000 to December 2013. The selection of participants in this study is shown in Fig. 1. There were 73,829 singleton pregnancies among the database cohort during the study period. The exclusion criteria were as follows (1) women with delivery before Dec 31st 2000 or after July 31st 2013 ($n = 11{,}480$); (2) women who were younger than 20 years old ($n = 2571$); (3) women who had a previous history of major depressive disorder ($n = 2449$); and (4) women with a follow-up period of less than 6 months ($n = 55$). In Taiwanese civil law, people in their twenty years of age are adult. We chose adult women in our study with approval by the Institutional Review Board. We selected women identified as having PPD according to a medical record of a PPD diagnosis made by a psychiatrist and by the use of antidepressants in the first 6 months after delivery (ICD-9-CM: 309, 311, 296.2, 296.3, 296.5, 300.4).

Each UTI was diagnosed by collecting a clean-voided, midstream urine sample for urinalysis and urine culture. A positive urine culture was defined by the isolation of at least one single microorganism with > 10,000 colonies/mL. An upper UTI was diagnosed according to physical examination, urinalysis, and urine culture results, with positive physical examination findings including flank pain, fever, chills, anorexia, nausea, and vomiting. The diagnosis of a lower UTI was also made via physical examination, urinalysis, and urine culture results, with the typical manifestations of a lower UTI including dysuria, frequency, urgency, and suprapubic pain.

Variables

Variables were selected based on clinical manifestations or complications during pregnancy. We retrospectively investigated different variables in women with or without PPD. In this study, antepartum UTIs were grouped into two categories: upper and lower UTIs. An upper UTI consists of an infection of the renal parenchyma and pelvicaliceal system. This includes cases of pyelonephritis, pyelitis, and perirenal infection or abscess (ICD-9-CM: 590.1, 590.2, 590.8, 590.9). Lower UTI infections are located in the lower urinary tract and include cystitis and urethritis (ICD-9-CM: 595.0, 595.1, 595.2, 595.3, 595.4, 595.8, 595.9, 597.8, 599.0). Additional factors of antepartum, peripartum, and postpartum complications that are related to PPD, according to a previous study [20], were also analyzed, including antepartum hemorrhage (ICD-9-CM: 641.8, 641.9), eclampsia or pre-eclampsia (ICD-9-CM: 642.4, 642.5, 642.6), premature separation of placenta (ICD-9-CM: 641.2), placenta previa (ICD-9-CM: 641.0, 641.1), oligohydramnios (ICD-9-CM: 658), polyhydramnios (ICD-9-CM: 657), poor fetal growth (ICD-9-CM: 656.5), excessive fetal growth (ICD-9-CM: 656.6), cervical incompetence (ICD-9-CM: 654.5), premature birth (ICD-9-CM: 644), chronic pulmonary disease (ICD-9-CM: 490–492, 494,496), hypertension (ICD-9-CM: 401.1401.9), hypertension-complicated pregnancy (ICD-9-CM: 642.0, 642.1, 642.2, 642.3, 642.9), diabetes complicating pregnancy childbirth (ICD-9-CM: 648.0), hyperlipidemia (ICD-9-CM: 272.4), heart disease (ICD-9-CM: 393–398, 402, 404.0, 404.1, 404.9, 410–414, 415.0, 416.1, 416.8, 416.9, 420–429), anemia (ICD-9- CM: 280–285), cerebrovascular disease (ICD-9-CM: 430–438), Parkinson disease (ICD-9-CM: 332), epilepsy (ICD-9-CM: 345), tuberculosis (ICD-9-CM: 011,012), asthma (ICD-9-CM: 493), chronic kidney disease (ICD-9-CM: 585,586,588). The monthly incomes of the study population, as per insurance information, were divided into four groups: < 20,000, 20,000–40,000, 40,000–60,000, and ≥60,000 new Taiwan dollars [21].

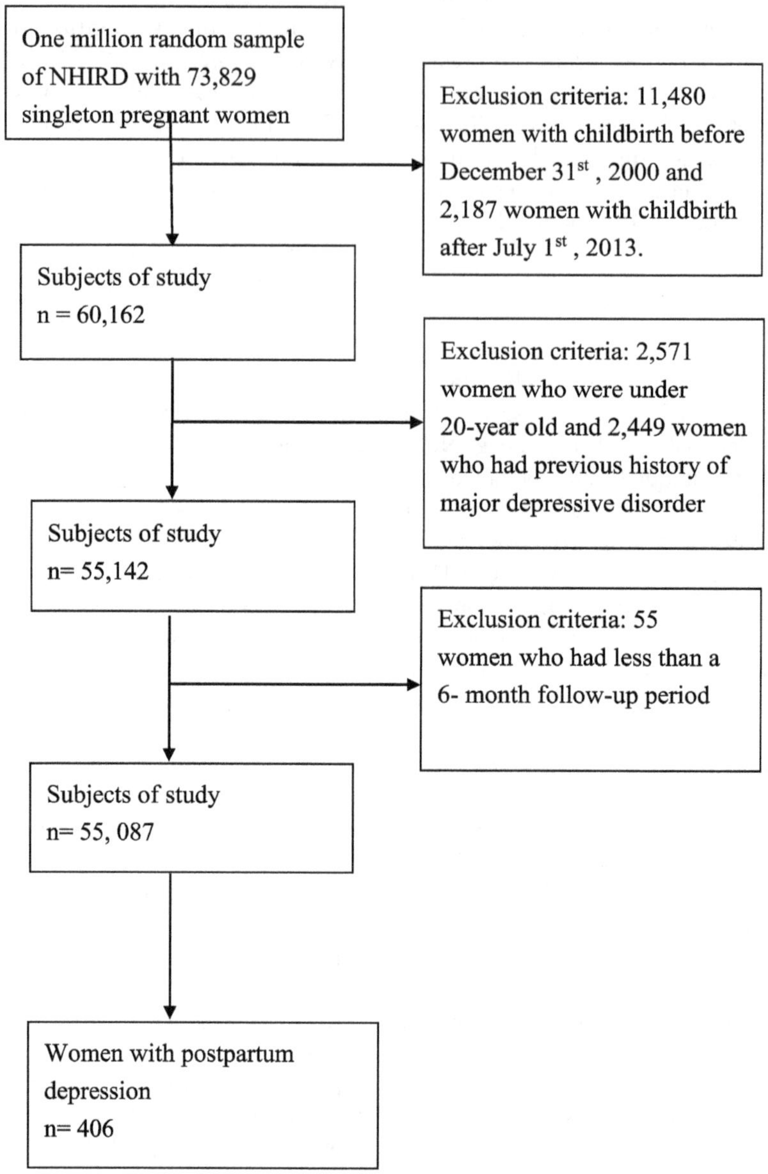

Fig. 1 Flowchart of the collection of subjects from the Longitudinal Health Insurance Database2000 (LHID2000), a sub-dataset of National Health Insurance Research Database (NHIRD), from January 2000 to December 2013

Statistical analysis

We used the Microsoft® SQL Server® 2008 to calculate and manage the patients' baseline data. The IBM SPSS statistics software v20 (IBM SPSS, 2013) was used for further data analysis. All the variables were calculated as percentages. Standard deviations and mean values were determined for the quantitative variables. Statistical significance was determined using Student's T test and the Chi-square test. Multivariate logistic regression analysis was used to determine any associations between antepartum UTIs, PPD, and additional factors. We selected risk factors into further multivariate logistic regression analysis by which total n≥5 in the PPD group. A two-sided p-value < 0.05 was regarded as statistically significant in all statistical tests.

Results

Demographics

Data for a total of 55,087 women who had singleton pregnancies between January 2001 and June 2013 was utilized in this study, including data for a total of 406 women who were newly diagnosed with PPD in the first 6 months postpartum. All the singleton pregnancy women were divided into two groups: a PPD group ($n = 406$) and a non-PPD group ($n = 54{,}691$). Table 1 shows the demographic characteristics of the two

Table 1 Demographic characteristics of study populations in Taiwan from 2000 to 2013

Demographic factor	Total pregnant women *n* (%)	Without PPD *n* (%)	PPD *n* (%)	*P* value[a]
No. of patients	55,087	54,681	406	
Age (mean ± standard deviation, years)	30 ± 6.2	29.9 ± 6.1	31.9 ± 10.4	0.003
Age_group				< 0.001**
20–24	7986(14.5)	7928(14.5)	58(14.3)	
25–29	19,548(35.5)	19,405(35.5)	143(35.2)	
30–34	19,092(34.7)	18,968(34.7)	124(30.5)	
35–39	6724(12.2)	6679(12.2)	45(11.1)	
≧40	1737(3.1)	1701(3.1)	36(8.9)	
Hospital stay (mean ± standard deviation)	4.8 ± 2.2	4.8 ± 1.6	4.2 ± 3.2	
Monthly income (TWD [b])				< 0.05*
< 20,000	36,586(66.4)	36,292(66.4)	294(72.4)	
20,000–40,000	14,340(26.0)	14,246(26.1)	94(23.2)	
40,000–60,000	3687(6.7)	3670(6.6)	17(4.2)	
≧60,000	474(0.9)	473(0.9)	1(0.2)	
Antepartum urinary tract infection				
Yes	7325(13.3)	7255(13.3)	70(17.2)	< 0.05*
Upper	255(0.5)	249(0.5)	6(1.5)	< 0.05*
Lower	7070(12.9)	7006(12.9)	64(16)	< 0.05*
No	47,762(86.7)	47,426(86.7)	336(82.8)	
Co-morbidity disease				
Antepartum hemorrhage	460(0.8)	456(0.8)	4(1.0)	0.739
Premature separation of placenta	320(0.6)	316(0.6)	4(1.0)	0.282
Placenta previa	854(1.6)	849(1.6)	5(1.2)	0.602
Eclampsia or pre-eclampsia	799(1.5)	792(1.4)	7(1.7)	0.643
Unstable lie	47(0.1)	47(0.1)	0	–
Polyhydramnios	37(0.1)	37(0.1)	0	–
Oligohydramnios	4118(7.5)	4082(7.5)	36(8.9)	0.285
Poor fetal growth	521(0.9)	518(0.9)	3(0.7)	0.666
Excessive fetal growth	532(1.0)	526(1.0)	6(1.5)	0.290
Cervical incompetence	56(0.1)	56(0.1)	0	–
Premature birth	3648(6.6)	3615(6.6)	33(8.1)	0.221
Chronic pulmonary disease	1383(2.5)	1366(2.5)	17 (4.2)	< 0.05*
Hypertension	879(1.6)	860(1.6)	19(4.7)	< 0.001**
Hypertension-complicated pregnancy	1151(2.1)	1140(2.1)	11(2.7)	0.381
Diabetes complicating pregnancy childbirth	2655(4.8)	2636(4.8)	19(4.7)	0.895
Hyperlipidemia	321(0.6)	314(0.6)	7(1.7)	< 0.05*
Heart disease	1551(2.8)	1517(2.8)	34(8.4)	< 0.001**
Anemia	5872(10.7)	5824(10.7)	48(11.8)	0.446
Cerebrovascular disease	250(0.5)	240(0.4)	10(2.5)	< 0.001**
Parkinson disease	24(0.04)	20(0.03)	4(1.0)	< 0.001**

Table 1 Demographic characteristics of study populations in Taiwan from 2000 to 2013 *(Continued)*

Demographic factor	Total pregnant women *n* (%)	Without PPD *n* (%)	PPD *n* (%)	*P* value[a]
Epilepsy	112(0.2)	108(0.2)	4(1.0)	< 0.001**
Tuberculosis	59(0.1)	59(0.1)	0	–
Asthma	892(1.6)	883(1.6)	9(2.2)	0.338
Chronic kidney disease	145(0.3)	140(0.3)	5(1.2)	< 0.001**

[a] *p*-values are two-sided
[b] TWD refers to New Taiwan dollars, of which 1 US dollar = 30TWD
** $p < 0.001$, * $p < 0.05$

study groups. Women with PPD had older ages (31.9 ± 10.4 years, $p < 0.001$) compared with the non-PPD group. There were many antepartum comorbidities that were found to be significantly associated with PPD, including chronic pulmonary disease, hypertension, peptic ulcer disease, chronic kidney disease, liver cirrhosis, hypertension-complicated pregnancy, heart disease, asthma, epilepsy, early delivery onset, premature birth, and UTI. Both upper and lower tract UTIs showed significant associations with PPD. The average hospital stay of all the women for childbirth was 4.8 ± 2.2 days. The average time to PPD diagnosis was 88.0 ± 51.0 days after delivery.

Multivariable logistic regression analysis of postpartum depression

Table 2 shows the logistic regression analysis results for certain risk factors of PPD. A monthly income of less than NT$ 20,000 and aged 20–24 were used as the reference. Heart disease (aOR 1.95 (1.26, 3.02), $p < 0.001$), antepartum UTI (aOR 1.27 (1.07, 1.65), $p < 0.05$), and age≥40 (aOR 1.98 (1.20, 3.29), $p < 0.01$) were all significant risk factors of PPD.

Among all antepartum UTIs, upper tract UTIs (aOR 2.97 (1.31,6.77)) had a higher OR than lower tract UTIs (aOR 1.21 (1.02, 1.58)). In addition, the aOR of monthly income NT$40,000–60,000 was 0.59 ((0.36, 0.97), $p < 0.05$).

Discussion

This is the first study that has focused on the relationship between antepartum UTIs and PPD. The results of this 14-year population based study show that antepartum UTIs are significantly associated with PPD. In addition, women with upper antepartum UTIs had near 3-fold greater risk of PPD than normal groups (aOR 2.97(1.31, 6.77)).

According to the study results, chronic kidney disease, epilepsy, heart disease, and upper UTI are the four greatest risk factors for PPD. These findings are consistent with those of previous studies that have also found that chronic kidney disease, epilepsy, and heart disease are associated with major depressive disorder or PPD [22–28]. In fact, the relationship between chronic kidney disease and major depressive disorder is well documented [22–24], with the decreased quality of life caused by chronic kidney disease having been found to affect mental health in both men and women [24]. Similarly, the relationship between epilepsy and higher rates of PPD is well documented [25–27]. Meanwhile, a prospective study revealed that the rate of neonatal complications is significantly higher in women with heart disease [28]. Therefore, it is reasonable that PPD is related to antepartum heart disease.

UTIs are among the most common bacterial infections in women, affecting approximately 10% of women. A previous study showed that 2–10% of pregnant women had suffered from a UTI [8], while another study found that 10% of all antepartum admissions were due to UTIs [29]. The higher UTI rate is caused by anatomical and physiological changes to the urinary tract system due to pregnancy [30]. Furthermore, pregnancy also causes asymptomatic bacteriuria changes to symptomatic UTI and reinfection [31].

The symptoms accompanying a UTI include urinary frequency and urgency, painful urination, and lower abdomen discomfort. Overactive bladder syndrome shares some of the same symptoms as UTIs, including urinary frequency and urgency, as well as urgency incontinence. In non-pregnant women, an association between overactive bladder syndrome and major depressive disorder has previously been reported [32–36]. Relatedly, van de Pol et al. demonstrated a significant relationship between PPD and overactive bladder syndrome [37]. Pregnant women who experience urinary frequency and urgency due to a UTI or overactive bladder syndrome may be embarrassed to talk about these symptoms with their physicians, which may further increase the mental stress experienced by these women. Abdollahi et al. demonstrated that recurrent UTIs are associated with PPD, but they did not further examine the relationship with respect to upper and lower UTIs [38].

Antepartum UTIs and PPD have several common risk factors such as obstetric, pediatric, and socioeconomic factors. Mazor-Dray et al. demonstrated that maternal UTIs are associated with preterm delivery, preeclampsia, intra-uterine growth restriction, and cesarean delivery [12]. Furthermore, the rates of PPD have been found to be as high as 40% among women with premature delivery [39], while Yang et al. demonstrated that cesarean delivery, preterm delivery, and preeclampsia were associated with

Table 2 The association between PPD and certain risk factors (in which total n≧5 in the PPD group) analyzed by multivariate logistic regression model

	Crude odds ratio	95% Confidence Interval	Adjusted odds ratio	95% Confidence Interval
Antepartum UTI	1.36	(1.05, 1.76)[a]	1.27	(1.07, 1.65)[a]
Upper UTI	3.28	(1.45, 7.41)[b]	2.97	(1.31, 6.77)[b]
Lower UTI	1.29	(1.04, 1.68)[a]	1.21	(1.02, 1.58)[a]
Age group (reference: 20–24)				
20–24	1		1	
25–29	1.00	(0.74, 1.37)	1.05	(0.77, 1.43)
30–34	0.89	(0.65, 1.22)	0.97	(0.71, 1.34)
35–39	0.92	(0.62, 1.36)	1.02	(0.69, 1.53)
≧40	2.89	(1.90, 4.40)[c]	1.98	(1.20, 3.29)[b]
Monthly income (TWD) (reference:< 20,000)				
20,000–40,000	0.82	(0.65, 1.03)	0.86	(0.68, 1.09)
40,000–60,000	0.57	(0.35, 0.93)[a]	0.59	(0.36, 0.97)[a]
≧60,000	0.26	(0.37, 1.86)	0.25	(0.04, 1.81)
Co-morbidity disease				
Chronic pulmonary disease	1.71	(1.05, 2.78)[a]	0.87	(0.50, 1.53)
Hypertension	3.07	(1.93, 4.89)[c]	1.11	(0.61, 2.04)
Hyperlipidemia	3.04	(1.43, 6.47)[b]	1.20	(0.52, 2.75)
Heart disease	3.20	(2.25, 4.57)[c]	1.95	(1.26, 3.02)[b]
Cerebrovascular disease	5.73	(3.02, 10.87)[c]	1.36	(0.58, 3.19)
Chronic kidney disease	4.86	(1.98, 11.92)[b]	1.19	(0.42, 3.38)

Note 1. a: $p < 0.05$, b: $p < 0.01$, c: $p < 0.001$
Note 2. TWD refers to New Taiwan dollars, of which 1 US dollar = 30 TWD

the development of PPD [21]. That being said, preeclampsia was not shown to be associated with PPD in our study. Otherwise, women of low socioeconomic status have a five-fold greater incidence of bacteriuria than normal populations. Low socioeconomic status has also been found to be a risk factor for both antepartum UTIs [40, 41] and PPD [42, 43], while antepartum UTIs are an independent risk factor of PPD.

In our study, upper antepartum UTIs had a higher aOR (OR 2.97 (1.31,6.77)) than lower UTIs. Upper antepartum UTIs are more common during the second half of pregnancy [44], are the most common severe complication of pregnancy [28], and cause approximately 12% of pregnancy associated sepsis complications that result in admission to an obstetric intensive care unit [45]. Approximately 20% of upper UTIs in pregnant women will lead to sepsis and multiple-system failure from endotoxemia [44, 46]. Upper antepartum UTIs reduce physical strength and increase mental stress in pregnant women. In addition, upper antepartum UTIs has 2.97-fold risk of preterm delivery [47], which is another important risk factor of PPD [21].

This study was a retrospective population-based study. Some data that can be useful in determining the severity of a UTI, such as the bacterial species involved, laboratory findings, asymptomatic bacteriuria status, and the side of pyelonephritis, were not available in the NHIRD. In addition, the number of upper and lower antepartum UTI patients in the study was relatively limited. Moreover, we collected PPD patients by coding ICD-9-CM coded which were diagnosed by psychiatrists who have individual concerns about PPD diagnosis. The incidence of PPD in the study cohort may have been underestimated as some women who experience depression after delivery do not seek medical help. Large-scale, prospective studies are needed to further evaluate the association between antepartum UTIs and PPD.

Conclusions

The results of this study demonstrate that antepartum UTIs, particularly upper antepartum UTIs, are significantly associated with PPD. Specifically, women with upper antepartum UTIs had 2.97-fold increased risk of PPD. As UTIs are among the most common bacterial infections in pregnant women, our results provide useful information for gynecologists, obstetricians, and health policy planners. Above all, they indicate that these health care professionals should pay greater attention to the mental health of mothers who have suffered upper UTIs during their pregnancies.

Abbreviations

CCI: Charlson comorbidity index; ICD-9-CM: International classification of diseases, 9th revision, clinical modification; LHID 2000: Longitudinal health insurance database 2000; NHIRD: National health insurance research database; OR: Odds ratio; PPD: Postpartum depression; UTI: Urinary tract infection

Acknowledgments

The implications and conclusions of this study do not represent the opinions of the Bureau of National Health Insurance, the Department of Health, or the National Health Research Institute.

Funding

This work was supported by grants from the Ministry of Science and Technology Taiwan (MOST 104–2320-B-016 -012 -MY3), the Tri-Service General Hospital of Taipei, Taiwan (TSGH-106-148 and TSGH-107-104-2320B-016-012-MY3), the grants from the Taoyuan General Hospital, Ministry of Health and Welfare (PYT10702), and the Teh-Tzer Study Group for Human Medical Research Foundation (A1061082). The funders had no role in the study design, data collection, analysis, decision to publish, or preparation of the manuscript.

Authors' contributions

JML wrote the proposal and prepared the manuscript. YPL contributed the conception and design of the manuscript. FWC revised the manuscript. SPC conducted the data analysis. HHC and SPC collected the data and helped prepare the manuscript. RJH prepared the manuscript and data analysis. JJY revised the manuscript. RJH revised the manuscript and data analysis. All the authors read and approved the final manuscript.

Competing interests

The authors declare that they have no competing interests.

Author details

[1]Division of Urology, Department of Surgery, Taoyuan General Hospital, Ministry of Health and Welfare, Taoyuan, Taiwan. [2]Department of Medicine, National Yang-Ming University, Taipei, Taiwan. [3]Graduate Institute of Life Sciences, National Defense Medical Center, Taipei, Taiwan. [4]American-Sino Women's & Children's, Hospital (SongYuan), Shanghai City, China. [5]Lihuili Eastern Hospital, Ningbo Medical Center, Ningbo City, Zhejiang province, China. [6]Department of emergency Medicine, National Taiwan University Hospital, Taipei, Taiwan. [7]Division of Genetics and endocrinology, Chang Gung Children's Hospital, Taoyuan, Taiwan. [8]Division of Urology, Department of Surgery, Yumin medical corporation Yumin hospital, Nantou, Taiwan. [9]Department of Psychiatry, Cardinal Tien Hospital, New Taipei City, Taiwan. [10]Institute of Biomedical Engineering, College of Medicine and College of Engineering, National Taiwan University, Taipei, Taiwan. [11]Superintendent, Tri-Service General Hospital Penghu Branch, National Defence Medical Center, Penghu Branch, Taiwan. [12]Biobank Management Center of the Tri-Service General Hospital, National Defense Medical Center, Taipei, Taiwan. [13]Department of Pathology and Graduate Institute of Pathology and Parasitology, the Tri-Service General Hospital, National Defense Medical Center, No. 161, Sec. 6, Minquan E. Road, Neihu District, Taipei 114, Taiwan.

References

1. O'Hara MW, Schlechte JA, Lewis DA, Varner MW. Controlled prospective study of postpartum mood disorders: psychological, environmental, and hormonal variables. J Abnorm Psychol. 1991;100(1):63.
2. Stowe ZN, Nemeroff CB. 1995. Women at risk for postpartum-onset major depression. Am J Obstet Gynecol. 1995;173(2):639–45.
3. Lee DT, Yip AS, Chiu HF, Leung TY, Chung TK. A psychiatric epidemiological study of postpartum Chinese women. Am J Psychiatry. 2001;158(2):220–6.
4. APA. Diagnostic and statistical manual of mental disorders DSM-V. Washington, DC: American Psychiatric Association; 2013.
5. O'Hara MW A, McCabe JE. Postpartum depression: current status and future directions. Annu Rev Clin Psychol. 2013;9:379–407.
6. Chang FW, Lee WY, Liu YP, Yang JJ, Chen SP, Cheng KC, Lin YC, Ho TW, Chiu FH, Hsu RJ, et al. The relationship between economic conditions and postpartum depression in Taiwan: a nationwide population-based study. J Affect Disord. 2016;204:174–9.
7. Huang YC, Mathers N. Postnatal depression – biological or cultural? A comparative study of postnatal women in the UK and Taiwan. J Adv Nurs. 2008;33:279–87.
8. Robertson E, Grace S, Wallington T, Stewart DE. Antenatal risk factors for postpartum depression: a synthesis of recent literature. Gen Hosp Psychiatry. 2004;26(4):289–95.
9. Norhayati MN, Hazlina NN, Asrenee AR, Emilin WW. Magnitude and risk factors for postpartum symptoms: a literature review. J Affect Disord. 2015; 175:34–52.
10. Le J, Briggs GG, McKeown A, Bustillo G. Urinary tract infections during pregnancy. Ann Pharmacother. 2004;38(10):1692–701.
11. Lee M, Bozzo P, Einarson A, Koren G. Urinary tract infections in pregnancy. Can Fam Physician. 2008;54:853–4.
12. Mazor-Dray E, Levy A, Schlaeffer F, Sheiner E. Maternal urinary tract infection: is it independently associated with adverse pregnancy outcome? J Matern Fetal Neonatal Med. 2009;22(2):124–8.
13. Sheffield JS, Cunningham FG. Urinary tract infection in women. Obstet Gynecol. 2005;106(5):1085–92.
14. Chen JY, Liu JM, Chang FW, Chang H, Cheng KC, Yeh CL, Wei YF, Hsu RJ. Scabies increased the risk and severity of COPD: a nationwide population-based study. Int J Chron Obstruct Pulmon Dis. 2016;11:2171–8.
15. Liu JM, Lin PH, Hsu RJ, Chang YH, Cheng KC, Pang ST, Lin SK. Complementary traditional Chinese medicine therapy improves survival in patients with metastatic prostate cancer. Medicine. 2016;95(31):e4475.
16. Liu JM, Wang HW, Chang FW, Liu YP, Chiu FH, Lin YC, Cheng KC, Hsu RJ. The effects of climate factors on scabies. A 14-year population-based study in Taiwan. Parasite. 2016;23:54.
17. Hsing AW, Ioannidis JP. Nationwide population science: lessons from the Taiwan National Health Insurance Research Database. JAMA Intern Med. 2015;175(9):1527–9.
18. National Health Insurance Institutes: National Health Insurance Research Database. http://nhird.nhri.org.tw/en/Data_Subsets.html# Accessed 10 Oct 2016.
19. Liu JM, Chiu FH, Lin CY, Chang FW, Hsu RJ. Incidence of autoimmune diseases in patients with scabies: a nationwide population-based study in Taiwan. Rheumatol Int. 2017;37(7):1125–34.
20. Yang SN, Shen LJ, Ping T, Wang YC, Chien CW. The delivery mode and seasonal variation are associated with the development of postpartum depression. J Affect Disord. 2011;132(1):158–64.
21. Lin CY, Chang FW, Yang JJ, Chang CH, Yeh CL, et al. Increased risk of bipolar disorder in patients with scabies: a nationwide population-based matched-cohort study. Psychiatry Res. 2017;257:14–20.
22. Hedayati SS, Minhajuddin AT, Afshar M, Toto RD, Trivedi MH, Rush AJ. Association between major depressive episodes in patients with chronic kidney disease and initiation of dialysis, hospitalization, or death. JAMA. 2010;303(19):1946–53.
23. Zalai D, Szeifert L, Novak M. Psychological distress and depression in patients with chronic kidney disease. Semin Dial. 2012;25(4):428–38.
24. Abdel-Kader K, Unruh ML, Weisbord SD. Symptom burden, depression, and quality of life in chronic and end-stage kidney disease. Clin J Am Soc Nephrol. 2009;4(6):1057–64.

25. Turner K, Piazzini A, Franza A, Fumarola C, Chifari R, Marconi AM, et al. Postpartum depression in women with epilepsy versus women without epilepsy. Epilepsy Behav. 2006;9(2):293–7.
26. Galanti M, Newport DJ, Pennell PB, Titchner D, Newman M, Knight BT, et al. Postpartum depression in women with epilepsy: influence of antiepileptic drugs in a prospective study. Epilepsy Behav. 2009;16(3):426–30.
27. Turner K, Piazzini A, Franza A, Marconi AM, Canger R, Canevini MP. Epilepsy and postpartum depression. Epilepsia. 2009;50(Suppl 1):24–7.
28. Siu SC, Sermer M, Colman JM, Alvarez AN, Mercier LA, Morton BC, et al. Cardiac disease in pregnancy (CARPREG) investigators. Prospective multicenter study of pregnancy outcomes in women with heart disease. Circulation. 2001;104(5):515–21.
29. Bacak SJ, Callaghan WM, Dietz PM, Crouse C. Pregnancy-associated hospitalizations in the United States, 1999–2000. Am J Obstet Gynecol. 2005;192(2):592–7.
30. Nowicki B. Urinary tract infection in pregnant women: old dogmas and current concepts regarding pathogenesis. Curr Infect Dis Rep. 2002;4:529–35.
31. Foxman B, Brown P. Epidemiology of urinary tract infections: transmission and risk factors, incidence, and costs. Infect Dis Clin N Am. 2003;17:227–41.
32. Zorn BH, Montgomery H, Pieper K, Gray M, Steers WD. Urinary incontinence and depression. J Urol. 1999;162:82–4.
33. Buchsbaum GM, Chin M, Glantz C, Guzick D. Prevalence of urinary incontinence and associated risk factors in a cohort of nuns. Obstet Gynecol. 2002;100:226–9.
34. Chiverton PA, Wells TJ, Brink CA, Mayer R. Psychological factors associated with urinary incontinence. Clin Nurse Spec. 1996;10:229–33.
35. Stewart WF, Van Rooyen JB, Cundiff GW, Abrams P, Herzog AR, Corey R, et al. Prevalence and burden of overactive bladder in the United States. World J Urol. 2003;20:327–36.
36. Melville JL, Delaney K, Newton K, Katon W. Incontinence severity and major depression in incontinent women. Obstet Gynecol. 2005;106:585–92.
37. van de Pol G, van Brummen HJ, Bruinse HW, Heintz AP, van der Vaart CH. Is there an association between depressive and urinary symptoms during and after pregnancy? Int Urogynecol J Pelvic Floor Dysfunct. 2007;18(12):1409–15.
38. Abdollahi F, Zarghami M, Azhar MZ, Sazlina SG, Lye MS. Predictors and incidence of post-partum depression: a longitudinal cohort study. J Obstet Gynaecol Res. 2014;40(12):2191–200.
39. Vigod SN, Villegas L, Dennis CL, Ross LE. Prevalence and risk factors for postpartum depression among women with preterm and low-birth-weight infants: a systematic review. BJOG. 2010;117(5):540–50.
40. Turck M, Goffe BS, Petersdorf RG. Bacteriuria of pregnancy. Relation to socioeconomic factors. N Engl J Med. 1962;266:857–60.
41. Golan A, Wexler S, Amit A, Gordon D, David MP. Asymptomatic bacteriuria in normal and high-risk pregnancy. Eur J Obstet Gynecol Reprod Biol. 1989; 33:101–8.
42. Inandi T, Bugdayci R, Dundar P, Sumer H, Sasmaz T. Risk factors for depression in the first postnatal year: a Turkish study. Soc Psychiatry Psychiatr Epidemiol. 2005;40:725–30.
43. Ozdemir H, Ergin N, Selimoglu K, Bilgel N. Postnatal depressive mood in Turkish women. Psychol Health Med. 2014;10:96–107.
44. Hill JB, Sheffield JS, McIntire DD, Wendel GD Jr. Acute pyelonephritis in pregnancy. Obstet Gynecol. 2005;105:18–23.
45. Zeeman GG, Wendel GD, Cunningham FG. A blueprint for obstetric critical care. Am J Obstet Gynecol. 2003;188(2):532–6.
46. Cunningham FG, Morris GB, Mickal A. Acute pyelonephritis of pregnancy: a clinical review. Obstet Gynecol. 1973;42(1):112–7.
47. Farkash E, Weintraub AY, Sergienko R, Wiznitzer A, Zlotnik A, Sheiner E. Acute antepartum pyelonephritis in pregnancy: a critical analysis of risk factors and outcomes. Eur J Obstet Gynecol Reprod Biol. 2012;162(1):24–7.

19

Huge fetal hepatic Hemangioma: prenatal diagnosis on ultrasound and prognosis

Li Jiao-ling[1*], Geng Xiu-ping[1], Chen Kun-shan[2], He Qiu-ming[3], Li Xiao-fen[1], Yang Bo-yang[1] and Fang Qian[1]

Abstract

Background: Although huge fetal hepatic hemangiomas are rare, they can cause fatal complications. The purpose of this study is to describe the imaging features and prognosis of these tumors.

Methods: Imaging data were collected for 6 patients with huge fetal hepatic hemangiomas treated at our hospital. Imaging modalities included prenatal magnetic resonance imaging and ultrasound and postnatal color Doppler ultrasound and contrast-enhanced computed tomography (CT).

Results: Among the 93,562 fetuses of 92,126 pregnant women examined at our hospital, 6 had huge hepatic hemangiomas (incidence rate, 0.64/10,000), as confirmed via postnatal color Doppler imaging and contrast-enhanced CT. Five fetuses had solitary lesions, whereas 1 (fetus 2) had multiple lesions. Four fetuses had lesions in the right liver lobe and 1 had a lesion in the left liver lobe, and 1 (fetus 2) had lesions in both lobes. All lesions showed centripetal enhancement on postnatal contrast-enhanced CT, which was more intense peripherally. Following postnatal treatment with oral propranolol, with or without dexamethasone or interventional therapy with the medical sclerosant pingyangmycin, all lesions decreased in size, with calcification plaques appearing 6 months after treatment.

Conclusions: Huge hepatic hemangiomas have typical ultrasonographic features and can be diagnosed prenatally. Treatment with propranolol, with or without dexamethasone, may result in a favorable prognosis.

Keywords: Liver tumor, Huge hepatic hemangioma, Prenatal diagnosis, Ultrasound, Magnetic resonance imaging, Contrast-enhanced computed tomography

Background

Fetal tumors are a diverse but rare group of conditions with significant implications for the health of both mother and fetus. Approximately 15% of fetal tumors are hemangiomas [1, 2], which usually appear on the face, neck and limbs. Fetal hepatic hemangiomas are benign vascular tumors present at birth and distinct from vascular malformations. They are characterized as either rapidly involuting or non-involuting based on their clinical progression [3, 4]. Fetal hepatic hemangiomas are rarely reported; hence, their exact incidence rate remains undetermined [5, 6].

Parents and clinicians are advised to regularly monitor congenital hepatic hemangiomas, which reach maximum size at birth and, in some cases, gradually disappear. Small hepatic hemangiomas are often asymptomatic and seldom require treatment. In contrast, huge hepatic hemangiomas (mean diameter > 4 cm) are less frequently reported than small hepatic hemangiomas [7] and can cause serious complications [8, 9]. Without prompt intervention, neonatal mortality rates reach 30–100% [10–12].

Hence, studies on the prenatal diagnosis of huge hepatic hemangiomas are important. Information gained by systematically monitoring fetuses for tumor progression and related complications will help obstetricians decide on timely delivery and appropriate neonatal treatments. This retrospective study examined the ultrasound characteristics and prognosis of 6 huge fetal hepatic hemangiomas in south China. To the best of our knowledge, this study is the first to report the incidence of this disease in south China and the successful use of propranolol as treatment.

* Correspondence: doctorlijiaolin@126.com
[1]Department of Ultrasound, GZ Women & Children Medical Centre, Jinsui Road 9, Guangzhou 510623, China
Full list of author information is available at the end of the article

Methods

This study was approved by the ethics committee of the GZ Women & Children Medical Centre. All pregnant women in the study provided informed consent for ultrasound.

Among the 93,562 fetuses of 92,126 pregnant women examined routinely via serial ultrasound at 22–24 weeks, 30–32 weeks, and 36–38 weeks between January 1, 2013 and February 28, 2016, only 6 fetuses, of 6 women, were prenatally diagnosed with huge hepatic hemangiomas, with the diagnosis confirmed postnatally. All 6 women were referred to our center due to suspicion of fetal anomalies on ultrasound examinations at other hospitals. The mean age of the pregnant women was 27 years (range, 22–31 years).

Five of the 6 fetuses were evaluated by prenatal magnetic resonance imaging (MRI) (Signa; GE Medical Systems, Milwaukee, WI, USA), except for fetus 6, and all were evaluated by using postnatal color Doppler ultrasound and contrast-enhanced computed tomography (CT). Fetal gestational age was estimated based on the mother's last menstrual period or via ultrasound scan performed early in the pregnancy.

A high-resolution ultrasound system equipped with a 3–5 MHz transducer (Sequoia 512; Acuson Siemens, Germany) was used to screen for fetal structural abnormalities in the middle of the second trimester. Fetuses diagnosed with hemangioma were assessed by follow-up ultrasound in our department daily, or weekly. The diagnosis of huge fetal hepatic hemangiomas was independently confirmed by 2 experienced physicians. Any complication and the mode and time of delivery were also recorded.

Neonates prenatally diagnosed with huge hepatic hemangiomas were examined immediately after birth via color Doppler ultrasound. These neonates were subsequently transferred to the neonatal intensive care unit (NICU), where they underwent contrast-enhanced CT for further evaluation. Shortly thereafter, blood concentrations of alpha-fetoprotein (AFP), neuron-specific enolase (NSE), vanillylmandelic acid (VMA), and other tumor markers were measured to rule out primary and metastatic malignant liver tumors. After performing routine blood tests and examining blood coagulation, liver and thyroid function tests, oral propranolol, with or without dexamethasone, or interventional therapy with the medical sclerosant pingyangmycin was administered [13]. The size, internal echo, and blood flow of the lesions were monitored via color Doppler ultrasound. During the neonatal follow-up period, the lesions became enlarged and surgical treatment was considered.

Results

A total of 6 of the 93,562 fetuses of 92,126 pregnant women examined at our hospital were diagnosed with huge hepatic hemangiomas. All were incidental findings on routine ultrasound scans of the third trimester (mean, 35 + 1 weeks [range, 31+ to 39+ weeks]) at other hospitals. Five of the 6 fetuses (fetus 6 was the exception) were examined via prenatal MRI, and all were evaluated by using prenatal ultrasound and postnatal color Doppler ultrasound and contrast-enhanced CT.

One fetus (fetus 2) had multiple lesions, with the other 5 having solitary lesions. Hemangiomas were present in the left liver lobe in fetus 1 and in the right liver lobe in fetuses 3–6 (Table 1). The lesions in fetus 2 varied in size, with the largest lesion in the left lobe and the smaller lesions scattered throughout the right lobe. The largest lesion in fetus 2 measured 92 × 56 × 80 mm, whereas the solitary lesions in fetus 1, 3, 4, 5, and 6 measured 86 × 81 × 103 mm, 45 × 23 × 41 mm, 56 × 42 × 41 mm, 50 × 47 × 43 mm, and 52 × 48 × 55 mm, respectively. The cardiothoracic ratio was normal in fetuses 1, 3, and 4, and above normal (<0.33) in fetuses 2, 5, and 6. The ultrasonographic features of fetuses 1, 2, and 4 are summarized in Figs. 1, 2 and 3. The boundaries of all lesions were well-defined. The internal echo was uniform in fetuses 5 and 6 and nonuniform (grid shaped) in the other 4 fetuses. The lesions in fetuses 2, 3, and 4 had a central necrotic hypoechoic area, the lesion in fetus 2 had a cystic cavity, and the lesion in fetus 4 also contained scattered punctate calcifications. Prenatal color Doppler ultrasound showed that the lesions were mainly supplied by branches of the hepatic artery and drained by 1 or 2 hepatic veins, which were usually tortuous and dilated. No abnormalities in the portal vein flow were detected on color Doppler flow images. Pulse Doppler ultrasound revealed low to medium blood flow resistance in the lesions.

All lesions had low signal intensity on prenatal T1-weighted MRI images and high signal intensity on T2-weighted images, relative to the signal intensity of the liver. Scattered punctate calcifications were again noted in the lesion in fetus 4. Flow voids, associated with intralesional high blood flow, were frequently seen. In addition to the large lesion in the left liver lobe in fetus 2, prenatal MRI also revealed multiple low-signal-intensity nodules of various sizes scattered throughout the right liver lobe. These nodules were spherical in shape, with clear boundaries and relatively uniform internal signal intensity. The signal intensity in the liver parenchyma between the nodules was normal. On postnatal contrast-enhanced CT, all lesions showed centripetal enhancement, which was more intense peripherally.

The obstetric information of the 6 fetuses is summarized in Table 1. Fetuses 1, 2 and 3 were delivered via cesarean section, because no signs of spontaneous labor were noted and the fetal heart rate was gradually slowing down (fetus 1), the cardiothoracic ratio had increased (fetus 2), or the uterus was scarred (fetus 3). Fetus 4 had

Table 1 Ultrasonographic diagnosis and follow-up of 6 fetuses with huge hepatic hemangiomas

Fetus	GA at diagnosis (weeks)	Lesion size (mm)	Site	Cardiothoracic ratio	Delivery mode	GA at delivery (weeks)	Apgar score	Wt (g)	Sex	Postnatal therapy	Post-treatment lesion size (mm)
1	36	86 × 81 × 103	LL	Normal	CS	40	9–9-9	3120	Male	MT	35 × 36 × 34
2	31 + 6	92 × 56 × 80	BL	High	CS	37	9–9-9	3220	Male	MT	19 × 19 × 10
3	36	45 × 23 × 41	RL	Normal	CS	39 + 2	9–9-10	3220	Male	MT	31 × 33 × 26
4	34 + 2	56 × 42 × 41	RL	Normal	SD	39 + 5	9–9-9	3160	Male	MT	28 × 25 × 27
5	36 + 3	50 × 47 × 43	RL	High, TVR, little PE	SD	37 + 2	9–9-9	2710	Male	MT	20 × 20 × 17
6	37 + 1	52 × 48 × 55	RL	High, little PE	SD	38 + 3	9–9-9	2800	Male	IT	27 × 25 × 22

Abbreviations: *GA* Gestational age, *LL* Left liver lobe, *RL* Right liver lobe, *BL* Both liver lobes, *CS* Cesarean section, *SD* Spontaneous delivery, *MT* Medical treatment, *IT* Interventional therapy, *TVR* Tricuspid valve regurgitation, *PE* Pericardial effusion

no complications and was delivered spontaneously. Fetuses 5 and 6 were delivered spontaneously, 2 days after the occurrence of mild pericardial effusion. Postpartum Apgar scores were normal in all neonates (>8 for 1, 5, and 10 min). Neonates 1–5 received oral propranolol with or without dexamethasone, and neonate 6 underwent interventional sclerotherapy with pingyangmycin due to a relative contraindication to beta blockers. All lesions gradually decreased in size, and internal calcification plaques could be detected after 6 months. Color Doppler ultrasound showed sparse blood flow in all lesions.

Discussion

Ultrasound is widely used in obstetrics, because it is safe for both the fetus and mother. Approximately 30% of the blood supply to the liver comes from the hepatic artery and approximately 70% from the portal vein [14], with blood drained from the liver via 3 hepatic veins. Hepatic lesions alter the pathways by which blood enters and exits the liver [15, 16], thereby aiding in the ultrasound detection of hepatic lesions.

The most likely differential diagnoses of fetal liver lesions include hepatic hemangioma, hepatoblastoma, and metastatic malignant tumor. In general, hepatic hemangiomas are well-defined mixed, solid lesions with hypervascularization and fine granular calcifications. Hepatoblastomas are spoke-wheel-like solid tumors with poor vascularization and coarse, dense calcifications. Metastatic liver tumors are solid masses with a bull's-eye configuration and primary lesions. Malignant lesions and some benign lesions such as

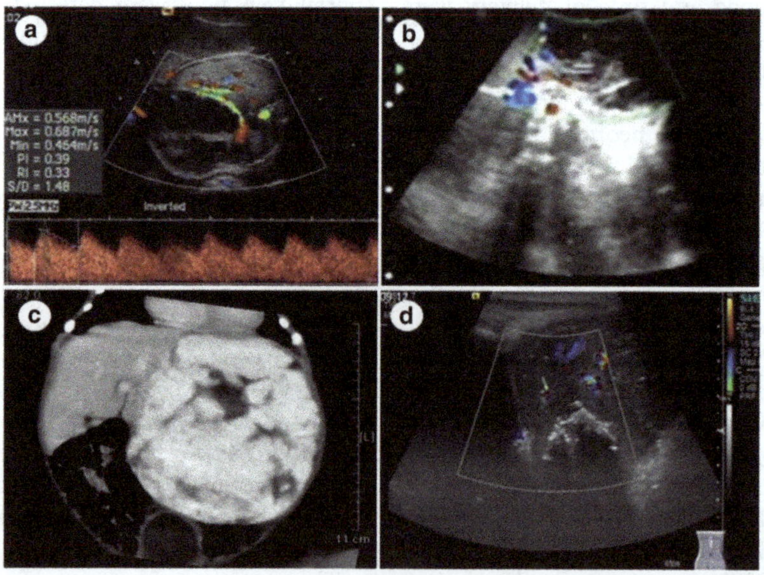

Fig. 1 Fetus with a hemangioma in the left liver lobe (fetus 1). **a** Circular hypoechoic lesion, measuring 86 × 81 × 103 mm. Color Doppler ultrasound shows a ring of blood flow at the edge of the lesion and stars intralesion. Pulse Doppler ultrasound suggests that the resistance index is 0.33. **b** Ultrasound on the day of birth shows that lesion has a clear border, an excentric growth pattern, and an internal grid-shaped region and bypasses the left hepatic vein. **c** Postnatal computed tomography (CT) shows the lesion in the left lobe. On contrast-enhanced CT, the lesion was centripetal enhancement. **d** Two years after treatment of the neonate with propranolol and dexamethasone, the lesion was 35 × 36 × 34 mm in size, with multiple strong echo spots in the center

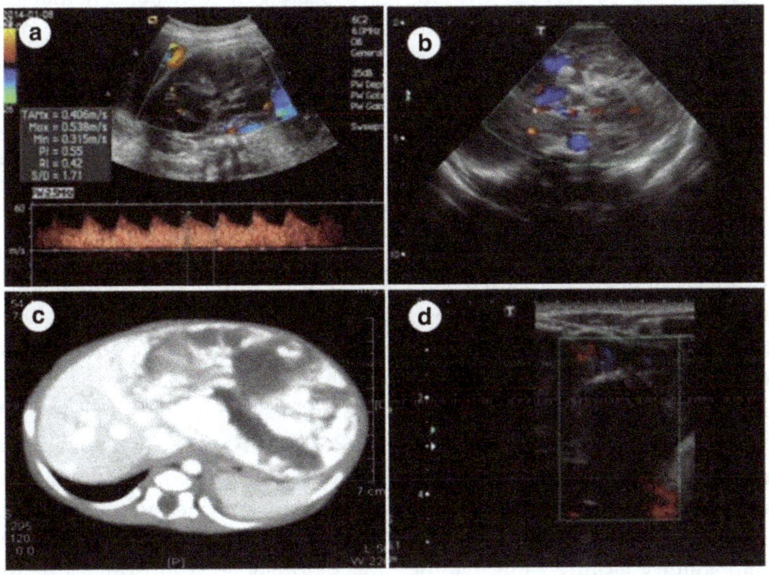

Fig. 2 Fetus with multiple hemangiomas in the whole liver (fetus 2). **a** Largest hypoechoic lesion, measuring 92 × 56 × 80 mm and located in the left liver lobe. Color Doppler ultrasound shows a ring of blood flow at the edge of the lesion and stars intralesion. Pulse Doppler ultrasound suggests that the resistance index is 0.42. **b** Ultrasound on the day of birth shows that the large lesion has a clear border and an internal grid-shaped region. The portal vein was unobstructed, and its inner diameter was normal. **c** Postnatal computed tomography (CT) shows the large lesion in the left lobe and several smaller lesions in the right lobe. The density of the mass was low but not uniform. On contrast-enhanced CT, the edge of the lesion increased in intensity in a lattice-like pattern in the early phase of the scan, and the center of the mass gradually increased in intensity during the delay phase; there was no enhancement in the low-density zone. **d** Two years after treatment of the neonate with propranolol and dexamethasone, the lesion was 19 × 19 × 10 mm in size. Calcification plaques were observed in the lesion, and the intrahepatic and the extrahepatic bile ducts were not dilated

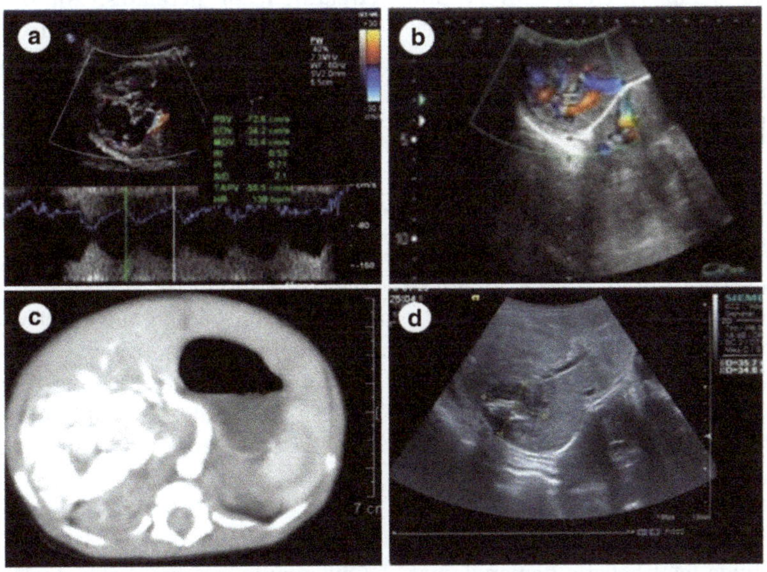

Fig. 3 Fetus with a hemangioma in the right liver lobe (fetus 4). **a** Hypoechoic lesion measuring 56 × 42 × 41 mm. Color Doppler ultrasound shows a strip of blood flow at the edge of the lesion and stars intralesion. Pulse Doppler ultrasound suggests that the resistance index is 0.53. **b** Ultrasound on the day of birth shows that the lesion is less clear, with nonuniform density and punctate calcifications. The hepatic vein was bypassed. **c** Postnatal computed tomography (CT) shows nonuniform density and punctate calcifications. On contrast-enhanced CT, the lesion was centripetal enhancement. It was supplied by a branch of the hepatic artery and drained via the hepatic veins; the right and middle hepatic veins were thickened. **d** Six months after treatment of the neonate with propranolol and dexamethasone, the lesion was 28 × 25 × 27 mm in size. Calcification plaques were observed, and the intrahepatic and the extrahepatic bile ducts were not dilated

huge hepatic hemangiomas can cause serious complications that endanger fetal survival. The reported neonatal mortality rate of fetuses diagnosed with liver lesions is 30–100%. If huge hepatic hemangiomas are prenatally diagnosed, they can be monitored in utero to identify these potential fatal complications.

Huge hepatic hemangiomas are vascular tumors with a diameter of over 4 cm. Because these tumors are rarely reported, their actual incidence is unclear. Our study found that only 6 of the 93,562 fetuses were prenatally diagnosed with huge hepatic hemangiomas, a diagnosis that was confirmed postnatally, making the incidence of huge hepatic hemangiomas 0.64/10,000. All 6 huge hepatic hemangiomas were prenatally detected on serial ultrasounds during the third trimester at different hospitals.

Hepatic hemangiomas can occur in either or both lobes of the liver. The lesions can be solitary or multifocal and vary in size [17]. In this study, 4 fetuses had right-lobe lesions and 5 had solitary lesions. Only 1 fetus (fetus 1) had a left-lobe lesion, and only 1 (fetus 2) had multiple lesions. Cases of fetal multiple hepatic hemangiomas have only been reported twice [12, 18]. Hence, fetus 2 in this study is the third reported case in literature. The small lesions in the right lobe of fetus 2 in this study were visible only on prenatal MRI, but not on prenatal ultrasound. Postpartum color Doppler ultrasound and contrast-enhanced CT confirmed the presence of multiple small lesions in the right lobe of this fetus.

Huge hepatic hemangiomas have well-defined borderlines on 2-dimensional sonography before delivery, and are hypoechoic compared with the normal liver. Although hemangiomas have been reported hyperechoic or isoechoic, none of our lesions had such characteristics. The lesions were either uniformly or non-uniformly hypoechoic. We also observed necrotic areas with or without calcification and a cystic cavity in these lesions. Postnatal ultrasound findings were concordant with the prenatal findings in all 6 cases, and the MRI findings (described in the results section) in all 6 were in agreement with those reported by Dong et al. [19].

Both antenatal ultrasound and MRI can demonstrate larger lesions and scattered punctate calcifications, whereas prenatal MRI can reveal smaller lesions not detected on prenatal ultrasound. When prenatal ultrasound showed abundant blood flow within the lesion, flow voids associated with intralesional high blood flow were frequently observed on prenatal MRI.

Fatal complications of huge fetal hepatic hemangiomas include congestive heart failure, consumptive coagulation dysfunction, and liver rupture [18, 20]. Hence, evaluation of intrauterine conditions via serial ultrasound examinations is important in making pregnancy-related decisions, including active management with in-utero treatment, expectant management, or expediting delivery. Fetuses with suspected huge hepatic hemangiomas in our study were monitored weekly for tumor progression and complications. When the cardiothoracic ratio increased and the fetus was full term, we chose a suitable delivery method, and the infant was delivered in a timely manner. By contrast, when the cardiothoracic ratio increased prior to full term, we usually monitored the fetus daily until 32 weeks gestation, with the fetus delivered immediately upon the appearance of a pericardial effusion.

Fetuses with hepatic hemangiomas have been successfully delivered vaginally [21]. This was also true in our study, with 3 fetuses being spontaneously delivered. The mode of delivery was unrelated to lesion size, number of lesions, lesion location (right or left liver lobe) or gestational age.

Postnatally, the 6 neonates had stable vital signs. Contrast-enhanced CT, blood tests, liver and thyroid function tests, and measurements of tumor marker levels (e.g., AFP, NSE, and VMA) were performed in the NICU. There was no evidence of primary or metastatic malignant liver tumors. Multiple hepatic hemangiomas have been reported to result in hypothyroidism, but it has not been determined whether patients with rapidly involuting congenital hemangioma also had hypothyroidism. Although fetus 2 in our study had multiple lesions, his thyroid function was normal.

CT has several advantages over other imaging modalities, including a fast scanning speed, the lack of need for sedation, and low system impact, suggesting that this modality may expedite the diagnosis and treatment of neonates. All 6 neonates in this study underwent contrast-enhanced CT, which showed centripetal enhancement of all lesions, an enhancement that was more intense peripherally.

Corticosteroids have been shown to shrink hepatic hemangiomas [22, 23]. For example, multimodal management of 17 neonates included steroid treatment. One of these neonates underwent embolization as supportive medical treatment, followed by propranolol administration, but died at 1 month of age. In our study, neonates received either oral propranolol with or without dexamethasone or interventional therapy with pingyangmycin. These treatments were effective, as shown by the gradual reductions in lesion size and internal blood flow and the presence of calcification plaques 6 months after treatment.

Conclusions

Our results suggest that accurate prenatal diagnosis and regular monitoring of fetuses with huge hepatic hemangiomas may improve prognosis and help avert serious complications. Basing postnatal treatments on prenatal imaging findings may help reduce the perinatal mortality rate due to this condition. Our findings may assist physicians in choosing the best mode and time of delivery as well as the appropriate treatment for these fetuses and neonates. To our knowledge, this study is the first to report the incidence rate (0.64/10,000) of huge congenital hepatic hemangiomas in south China. We intend to perform a prospective, controlled study to further investigate whether oral propranolol with or without dexamethasone is effective for the management of huge congenital hepatic hemangiomas.

Abbreviations

AFP: Alpha-fetoprotein; CT: Computed tomography; MRI: Magnetic resonance imaging; NICU: Neonatal intensive care unit; NSE: Neuron-specific enolase; VMA: Vanillylmandelic acid

Acknowledgments

We would like to thank Yang Yixin of the University of Quebec, Canada for English language editing.

Funding

The study was funded by our hospital, a total of 10,000 yuan, 4000 yuan was used in the design of the study and collection, analysis, and interpretation of data, and 6000 yuan was used in writing the manuscript.

Authors' contributions

LJL, GXP, and LXF were involved in prenatal ultrasound diagnosis of huge hepatic hemangiomas, and analyzed and interpreted the 6 fetuses data regarding huge hepatic hemangioma. CKSh performed interventional therapy on 1 newborn with hepatic hemangioma, and analyzed and interpreted the newborn data. HQM was responsible for the conservative treatment of 5 neonates with hepatic hemangioma, and analyzed and interpreted the 5 neonates data. YBY and FQ performed abdominal ultrasonography in all cases, and analyzed and interpreted the 6 neonates data. All authors contributed to the preparation of the manuscript and approve of the final version of the paper to be submitted. Each author can respond to any questions in regard to this study in their area of expertise.

Competing interests

The authors declare that they have no competing interests.

Author details

[1]Department of Ultrasound, GZ Women & Children Medical Centre, Jinsui Road 9, Guangzhou 510623, China. [2]Department of Invasive Technology, GZ Women & Children Medical Centre, Guangzhou 510623, China. [3]Neonatal Intensive Care Unit, GZ Women & Children Medical Centre, Guangzhou 510623, China.

References

1. Kamil D, Tepelmann J, Berg C, Heep A, Axt-Fliedner R, Gembruch U, et al. Spectrum and outcome of prenatally diagnosed fetal tumors. Ultrasound Obstet Gynecol. 2008;31(3):296–302.
2. Boull C, Maguiness SM. Congenital hemangiomas. Semin Cutan Med Surg. 2016;35(3):124–7.
3. Mulliken JB, Enjolras O. Congenital hemangiomas and infantile hemangioma: missing links. J Am Acad Dermatol. 2004;50(6):875–82.
4. Cohen MM Jr. Hemangiomas: their uses and abuses. Am J Med Genet A. 2007;143(3):235–40.
5. Dreyfus M, Baldauf JJ, Dadoun K, Becmeur F, Berrut F, Ritter J. Prenatal diagnosis of hepatic hemangioma. Fetal Diagn Ther. 1996;11(1):57–60.
6. Helmberger TK, Ros PR, Mergo PJ, Tomczak R, Reiser MF. Pediatric liver neoplasms: a radiologic-pathologic correlation. Eur Radiol. 1999;9(7):1339–47.
7. Pott Bartsch EM, Paek BW, Yoshizawa J, Goldstein RB, Ferrell LD, Coakley FV, et al. Giant fetal hepatic hemangioma: case report and literature review. Fetal Diagn Ther. 2003;18(1):59–64.
8. Chuileannain FN, Rowlands S, Sampson A. Ultrasonographic appearances of fetal hepatic hemangioma. J Ultrasound Med. 1999;18(5):379–81.
9. Aslan H, Dural O, Yildirim G, Acar DK. Prenatal diagnosis of a liver cavernous hemangioma. Fetal Pediatr Pathol. 2013;32(5):341–5.
10. Sur A, Manraj H, Lavoie PM, Lim K, Courtemanche D, Brooks P, et al. Multiple successful angioembolizations for refractory cardiac failure in a preterm with rapidly involuting congenital hemangioma. AJP Rep. 2016;6(1):99–103.
11. Morimura Y, Fujimori K, Ishida T, Ito A, Nomura Y, Sato A. Fetal hepatic hemangioma representing non-reassuring pattern in fetal heart rate monitoring. J Obstet Gynaecol Res. 2003;29(5):347–50.
12. Franchi-Abella S, Gorincour G, Avni F, Guibaud L, Chevret L, Pariente D. SFIPP-GRRIF (Société Francophone d'Imagerie Pédiatrique et Périnatale-Groupe de Recherche Radiopédiatrique en Imagerie Foetale). Hepatic haemangioma-prenatal imaging findings, complications and perinatal outcome in a case series. Pediatr Radiol. 2012;42(3):298–307.
13. Hou J, Wang M, Tang H, Wang Y, Huang H. Pingyangmycin sclerotherapy for infantile hemangiomas in oral and maxillofacial regions: an evaluation of 66 consecutive patients. Int J Oral Maxillofac Surg. 2011;40(11):1246–51.
14. Wang H. editor-in-chief. Topographic anatomy. Shelton: People's Medical Publishing House; 2005. p. 187.
15. Isaacs H Jr. Fetal and neonatal hepatic tumors. J Pediatr Surg. 2007;42(11): 1797–803.
16. Makin E, Davenport M. Fetal and neonatal liver tumours. Early Hum Dev. 2010;86(10):637–42.
17. Lutgendorf MA, Magann EF, Yousef M, Hill JB, Foster DT. Hepatic epithelial hemangioendothelioma in pregnancy. Gynecol Obstet Investig. 2009;67(4): 238–40.
18. Gembruch U, Baschat AA, Gloeckner-Hoffmann K, Gortner L, Germer U. Prenatal diagnosis and management of fetuses with liver hemangiomata. Ultrasound Obstet Gynecol. 2002;19(5):454–60.
19. Dong SZ, Zhu M, Zhong YM, Yin MZ. Use of foetal MRI in diagnosing hepatic hemangioendotheliomas: a report of four cases. Eur J Radiol. 2010; 75(3):301–5.
20. Meirowitz NB, Guzman ER, Underberg-Davis SJ, Pellegrino JE, Vintzileos AM. Hepatic hemangioendothelioma: prenatal sonographic findings and evolution of the lesion. J Clin Ultrasound. 2000;28(5):258–63.
21. Chou SY, Chiang HK, Chow PK, Wu CF, Liang SJ, Hsu CS. Fetal hepatic hemangioma diagnosed prenatally with ultrasonography. Acta Obstet Gynecol Scand. 2005;84(3):301–2.
22. Schmitz R, Heinig J, Klockenbusch W, Kiesel L, Steinhard J. Antenatal diagnosis of a giant fetal hepatic hemangioma and treatment with maternal corticosteroid. Ultraschall Med. 2009;30(3):223–6.
23. Morris J, Abbott J, Burrows P, Levine D. Antenatal diagnosis of fetal hepatic hemangioma treated with maternal corticosteroids. Obstet Gynecol. 1999; 94(5):813–5.

20

Prenatal micronutrient supplementation and postpartum depressive symptoms in a pregnancy cohort

Brenda MY Leung[1], Bonnie J Kaplan[1,2*], Catherine J Field[3], Suzanne Tough[1,2], Misha Eliasziw[1,4], Mariel Fajer Gomez[3], Linda J McCargar[3] , Lisa Gagnon[5]and the APrON Study Team

Abstract

Background: Postpartum depression is a serious problem for women and their offspring. Micronutrient supplements are recommended for pregnant women because of their documented protective effects for the offspring, but their potential beneficial effects on maternal mental health are unknown. This study investigated the association between prenatal micronutrient supplementation and the risk for symptoms of postpartum depression in a longitudinal pregnancy cohort from the Alberta Pregnancy Outcomes and Nutrition (APrON) study.

Methods: Participants came from a cohort of the first 600 APrON women. Supplemental nutrient intake and symptoms of depression (measured with the Edinburgh Postnatal Depression Scale (EPDS)) were collected at each trimester and 12 weeks postpartum.

Results: Of the 475 participants who completed the EPDS at least twice in pregnancy and at 12 weeks postpartum, 416 (88%) scored <10 and 59 (12%) scored ≥10, where an EPDS ≥10 is considered to be "at least probable minor depression". Mean nutrient intakes from supplements were higher in women with lower EPDS scores, particularly selenium ($p = 0.0015$) and omega-3s ($p = 0.01$). Bivariate analyses showed that several demographic and social/ lifestyle variables were associated with EPDS ≥10: not having been born in Canada ($p = 0.01$), greater number of chronic conditions ($p = 0.05$), greater number of stressful life events during this pregnancy ($p = 0.02$), and lower prenatal and postnatal support ($p = 0.0043$ and $p = 0.0001$, respectively). Adjusting for covariates and nutrients known to be associated with postpartum depression, logistic regression showed that having a prenatal EPDS ≥ 10 increased the odds of postpartum depressive symptoms (second and third trimester OR = 3.29, 95% CI = 1.55 - 7.01, $p = 0.004$ and OR = 4.26, 95% CI = 2.05 - 8.85, $p < 0.0001$, respectively), while prenatal supplemental selenium (per 10 mcg, OR = 0.76, 95% CI = 0.74 - 0.78, $p = 0.0019$) and postnatal social support (OR = 0.87, 95% CI = 0.78 - 0.97, $p = 0.0015$) were protective.

Conclusions: Multiple factors, including supplementary selenium intake, are associated with the risk of postpartum depressive symptoms. Future research on dietary supplementation in pregnancy with special attention to selenium intake is warranted.

Keywords: Postpartum depression, Dietary supplements, Selenium, Omega-3

* Correspondence: kaplan@ucalgary.ca
[1]Department of Community Health Sciences, University of Calgary, Calgary, AB, Canada
[2]Department of Paediatrics, University of Calgary, 2888 Shaganappi Trail SW, Calgary, AB, Canada
Full list of author information is available at the end of the article

Background

Postpartum depression is a serious mental health problem that has been estimated to affect 10 - 15% of women after the birth of a child [1], and can occur anywhere from shortly after birth to one year postpartum. A review by Gavin and colleagues stated the prevalence may be as high as 19% within the first three months of giving birth [2]. The difference in rates may be due to the diagnostic criteria, timing of screening, and screening instruments used [1]. Regardless of the precise prevalence rate, it is clear that postpartum depression poses a significant public health issue because of its impact not only on the lives of the women themselves, but also on their children's growth and development (cognitive, social, behavioural) [3,4].

A number of social and biological factors are known to be associated with an increased risk for developing postpartum depression. Social risk factors include a history of depression/anxiety, lack of a marital partner, marital difficulties, poverty, and lack of social support [5], as well as family violence, life stress, and substance abuse [6]. Biological risk factors associated with postpartum depression include hormonal influences [7] and nutrient deficiencies from malnutrition or poor diet quality [8-10]. Research has shown a number of nutrient deficiencies associated with depression in the non-pregnant or postpartum population, including folate and vitamin B12 [11,12] , calcium [12,13], iron [11,12,14], selenium [11,15], zinc [11,16] and omega-3 polyunsaturated fatty acids [11,17-23]. Postpartum depression is not qualitatively different from depression that is not linked to pregnancy, but only recently has research on the role of nutrients in postpartum depression begun to emerge [24]. A summary has been published elsewhere describing some of the known biochemical effects of these nutrients on brain and neurological function, pointing toward the neurophysiological mechanisms by which insufficient nutrients could influence mood [24].

It is well-documented that proper nutrition during pregnancy is vital to the health of a woman and her fetus [25,26]. Today, it is common for health professionals to recommend that pregnant women take micronutrient supplements, the benefits of which have been established for the offspring. For instance, a meta-analysis by Goh and colleagues reported that offspring of women who took prenatal multivitamins were less likely to have leukemia (odds ratio (OR)=0.61, 95% confidence interval (CI)=0.50-0.74), pediatric brain tumors (OR=0.73, 95% CI=0.60-0.88) and neuroblastoma (OR=0.53, 95% CI=0.42-0.68), compared to children whose mothers did not take supplements [27]. Another meta-analysis found prenatal supplements to be associated with decreased risk for a number of congenital anomalies (e.g. cardiovascular defects, limb defects, urinary tract anomalies, and cleft palate or oral cleft anomalies), in addition to neural tube defects [28]. A meta-analysis of research in developing countries showed that multiple micronutrient supplementation was more effective than iron and folic acid supplementation at reducing the risk of low birth weight (RR=0.86, 95% CI=0.79-0.93) and of small size for gestational age (RR=0.85; 95% CI=0.78-0.93), but had no effect on perinatal mortality [29].

These results demonstrate important protective effects for the offspring from maternal use of prenatal multiple micronutrient supplementation. The effect of prenatal supplementation on maternal mental health, however, has not been established. The *purpose* of this study was to investigate the association between prenatal micronutrient supplementation and the risk for postpartum depressive symptoms in pregnant women from the Alberta Pregnancy Outcomes and Nutrition (APrON) study. We evaluated the nutrients ingested through supplements to determine whether any individual supplementary nutrients were associated with postpartum depressive symptoms as measured by the Edinburgh Postnatal Depression Scale (EPDS).

Methods

Study design and participants

Participants for this study are the first 600 pregnant women from the APrON study, which is a longitudinal prospective study in Alberta, Canada. Participants were at least 16 years old with gestational age ≤27 weeks. Women must be in the first (T1) or second (T2) trimester to be in this study; we did not include any woman who was 28 weeks or beyond. Non-English speakers, known drug and alcohol abusers, and those planning to move out of the region within 6 months were excluded. Data were collected using questionnaires and interviews at each trimester and 12 weeks postpartum. Windows for data collection were defined *a priori* as week 10 ±2 for first trimester, week 18 ± 2 for second trimester, and week 32 ± 2 for third trimester. Every attempt was made to meet these specific timepoints as closely as possible (see Figure 1). Details of recruitment and data collection are available elsewhere [30]; also refer to the APrON website at www.ApronStudy.ca.

Participant background and covariates

Data on sociodemographic background and variables such as stressful life events and perceived social support known to be associated with increased risk for postpartum depression were collected using a questionnaire developed specifically for the APrON study (see Table 1). Perceived social support was measured with questions from the National Population Health Survey (NPHS) – Social Support section (Statistics Canada, 1994/95 & 1996/97 cycles) [31] with response options modified for the APrON study. The NPHS-Social Support section is comprised of four statements about having "someone to confide in", "someone one can count on in a crisis",

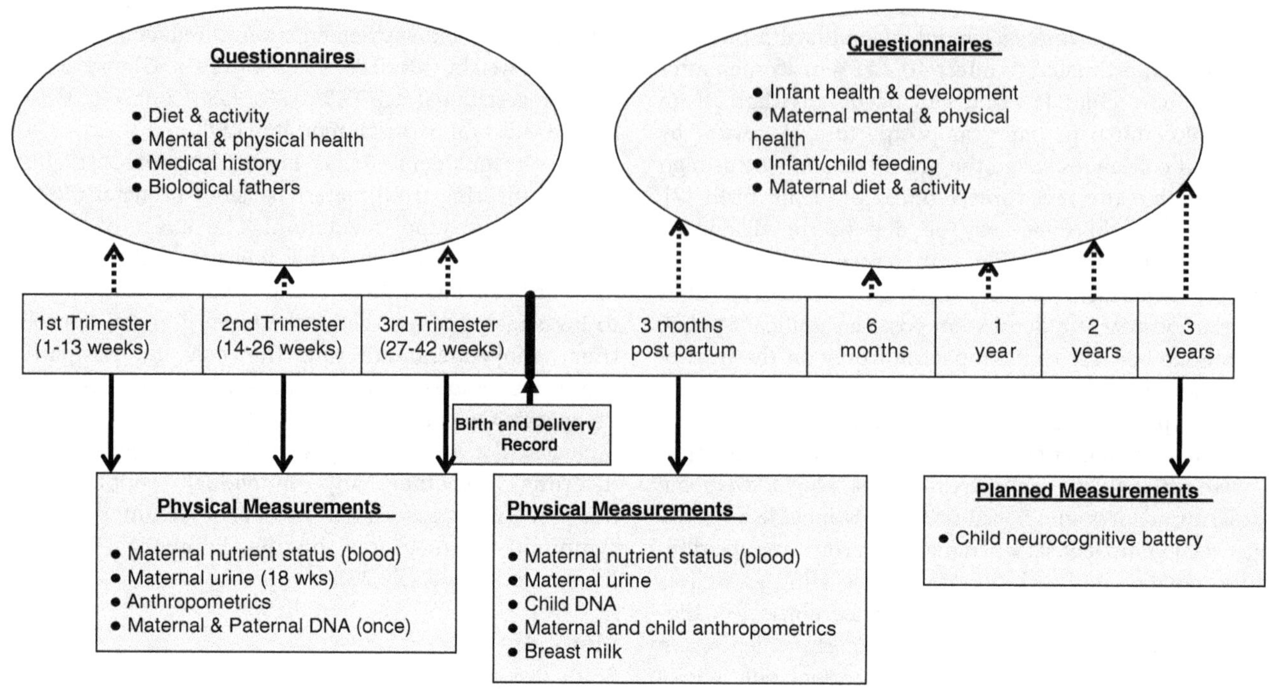

Figure 1 APrON timeline.

"someone one can count on for advice", and "someone who makes one feel loved and cared for", with Yes/No response options. Guided by expert advice from team members, the APrON study kept the wording of the statements, but modified the response options to five possible answers: none of the time, a little of the time, about half of the time, most of the time, all of the time. Each response option was then assigned a numerical value, "none of the time" was assigned a value of 0 and ranged up to a value of 4 for "all of the time". By summing the scores of each statement, an overall score of 16 indicated the highest possible level of perceived social support, while an overall score of 0 was the lowest possible level of perceived social support.

Prenatal nutrient intake from supplements

The Supplement Intake Questionnaire was developed for APrON to assess natural health product (NHP) intake. The structure of the Supplement Intake Questionnaire was adapted from questionnaires used in other studies of supplement intake, such as the National Cancer Institute and the Canadian Community Health Survey [32,33]. The Supplement Intake Questionnaire was pilot tested with a panel of nutrition experts as well as 50 pregnant women to determine whether it captured NHP data efficiently and accurately. Wording, formatting, and other modifications were made based on the feedback from the pilot study.

The final version of the Supplement Intake Questionnaire consisted of three sections: 1) section 1 listed options for multivitamins/minerals, 2) section 2 listed single nutrient supplements, and 3) section 3 consisted of herbal products, probiotics, homeopathic remedies, and other products such as amino acids, essential fatty acids and traditional medicines. Commonly used formulations were presented in a checklist. For products used by participants but not in the checklist, space was provided to record the name and manufacturer of the NHP as well as the Natural Product Number (NPN) or Drug Identification Number (DIN). Where possible, the products were verified using their NPNs and DINs against those within Health Canada's Natural Health Products Database, to confirm their formulations; then they were entered into the APrON database. A NPN or a DIN is assigned to all NHPs that have met standards for quality, safety and efficacy set by Health Canada [34]. Products that did not have a NPN or DIN were verified by obtaining ingredients from product labels or by finding the information from the manufacturer/supplier websites.

At each visit during pregnancy and postpartum, women were asked to describe in detail the quantity (i.e., frequency of intake and dosage) and type (e.g., prenatal multivitamins) of NHP consumed, using open-ended questions. To determine dose, women were asked "how much do you take?" and for frequency, women were asked "how often do you take it?" Typical responses were daily or times per week (e.g., 5 x/week). There was no

Table 1 Associations between socio-demographic characteristics of women and their postpartum EPDS

Characteristic	EPDS<10*	EPDS≥10*	p-value**	Odds ratio***(95% CI)
Demographics				
Age (mean (95% CI))	31.2 (30.8 - 31.6)	31.6 (30.3 - 32.8)	0.51	1.0 (0.9 - 1.1)
BMI (mean (95% CI))	24.1 (23.6 - 24.5)	24.2 (22.9 - 25.4)	0.90	1.0 (0.9 - 1.0)
Marital status (n (%))				
Married/common-law	406 (88.0)	55 (11.9)	0.17	1.0
Single/divorced	9 (75.0)	3 (25.0)		2.4 (0.6 - 9.3)
Education (n (%))				
High school	36 (87.8)	5 (12.2)	0.96	1.0
Trade/undergrad	286 (87.7)	40 (12.2)		0.6 (0.1 - 7.0)
Graduate	93 (87.7)	13 (12.2)		0.6 (0.1 - 5.9)
Household Income (n (%))				
< $20K	5 (83.3)	1 (16.7)	0.13	1.0
$20-$39K	12 (80.0)	3 (20.0)		1.2 (0.1 - 15.1)
$40-$69K	47 (78.3)	13 (21.7)		1.4 (0.1 - 12.9)
$70-$99K	107 (87.7)	15 (12.3)		0.7 (0.1 - 6.4)
≥$100K	236 (90.1)	26 (9.9)		0.5 (0.1 - 4.9)
Born in Canada (n (%))				
Yes	349 (89.9)	39 (10.0)	0.01	1.0
No	63 (79.7)	16 (20.2)		2.3 (1.2 - 4.3)
Ethnicity (n (%))				
Caucasian	363 (88.3)	48 (11.6)	0.30	1.0
Non-causasian	51 (83.6)	10 (16.4)		1.5 (0.7 - 3.1)
# of children (n (%))				
0	57 (87.7)	8 (13.3)	0.28	1.0
1-2	172 (88.2)	23 (11.8)		1.0 (0.5 - 1.9)
3-4	4 (66.7)	2 (34.3)		7.3 (1.0 - 53.7)
Social/lifestyle				
# of chronic conditions (n (%))				
0	206 (85.1)	36 (14.9)	0.05	1.0
1	91 (91.9)	8 (8.1)		0.5 (0.2 - 1.1)
2	15 (78.9)	4 (21.0)		1.5 (0.5 - 4.8)
3	5 (62.5)	3 (37.5)		3.4 (0.8 – 15.0)
# of life event stresses (n (%))				
During this pregnancy				
0	207 (89.6)	24 (10.4)	0.02	1.0
1-2	184 (88.0)	25 (11.9)		1.2 (0.6 - 2.1)
>3	24 (72.7)	9 (27.2)		3.2 (1.3 - 7.7)
12 mos before pregnancy				
0	196 (89.9)	22 (10.1)	0.08	1.0
1-2	149 (88.2)	20 (11.8)		1.2 (0.6 - 2.3)
>3	13 (72.2)	5 (27.8)		3.4 (1.1 - 10.5)
Before age 17				
0	126 (89.3)	15 (10.6)	0.06	1.0
1-2	224 (89.2)	27 (10.7)		1.2 (0.6 - 2.6)
>3	11 (68.7)	5 (31.2)		3.8 (1.1 - 12.5)
Social support (mean (95% CI))				
Prenatal	14.8 (14.7 - 15.0)	13.8 (13.1 - 14.5)	0.0043	0.8 (0.7 - 0.9)

Table 1 Associations between socio-demographic characteristics of women and their postpartum EPDS *(Continued)*

Postpartum	14.7 (14.5 - 14.9)	13.0 (12.2 - 13.8)	0.0001	0.8 (0.7 - 0.9)
EPDS score by time points				
(mean (95% CI)				
Time A (1st trimester)	4.8 (4.1 - 5.6)	8.0 (6.5 - 9.5)	0.0006	1.31 (1.11-1.55)
Time B (2nd trimester)	5.0 (4.7 - 5.4)	8.4 (7.2 - 9.5)	<0.0001	1.21 (1.13-1.30)
Time C (3rd trimester)	4.5 (4.2 - 4.8)	9.0 (7.9 - 10.1)	<0.0001	1.33 (1.23-1.44)
Time E (12 weeks postpartum)	3.6 (3.4 - 3.8)	12.1 (11.4 - 12.9)	<0.0001	n/a

* EPDS≥10 = "at least probable minor depression". The frequency calculations differed by variable because of missing values in some cases (e.g. participant did not answer a question).

**Assessment of associations with Chi-square test for categorical variables or t-test for continuous variable.

***OR from univariate logistic regression.

menu of responses from which to choose. For example, if a woman said she consumed 700 mg/week of a nutrient, it was calculated as 100mg/day for that specific trimester. The daily value was calculated for the specific trimester, and only for that trimester, and not extrapolated for the entire pregnancy.

A trained Research Assistant conducted the interview with each woman to elicit the information. All information provided by the participants was reviewed with them to ensure the items were correctly recorded. Women were also asked to bring in bottles and other containers of the supplements they were taking. Brand names, individual nutrients and their amounts, as well as dosage (i.e. number of pills/capsules/tablets taken per day) were recorded. Prior to each visit, an email was sent to the women, reminding them to bring in the NHP container(s) and other materials to the next clinic visit. When a woman did not bring in the container(s) of the NHPs, the research assistant followed the visit with a phone call to obtain the information.

For the purpose of this study, only supplements of vitamins, minerals, and fatty acids were analyzed. Supplement data was collected a minimum of two times, and maximum of three times during pregnancy. To obtain an average intake of each nutrient in the supplements, reported intake was averaged over the number of times data were collected. For example, if information on vitamin D supplement intake was collected at each trimester (i.e., three times), then the total amount consumed was divided by three; if information was collected at only two times, then the total was divided by two. The nutrients chosen for analysis in this study (listed in Table 2) were informed by the literature that has previously demonstrated a relationship with mood [8]. The Recommended Dietary Allowance (RDA) values from the Institute of Medicine [35] were used as the reference values for calculating the percentage of women above or below RDA for consuming the individual micronutrients from supplements. The comparison to RDA in this study did not include nutrients from dietary intake, but from supplement intake only.

Depression symptom measure – EPDS

The EPDS is a 10-item scale that measures mood, and requires about five minutes to complete. It has been widely validated, widely utilized, has a moderate to good reliability and test-retest reliability and has a good to moderate correlation with other depression measures [36]. It has a maximum score of 30; a score of 10 or more indicates possible depression of varying severity. The standardized and validated EPDS has been used extensively worldwide, and has been evaluated for its psychometric rigor [37-39]. It has been found to have high sensitivity and specificity (79% and 97% for first trimester at cut-off of 11, 70% and 96% for second trimester with cut-off of 10, and 76% and 94% for third trimester with cut-off of 10 [40]) in identifying those at risk of, or potentially suffering from prenatal depression.

The EPDS has been used for both clinical and research purposes, and cut-off scores have been obtained through empirical assessment [40,41]. These cut-offs provide rates of probable depression for referral or treatment, and can also be used to track the course of depression from antenatal to postpartum periods. As with other screening measures, sensitivity and positive predictive value may be variable when used in selected populations versus community populations [36,38]. For the purpose of this study, we used a cut-off score of 10 for probable depression [41]. Using the sample size of 397 we had 90% power to detect a relative risk of 1.5 or more for EPDS >10 in women consuming lower vs. adequate RDA of a nutrient from supplements.

Assessing predictors of depressive symptoms on the EPDS

From the first model, only *born in Canada* was statistically significant (OR = 2.27, 95% CI = 1.20 - 4.31, p = 0.012). In the second model, only postpartum social support was statistically significant (OR = 0.83, 95% CI = 0.72 - 0.95,

Table 2 Mean (SD), range and percentage below and above RDA for prenatal micronutrient intake from supplementation in pregnant women with postpartum EPDS<10 & EPDS≥10

Nutrient	EPDS<10 (n=416)	EPDS≥10 (n=59)	p-value*
Vitamin B1 (mg)			
Mean (SD)	5.5 (14.7)	3.5 (8.1)	0.12
Range	0 – 103	0 – 62.5	
Below RDA (n (%))	55 (84.6)	10 (15.4)	
Above RDA (n (%))	361 (88.1)	49 (11.9)	
Vitamin B3 (mg)			
Mean (SD)	22 (23)	19 (10)	0.10
Range	0 – 335	0 – 66	
Below RDA (n (%))	55 (82.1)	12 (17.9)	
Above RDA (n (%))	361 (88.5)	47 (11.5)	
Vitamin B6 (mg)			
Mean (SD)	9.1 (15.9)	7.8 (10.7)	0.43
Range	0 – 110	0 – 62.5	
Below RDA (n (%))	23 (79.3)	6 (20.7)	
Above RDA (n (%))	363 (88.1)	49 (11.9)	
Vitamin B9 (mcg)			
Mean (SD)	1259 (924)	1297 (962)	0.78
Range	0 – 6000	0 – 5000	
Below RDA (n (%))	30 (81.1)	7 (18.9)	
Above RDA (n (%))	386 (88.1)	52 (11.9)	
Vitamin B12 (mcg)			
Mean (SD)	31 (116)	18 (65)	0.23
Range	0 – 1210	0 – 502	
Below RDA (n (%))	19 (79.2)	5 (20.8)	
Above RDA (n (%))	397 (88.0)	54 (12.0)	
Vitamin D (IU)			
Mean (SD)	618 (539)	567 (512)	0.48
Range	0 – 4200	0 – 2750	
Below RDA (n (%))	292 (87.7)	41 (12.3)	
Above RDA (n (%))	124 (87.3)	18 (12.7)	
Iodine (mcg)			
Mean (SD)	173 (68)	158 (76)	0.15
Range	0 – 636	0 – 330	
Below RDA (n (%))	227 (85.7)	38 (14.3)	
Above RDA (n (%))	189 (90.0)	21 (10.0)	
Iron (mg)			
Mean (SD)	33 (20)	32 (20)	0.84
Range	0 – 127	0 – 87	
Below RDA (n (%))	68 (82.9)	14 (17.1)	
Above RDA (n (%))	348 (88.5)	45 (11.5)	
Magnesium (mg)			
Mean (SD)	67 (65)	59 (39)	0.19
Range	0 – 1025	0 – 208	
Below RDA (n (%))	415 (87.5)	59 (12.5)	
Above RDA (n (%))	1 (100.0)	0	
Selenium (mcg)			
Mean (SD)	25 (17)	19 (13)	0.0015
Range	0 – 125	0 – 45	
Below RDA (n (%))	401 (87.2)	59 (12.8)	
Above RDA (n (%))	15 (100.0)	0	
Zinc (mg)			
Mean (SD)	13 (8)	12 (8)	0.38
Range	0 – 48	0 – 32	
Below RDA (n (%))	233 (87.9)	32 (12.1)	
Above RDA (n (%))	183 (87.1)	27 (12.9)	
Omega-3 (mg)			
Mean (SD)	180 (440)	90 (208)	0.01
Range	0 – 4050	0 – 1000	
Below RDA (n (%))	RDA not determined	RDA not determined	
Above RDA (n (%))			

Note: RDA (Recommended Dietary Allowance) for pregnant women is "the average daily nutrient intake level sufficient to meet the nutrient requirement of nearly all (97– 98%) healthy individuals in a particular life stage and gender group" as defined by the Institute of Medicine (55). The percentages below and above RDA are calculated from supplements alone and does not account for dietary intake.
SD = Standard deviation.
* p values derived from t-tests.

p = 0.007). A third model with the nutrient variables resulted in only selenium being statistically significant (OR = 0.97, 95% CI = 0.94 - 0.99, p = 0.030). Although omega-3 was not significant in the logistic regression (OR = 1.00, 95% CI = 0.99 - 1.00, p = 0.07), given the strong association of omega-3 with depressive symptoms, both selenium and omega-3 were included in the next model with the significant variables from the first two models.

The fourth model was constructed to include *born in Canada, prenatal and postnatal social support, prenatal EPDS* (at 2nd and 3rd trimesters) and *prenatal omega-3* and *selenium* supplement. Prenatal EPDS scores were included because the literature has reported that prenatal depressive symptoms were predictive of postpartum depressive symptoms. Born in Canada, prenatal social support, and omega-3 were removed from the fourth model as they exceeded the pre-set p value of 0.05. Potential confounding of the remaining model by sociodemographic and lifestyle variables was assessed.

No meaningful differences were found between the crude and adjusted ORs. Therefore, the final model consisted of predictors that were statistically significant (see Table 3). Hosmer and Lemeshow's goodness-of-fit test resulted in $chi^2(7) = 8.08$, and $p = 0.33$, indicating that our model fits the data well. The mean VIF = 1.13, with VIF for individual variable ranged from 1.03 to 1.17 (and tolerance from .84 to .97), indicating that multicollinearity is not likely to be a problem in the model.

Missing values

To assess whether the 125 "missing" postpartum EDPS participants differed from those who responded, various statistical tests were used, including 1) exclusion of cases with missing postpartum EPDS, 2) re-categorization of missing as "not depressed", 3) re-categorization of missing as "depressed", 4) last observation carried forward using third trimester data, 5) creation of a category called "missing" to see what predicted "missing", and 6) comparison of participant characteristics with those without postpartum EPDS data.

Statistical methods

All statistical analyses were performed using STATA11 software. Values were expressed as mean and standard deviation, range, or proportions (n and %). Comparisons between groups (those having EPDS scores <10 and those with EPDS scores ≥10) were assessed for statistical significance by a Chi-square test for categorical variables and a t-test for continuous variables. Bonferroni correction was used for multiple test comparisons. Several logistic regression models were constructed to identify predictors of postpartum depression. Using multivariate logistic regression, the first model consisted of all the demographic variables; model two included social/lifestyle variables plus the significant variable from model one. The third model assessed nutrients from supplement intake (listed in Table 2), and the fourth model incorporated significant (and close to significant) variables from models one, two, and three (all the models with the covariates and nutrients and their respective outputs are provided in Table 3). For the final model, we tested the fit of the model with Hosmer and Lemeshow's goodness-of-fit test, and we computed the variance inflation factor (VIF) to test for collinearity. Odds ratios (OR) and the 95% CI for predictors of the EPDS depressive symptoms were calculated. A two-tailed p-value of 0.05 was considered statistically significant.

Ethics approval

The APrON study was approved by the Conjoint Health Research Ethics Board at the University of Calgary, and the Health Research Ethics Board at the University of Alberta. Each participant signed a consent form at the first clinic visit.

Table 3 Full and final models of predictors for EPDS depressive symptoms (EPDS≥10)

Predictor	Odds ratio	95% CI	p-value
Model 1			
Age	.98	.88-1.09	.69
Parity	.98	.56-1.71	.94
Marital status	.49	.19-1.24	.14
Education	.98	.63-1.51	.92
Income	5.32	.85-33.35	.07
Born outside Canada	2.41	.81-7.19	.11
Ethnic background	.73	.19-2.79	.65
BMI	1.00	.88-1.15	.90
Model 2			
Life stressors during this pregnancy	1.21	.87-1.69	.26
Life stressors 12 mons before this pregnancy	1.08	.77-1.50	.65
Life stressors prior to age 17	1.22	.85-1.75	.29
Social support	.85	.74-.97	.015
Model 3			
Vitamin B1	.98	.94-1.02	.33
Vitamin B3	.99	.97-1.01	.41
Vitamin B6	1.01	.98-1.05	.41
Vitamin B9 (folic acid)	1.00	.99-1.00	.96
Vitamin B12	1.00	.99-1.00	.76
Vitamin D	1.00	.99-1.00	.92
Iodine	.99	.99-1.00	.11
Iron	1.00	.98-1.01	.91
Magnesium	.99	.99-1.00	.37
Selenium	.97	.95-0.99	.03
Zinc	.98	.95-1.02	.41
Omega 3	1.00	.99-1.00	.20
Final model			
Prenatal EPDS (2nd trimester)	3.29	1.55 – 7.01	0.004
Prenatal EPDS (3rd trimester)	4.26	2.05 – 8.85	0.000
Postpartum Social Support	0.87	0.78 - 0.97	0.015
Prenatal Selenium supplement intake (per 10 mcg)	0.76	0.74 - 0.78	0.019

Results

Of the 600 pregnant women in the study cohort, 475 completed the EPDS questionnaire at least twice during pregnancy and at 12 weeks postpartum. Of the 125 with no EPDS data postpartum, nine miscarried, 36 withdrew from the study, 38 were non-respondent (i.e., could not be contacted), and 36 did not complete the EPDS. No differences in characteristics were found between those with postpartum EDPS data and those without.

Of the 475 available participants, 416 (88%) scored <10 on the EPDS and 59 (12%) scored ≥10. For demographic characteristics, women not *born in Canada* were more likely to have an EPDS ≥10 (p = 0.01); no other potential covariates were statistically significant (see Table 1). For the social/lifestyle characteristics, the *number of chronic conditions, stressful life events during this pregnancy,* and *pre/post-natal support* were all statistically significant (see Table 1); i.e. EPDS was associated with these characteristics. Women with higher number of stressful life events 12 months before pregnancy and before the age of 17 were more likely to have EPDS ≥10, with p-values close to significance (p = 0.08 and 0.06 respectively). Not presented were regressions for prenatal depression and the key nutrients found to be significantly associated with postpartum depression: the results (not shown) were that selenium was not a predictor of prenatal depression at second or third trimesters. Although not statistically significant, a trend was shown for women being single/divorced, had lower income, or had higher number of children to be associated with EPDS ≥10.

Nutrient data

Almost all women (99%) took some type of micronutrient supplement during the prenatal period. For this cohort, the nutrients most commonly consumed were vitamins B6, B9 (folate), B12, and E, with more than 90% above RDA. The supplement taken the least was omega-3, where 68.5% of women with EPDS <10 and 78.0% of women with EPDS ≥10 did not take any omega-3. The mean intake of *selenium* and *omega-3* differed significantly (p = 0.0015 and 0.01, respectively) between women with EPDS <10 and those with EPDS ≥10. As well, the mean intakes for all the other nutrients listed in Table 2 were more likely to be higher in women with EPDS <10 than those with EPDS ≥10, although not statistically significant. In fact, the upper ranges for intake were higher in almost all nutrients (except for folic acid) in women with EPDS <10 than women with EDPS ≥10. Finally, all the other nutrients listed (except vitamin D and zinc) showed an overall nonsignificant trend for those consuming below RDA levels to be more likely to have EPDS ≥10 (see Table 2). Supplement intake for many of the nutrients was not normally distributed. SIQ data was available for n=136 in the first trimester, n=575 in the second trimester and n=516 in the third trimester.

Table 3 showed the (statistically significant) predictors for postpartum depressive symptoms (i.e. EPDS ≥10) from the final model. Selenium use above RDA levels and postnatal social support reduced the odds of the EPDS ≥10, while prenatal EPDS (at 2nd and 3rd trimesters) increased the risk of EPDS ≥10.

Discussion

The results of this research support previous studies on the nutritional and social factors associated with depression [5,42,43]. In this study, women with an EPDS score ≥10 were more likely to be born outside of Canada; to report having more chronic health conditions, more life stress and less social support during the current pregnancy; and to have consumed fewer micronutrients from supplements, most notably selenium and omega-3. The logistic regression showed that prenatal EPDS ≥10 (at second and third trimesters) increased the odds of postpartum depressive symptoms, while prenatal selenium intake from supplements and postnatal social support were protective (decreased the odds) of postpartum depressive symptoms. Of the nutrients evaluated, all intakes were likely to be higher in women with EPDS <10 than those with EPDS ≥10.

The role of selenium in relation to mood is not as well studied as some other nutrients (e.g. omega-3s, folate, and zinc) that have been associated with depression. A recent nested case–control study by Pasco and colleagues found low intake of selenium (<8.9 μg/MJ/day) was associated with almost a three-fold increase in the likelihood of major depressive disorder (OR 2.95, 95% CI 1.00-8.72) after adjusting for age and socio-economic status [44]. A randomized trial by Mokhber and colleagues reported significantly lower mean EPDS scores in the group of primigravid pregnant Iranian women, aged 16 to 35, taking selenium supplements compared to a comparison group after controlling for sociodemographic and health history variables [42]. Hawkes and Hornbostel in a study of eleven healthy men found lower selenium status associated with worse mood scores [45].

This study reinforced the importance of social support for pregnant women in the prenatal and postnatal periods, the benefits of which have been well-documented for the reduction of the risk and symptoms of mood disorders and depression [43,46,47]. While there is little research into the mechanism by which environmental factors such as social support affect brain biochemistry in humans, animal studies indicate that improving external stimuli through an enriched environment may reverse the effects of stress-related events, at the behavioral, endocrine, and biochemical levels [48].

The findings from this study also revealed the need for evaluation for prenatal depressive symptoms. While there are programs in many jurisdictions to evaluate new mothers for the risk of this condition, prenatal mental health still receives little attention as part of prenatal care [49,50]. Since antenatal depression may be more common than postnatal depression, and women with antenatal depression are more likely to be depressed postnatally [51], prenatal depression screening should be as widely practiced as postpartum screening.

One limitation of this study was the effect of multicollinearity, which is a common problem in nutrition studies, particularly those that examine the intake of nutrients from supplements as supplements include multiple nutrients and many are in similar amounts and combinations due the nutrient recommendations by health agencies. Another limitation is that the present study did not have access to serum levels of selenium or any of the other nutrients discussed in this paper, thus there is no information as to whether supplementation affected biological levels. A third limitation was that dietary (food) intake was not included in the analysis. Although dietary intake was estimated in these women at two or three trimesters during pregnancy (data which will be available at some future date), selenium intake is difficult to estimate due to variations in the food supply and the inaccuracy of nutrient databases. The high supplement intake may mitigate dietary intake in this case, and would not be likely to change our findings. We did not have lab values at present to assess anemia in our sample. Although anemia is known to be a risk factor for depression, we also know that women are routinely supplemented with iron when anemia is diagnosed during pregnancy. In this study, for women below RDA, 82.9% scored <10 EPDS, 17.1% scored ≥10 EPDS; for women above RDA, 88.5% <10 EPDS, and 11.5% were ≥10, p = 0.84 (see Table 2), indicating that there was no difference of scoring ≥10 EPDS between being above or below the RDA for iron. While we recognize this is not the ideal measure for iron associated form of anemia, it served as a proxy for iron status. Another limitation was possible reporting error associated with recall of supplement intake (e.g. dosage and frequency). Recording of brand names and labels of supplements (e.g. types and amounts of nutrients) by research assistants, as well as the use of repeated measures, helped to minimized potential reporting bias. However, we acknowledge a major limitation with the Supplement Intake Questionnaire is self-reporting; thus we did not know whether the women actually consumed their supplements as they said they did. Furthermore, if a woman missed her trimester visit then this was treated as missing data and no estimation was made. Thus, there was some degree of projection as the women were asked for information for the entire trimester at the trimester midpoint and not the end, making this a limitation to our estimates. A limitation in the analysis was that we did not assess for interaction among the nutrients due to the absence of any *a priori* rationale from the literature. In addition, as data on prenatal nutrition status was not available, we were unable to test whether the effect of prenatal micronutrient supplementation on postpartum depression varied by prenatal nutritional status. For future research, we would like to assess whether specific nutrients interact to impact postpartum depression, and also whether prenatal nutritional status modified the association of supplementation and postpartum depression.

One of the strengths of this study was the temporal relationship of supplement intake and postpartum depressive symptoms could be established. Another strength was that supplement intake was collected repeatedly over time to obtain an average usual intake of the nutrients in the prenatal period, rather than using a single measure as in most studies. A third strength was the ability to control for a large number of factors associated with postpartum depressive symptoms in our analyses because of the variables (demographic, social, lifestyle) collected prospectively.

Implications for future research include examining objective measures of pre- and postnatal micronutrient status for: 1) relations between pre/postnatal blood nutrient levels (or changes in pre/postnatal blood levels) and postpartum depression, 2) moderating effect of prenatal blood nutrient levels on the relations between prenatal micronutrient supplementation and postpartum depression, and 3) interactions amongst nutrients and their effects on postpartum depression.

Conclusions

This study found multiple factors, including selenium intake from supplements, history of depression, and social support, are associated with the risk of postpartum depressive symptoms. The evidence suggests that there is likely no single casual factor to depression, and nutrients play an important role in the development of depressive symptoms. Thus, a future research focus on dietary supplementation with special attention to the intake of selenium in the pregnant population is warranted.

Competing interest

All authors declare no conflict of interest, financial or otherwise.

Authors' contributions

BMYL carried out the data analyses and drafted the manuscript. BJK reviewed and revised the manuscript. LJM and MFG provided methodological information on the supplement intake questionnaire. CJF, ST, and LG consulted on measures of nutrition, sociodemographics, and mental health. ME provided input on statistical analysis. All authors read and approved the final manuscript.

Acknowledgments

We are extremely grateful to all the families who took part in this study and the whole APrON team (www.ApronStudy.ca), including our research assistants, graduate and undergraduate students, volunteers, clerical staff and managers. This cohort was established by an interdisciplinary team grant from Alberta Innovates – Health Solutions (formerly Alberta Heritage Foundation for Medical Research). BL is the recipient of the Scobey Hartley Doctoral Award from the Alberta Centre for Child, Family and Community Research.

The individual members of the APrON research team are Bonnie J. Kaplan, Catherine J. Field, Deborah Dewey, Rhonda C. Bell, Francois P. Bernier, Marja Cantell, Linda M. Casey, Misha Eliasziw, Anna Farmer, Lisa Gagnon, Gerald F. Giesbrecht, Laki Goonewardene, David W. Johnston, Libbe Kooistra, Nicole Letourneau, Donna P. Manca, Jonathan W. Martin, Linda J. McCargar, Maeve O'Beirne, Victor J. Pop, Nalini Singhal

Author details
[1]Department of Community Health Sciences, University of Calgary, Calgary, AB, Canada. [2]Department of Paediatrics, University of Calgary, 2888 Shaganappi Trail SW, Calgary, AB, Canada. [3]Department of Agricultural, Food and Nutritional Science, University of Alberta, Edmonton, AB, Canada. [4]Department of Public Health and Community Medicine, Tufts University, Boston, MA, USA. [5]Department of Psychiatry, University of Calgary, Calgary, AB, Canada.

References

1. Marcus SM: **Depression during pregnancy: rates, risks and consequences–Motherisk Update 2008.** *Can J Clin Pharmacol* 2009, **16**:e15–22.
2. Gavin NI, Gaynes BN, Lohr KN, Meltzer-Brody S, Gartlehner G, Swinson T: **Perinatal depression: a systematic review of prevalence and incidence.** *Obstet Gynecol* 2005, **106**:1071–1083.
3. Stewart RC: **Maternal depression and infant growth - a review of recent evidence.** *Matern Child Nutr* 2007, **2**:94–107.
4. Logsdon MC, Wisner KL, Pinto-Foltz MD: **The impact of postpartum depression on mothering.** *JOGNN* 2006, **35**:652–8.
5. Verkerk GJ, Pop VJ, Van Son MJ, Van Heck GL: **Prediction of depression in the postpartum period: a longitudinal follow-up study in high-risk and low-risk women.** *J Affect Disord* 2003, **77**:159–66.
6. Ross LE, Dennis CL: **The prevalence of postpartum depression among women with substance use, an abuse history, or chronic illness: a systematic review.** *J Womens Health (Larchmt)* 2009, **18**:475–486.
7. Parry BL, Sorenson DL, Meliska CJ, Basavaraj N, Zirpoli GG, Gamst A, Hauger R: **Hormonal basis of mood and postpartum disorders.** *Curr Womens Health Rep* 2003, **3**:230–5.
8. Kaplan BJ, Crawford SG, Field CJ, Simpson JS: **Vitamins, minerals, and mood.** *Psychol Bull* 2007, **133**:747–760.
9. Bourre JM: **Effects of nutrients (in food) on the structure and function of the nervous system: update on dietary requirements for brain. Part 1: micronutrients.** *J Nutr Health Aging* 2006, **10**:377–385.
10. Bourre JM: **Effects of nutrients (in food) on the structure and function of the nervous system: update on dietary requirements for brain. Part 2: macronutrients.** *J Nutr Health Aging* 2006, **10**:386–399.
11. Bodnar LM, Wisner KL: **Nutrition and depression: implications for improving mental health among childbearing-aged women.** *Biol Psychiatry* 2005, **58**:679–685.
12. Pick ME, Edwards M, Moreau D, Ryan EA: **Assessment of diet quality in pregnant women using the Healthy Eating Index.** *J Am Diet Assoc* 2005, **105**:240–6.
13. Harrison-Hohner J, Coste S, Dorato V, Curet LB, McCarron D, Hatton D: **Prenatal calcium supplementation and postpartum depression: an ancillary study to a randomized trial of calcium for prevention of preeclampsia.** *Arch Womens Ment Health* 2001, **3**:141–146.
14. Corwin EJ, Murray-Kolb LE, Beard JL: **Low hemoglobin level is a risk factor for postpartum depression.** *J Nutr* 2003, **133**:4139–42.
15. Benton D: **Selenium intake, mood and other aspects of psychological functioning.** *Nutr Neurosci* 2002, **5**:363–374.
16. Nowak G, Siwek M, Dudek D, Zieba A, Pilc A: **Effect of zinc supplementation on antidepressant therapy in unipolar depression: a preliminary placebo-controlled study.** *Pol J Pharmacol* 2003, **55**:1143–1147.
17. Edwards R, Peet M, Shay J, Horrobin D: **Omega-3 polyunsaturated fatty acid levels in the diet and in red blood cell membranes of depressed patients.** *J Affect Disord* 1998, **48**:149–155.
18. Rees AM, Austin MP, Parker G: **Role of omega-3 fatty acids as a treatment for depression in the perinatal period.** *Aust N Z J Psychiatry* 2005, **39**:274–80.
19. De Vriese SR, Christophe AB, Maes M: **Lowered serum n-3 polyunsaturated fatty acid (PUFA) levels predict the occurrence of postpartum depression: further evidence that lowered n-PUFAs are related to major depression.** *Life Sci* 2003, **73**:3181–7.
20. Su KP, Huang SY, Chiu CC, Shen WW: **Omega-3 fatty acids in major depressive disorder. A preliminary double-blind placebo-controlled trial.** *Eur Neuropsychopharmacol* 2003, **13**:267–271.
21. Peet M, Murphy B, Shay J, Horrobin D: **Depletion of omega-3 fatty acid levels in red blood cell membranes of depressive patients.** *Biol Psychiatry* 1998, **43**:315–319.
22. Hibbeln JR: **Seafood consumption, the DHA content of mothers' milk and prevalence rates of postpartum depression: a cross-national, ecological analysis.** *J Affect Disord* 2002, **69**:15–29.
23. Mischoulon D, Fava M: **Docosahexanoic acid and omega-3 fatty acids in depression.** *Psychiatr Clin North Am* 2000, **23**:785–94.
24. Leung BM, Kaplan BJ: **Perinatal depression: prevalence, risks, and the nutrition link–a review of the literature.** *J Am Diet Assoc* 2009, **109**:1566–1575.
25. Kontic-Vucinic O, Sulovic N, Radunovic N: **Micronutrients in women's reproductive health: II. Minerals and trace elements.** *Int J Fertil Womens Med* 2006, **51**:116–24.
26. Kontic-Vucinic O, Sulovic N, Radunovic N: **Micronutrients in women's reproductive health: I. Vitamins.** *Int J Fertil Womens Med* 2006, **51**:106–115.
27. Goh YI, Bollano E, Einarson TR, Koren G: **Prenatal multivitamin supplementation and rates of pediatric cancers: a meta-analysis.** *Clin Pharmacol Ther* 2007, **81**:685–91.
28. Goh YI, Bollano E, Einarson TR, Koren G: **Prenatal multivitamin supplementation and rates of congenital anomalies: a meta-analysis.** *J Obstet Gynaecol Can* 2006, **28**:680–689.
29. Kawai K, Spiegelman D, Shankar AH, Fawzi WW: **Maternal multiple micronutrient supplementation and pregnancy outcomes in developing countries: meta-analysis and meta-regression.** *Bull World Health Organ* 2011, **89**:402–411B.
30. Kaplan BJ, Giesbrecht GF, Leung BM, Field CJ, Dewey D, Bell RC, Manca DP, O'Beirne M, Johnston DW, Pop VJ, Singhal N, Gagnon L, Bernier FP, Eliasziw M, McCargar LJ, Kooistra L, Farmer A, Cantell M, Goonewardene L, Casey LM, Letourneau N, Martin JW, the APrON Study Team: **The Alberta Pregnancy Outcomes and Nutrition (APrON) cohort study: rationale and methods.** *Matern Child Nutr* 2012, doi:10.1111/j.1740-8709.2012.00433.x [Epub ahead of print].
31. National Population Health Survey: *Content for Main Survey, May 1, 1994*; Unpublished information accessible at: http://www.statcan.gc.ca/imdb-bmdi/instrument/3225_Q1_V1-eng.pdf.
32. Canadian Community Health Survey, Cycle 2.2, Nutrition (2004): *A Guide to Accessing and Interpreting the Data.*
33. Csizmadi I, Kahle L, Ullman R, Dawe U, Zimmerman TP, Friedenreich CM, Bryant H, Subar AF: **Adaptation and evaluation of the National Cancer Institute's Diet History Questionnaire and nutrient database for Canadian populations.** *Public Health Nutr* 2007, **10**:88–96.
34. *Canada Gazette.* http://gazette.gc.ca/archives/p2/2003/2003-06-18/html/sor-dors196-eng.html.
35. Otten JJ, Hellwig JP, Meyers LD: *The Dietary Reference Intakes: The Essential Guide to Nutrient Requirements.* Washington: National Academic Press; 2006.
36. Boyd RC, Le HN, Somberg R: **Review of screening instruments for postpartum depression.** *Archives of Women's Mental Health* 2005, **8**:141–53.
37. Navarro P, Ascaso C, Garcia-Esteve L, Aguado J, Torres A, Martin-Santos R: **Postnatal psychiatric morbidity: a validation study of the GHQ-12 and the EPDS as screening tools.** *Gen Hosp Psychiatry* 2007, **29**:1–7.
38. Eberhard-Gran M, Tambs K, Opjordsmoen S, Skrondal A, Eskild A: **Depression during pregnancy and after delivery: a repeated measurement study.** *Psychosom Obstet Gynaecol* 2004, **25**:15–21.
39. Cox JL, Holden JM, Sagovsky R: **Detection of postnatal depression. Development of the 10-item Edinburgh Postnatal Depression Scale.** *Br J Psychiatry* 1987, **150**:782–786.
40. Bergink V, Kooistra L, den Berg MP L-v, Wijnen H, Bunevicius R, van Baar A, Pop V: **Validation of the Edinburgh Depression Scale during pregnancy.** *J Psychosom Res* 2011, **70**:385–389.
41. Matthey S, Henshaw C, Elliott S, Barnett B: **Variability in use of cut-off scores and formats on the Edinburgh Postnatal Depression Scale: implications for clinical and research practice.** *Arch Womens Ment Health* 2006, **9**:309–315.
42. Mokhber N, Namjoo M, Tara F, Boskabadi H, Rayman MP, Ghayour-Mobarhan M, Sahebkar A, Majdi MR, Tavallaie S, Azimi-Nezhad M, Shakeri MT, Nematy M, Oladi M, Mohammadi M, Ferns G: **Effect of supplementation with selenium on postpartum depression: a randomized double-blind placebo-controlled trial.** *J Matern Fetal Neonatal Med* 2011, **24**:104–108.

43. Leahy-Warren P, McCarthy G, Corcoran P: **Postnatal depression in first-time mothers: prevalence and relationships between functional and structural social support at 6 and 12 weeks postpartum.** *Arch Psychiatr Nurs* 2011, **25:**174–184.
44. Pasco JA, Jacka FN, Williams LJ, Evans-Cleverdon M, Brennan SL, Kotowicz MA, Nicholson GC, Ball MJ, Berk M: **Dietary selenium and major depression: a nested case–control study.** *Complement Ther Med* 2012, **20:**119–123.
45. Hawkes WC, Hornbostel L: **Effects of dietary selenium on mood in healthy men living in a metabolic research unit.** *Biol Psychiatry* 1996, **39:**121–128.
46. Evans M, Donelle L, Hume-Loveland L: **Social support and online postpartum depression discussion groups: A content analysis.** *Patient Educ Couns* 2012, **87:**405–410.
47. Joseph NT, Myers HF, Schettino JR, Olmos NT, Bingham-Mira C, Lesser IM, Poland RE: **Support and undermining in interpersonal relationships are associated with symptom improvement in a trial of antidepressant medication.** *Psychiatry* 2011, **74:**240–254.
48. Ilin Y, Richter-Levin G: **Enriched environment experience overcomes learning deficits and depressive-like behavior induced by juvenile stress.** *PLoS One* 2009, **4:**e4329.
49. Alder J, Fink N, Urech C, Hosli I, Bitzer J: **Identification of antenatal depression in obstetric care.** *Arch Gynecol Obstet* 2011, **284:**1403–1409.
50. Breedlove G, Fryzelka D: **Depression screening during pregnancy.** *J Midwifery Womens Health* 2011, **56:**18–25.
51. Edwards B, Galletly C, Semmler-Booth T, Dekker G: **Does antenatal screening for psychosocial risk factors predict postnatal depression? A follow-up study of 154 women in Adelaide, South Australia.** *Aust N Z J Psychiatry* 2008, **42:**51–55.

21

Impact of prenatal care provider on the use of ancillary health services during pregnancy

Amy Metcalfe[1], Kristen Grabowska[2], Carol Weller[3] and Suzanne C Tough[4*]

Abstract

Background: Recent declines in the provision of prenatal care by family physicians and the integration of midwives into the Canadian health care system have led to a shift in the pattern of prenatal care provision; however it is unknown if this also impacts use of other health services during pregnancy. This study aimed to assess the impact of the type of prenatal care provider on the self-reported use of ancillary services during pregnancy.

Methods: Data for this study was obtained from the *All Our Babies* study, a community-based prospective cohort study of women's experiences during pregnancy and the post-partum period. Chi-square tests and logistic regression were used to assess the association between type of prenatal care provider and use of ancillary health services in pregnancy.

Results: During pregnancy, 85.8% of women reported accessing ancillary health services. Compared to women who received prenatal care from a family physician, women who saw a midwife were less likely to call a nurse telephone advice line (OR = 0.30, 95% CI: 0.18-0.50) and visit the emergency department (OR = 0.47, 95% CI: 0.24-0.89), but were more likely receive chiropractic care (OR = 4.07, 95% CI: 2.49-6.67). Women who received their prenatal care from an obstetrician were more likely to visit a walk-in clinic (OR = 1.51, 95% CI: 1.11-2.05) than those who were cared for by a family physician.

Conclusions: Prenatal care is a complex entity and referral pathways between care providers and services are not always clear. This can lead to the provision of fragmented care and create opportunities for errors and loss of information. All types of care providers have a role in addressing the full range of health needs that pregnant women experience.

Keywords: Physician practice patterns, Pregnancy, Health services research

Background

Prenatal care is a publically funded health service available to all Canadian women; however, the provision of prenatal care in Canada is changing as a result of a decrease in the proportion of family physicians who provide prenatal and intra-partum care and the introduction of public funding of midwifery in some Canadian provinces [1-4]. Yet it is unknown how, or if, changes in prenatal care provision for low-risk pregnant women affect use of other ancillary services. The impact on what Chan refers to as 'the declining comprehensiveness of primary care' on other parts of the health care system is unknown [3]. Although, Coco hypothesized that the reduction in the number of family physicians providing prenatal care may impact access to ancillary services for women, such as use of walk-in clinics, visits to other health professionals, and calls to nurse-telephone advice lines [5]. If non-obstetric issues are not routinely addressed in the context of prenatal care or are treated in an inconsistent manner through disjointed episodes of care in walk-in clinics and emergency departments, this may lead to increased costs to the health care system due to duplication of services and the provision of inconsistent health information from multiple care providers. A smooth transition between care providers has been identified as an aspect of quality prenatal care [6], yet studies have shown that multiple prenatal care providers give different information to women, which results in confusion and anxiety [7].

* Correspondence: suzanne.tough@albertahealthservices.ca
[4]Departments of Pediatrics and Community Health Sciences, University of Calgary Child Development Centre, c/o 2888 Shaganappi Trail NW, Calgary, AB T3B 6A8, Canada
Full list of author information is available at the end of the article

The literature indicates that family physicians, midwives and obstetricians provide different intra-partum services to their patients, with obstetricians more frequently using medical and surgical interventions such as labour induction, episiotomies, assisted vaginal deliveries and cesearean sections [8-15]. Despite these different practice styles, few appreciable differences are seen in birth outcomes for women with low risk pregnancies [1,9,13,14,16]. Bai et al. postulate that obstetricians may be more likely to intervene as they are alert to managing women with high risk pregnancies [8], while Matthias asserts that practice differences are the result of different underlying philosophies about how risky birth can be [11]. While much work has focused on understanding reasons for, and implications of, intra-partum practice pattern differences, few studies report on the impact of practice pattern variation in a prenatal setting. While the number and frequency of prenatal visits for low-risk patients is common across specialties, the number of contact hours differs with typical prenatal visits for uncomplicated patients taking approximately 30–45 minutes with a midwife, compared to 15 minutes with family physicians and 10 minutes with obstetricians [17]. Another study shows that prenatal care provided by midwives tends to be less medicalized than care provided by physicians [6].

This study aimed to assess the impact of the type of prenatal care provider (family physician vs. midwife vs. obstetrician) on the self-reported use of ancillary services during pregnancy for a group of women at low medical risk. To our knowledge, this is the first study to evaluate the relationship between the type of prenatal care provider on service use during pregnancy other than for prenatal care in the context of a publically funded health care system.

Methods

Study participants

The All Our Babies study is a prospective community-based cohort study of women's experiences during pregnancy and the early post-partum period. Women were recruited from physician's offices, posters in the community and through follow-up phone calls after receiving pregnancy-related blood work. Women were eligible to participate if they were able to communicate in English, were accessing prenatal care in Calgary, Alberta, Canada and were less than 24 weeks pregnant. Women were asked to complete three written questionnaires – one prior to 24 weeks of gestation, one between 34 and 36 -weeks of gestation, and one at 4 months post-partum. Questionnaires consisted of validated scales and investigator derived questions. Following verbal consent to participate, participants were sent a package that included an information letter, a written consent form, a contact information form, the questionnaire and a postage-paid self-addressed return envelope. Participants who did not return their questionnaires within three weeks were contacted by telephone and email to remind them to complete the questionnaire and to provide them the opportunity to complete the questionnaire over the phone or to be mailed another questionnaire. Participants received a gift card to a grocery store for completion of each questionnaire and were sent congratulation cards following the birth of their baby and semi-annual newsletters to promote continual engagement with the study. Data were collected between May 2008 and May 2010 following pilot testing and revision of the questionnaires for clarity. This study was approved by the Conjoint Health Research Ethics Board at the University of Calgary and all participants provided written informed consent prior to participation. Please see http://www.ucalgary.ca/stough/allourbabies and McDonald et al. [18] for additional information on questionnaire content and survey methods or Appendix 1 for specific questions used in this analysis.

Overall, 1654 women participated in the All Our Babies cohort with a retention rate of 81%. Individuals with multiple gestation pregnancies (n = 24), who delivered preterm (gestational age <37 weeks) (n = 70), who had a caesarean delivery (n = 270), and who did not complete all three questionnaires (n = 383) were excluded from this analysis leaving a final sample size of 907. Completion of all three questionnaires was essential for this research question, as each questionnaire asked about the type of prenatal care provider and use of ancillary health services during pregnancy.

Type of prenatal care provider

Prenatal care in Calgary is typically provided by family physicians practicing alone or in the context of a low-risk maternity care clinic, although women can also self-refer to a midwife to obtain prenatal care. Since April 2009, midwifery has been publically funded in Alberta; prior to this, if women wanted to access midwifery care they were required to pay out of pocket [1,2].

The majority of midwives in Alberta practice in community-based settings and attend to women at low medical risk. Many women are seen by their own family physician early in pregnancy and are then referred to a low risk maternity clinic later in gestation. Women typically require a referral to see an obstetrician, and if referred, this transition of care would typically occur in the late second trimester.

Women were asked on each questionnaire from whom they received prenatal care – a family physician in an appointment-based office, a family physician in a low risk maternity clinic, an obstetrician, a midwife, a walk-in clinic physician or other. Women were categorized as having an obstetrician as their prenatal care provider if they ever selected this option. They were categorized as seeing a midwife if they ever reported this option and did not report seeing an obstetrician. They were categorized as having another prenatal care provider if they never reported seeing an obstetrician, a midwife, a family physician in an appointment-based office, or a family physician from a low risk maternity clinic. The remaining women were categorized as having their prenatal care provided by a family physician practicing either in an appointment-based office or in a low-risk maternity clinic. It was not possible to confirm the accuracy of women's assessments of their type of prenatal care provider or which type of care provider was the 'main' prenatal care provider for women who reported seeing multiple types of prenatal care providers.

Use of ancillary health services during pregnancy

For the purposes of this study the term 'ancillary health services' was defined as health services accessed during pregnancy for purposes other than regular prenatal care. On each survey, participants were asked if they had accessed any of the following services for any reason other than for prenatal care, and the number of visits to each service: chiropractor, emergency department, family physician, nurse telephone advice line (Telehealth), nutritionist/dietician, physiotherapist, psychologist/psychiatrist, social worker, specialist physician (other than an obstetrician), walk-in clinic or any other health care provider. They were also asked if they had been hospitalized overnight. Please see Table 1 for a brief overview of how women can access these services.

Statistical analysis

Descriptive statistics were used to characterize the sample. Chi-square tests and the Kruskal-Wallis test were used to assess for differences in demographic factors. Unadjusted logistic regression models were applied to the data first; these contained only the variable related to type of prenatal care provider. Subsequently, multivariable logistic regression models that also contained demographic (maternal age, education, ethnicity) and pregnancy-related (gravidity, use of prescription medications) covariates. Likelihood ratio tests were significant ($p < 0.001$) for all fully-adjusted models indicating that the covariates were significant predictors of the outcome of interest. All analyses were conducted using Stata SE Version 11.

Two sensitivity analyses were conducted. The first examined ancillary service utilization early (prior to 24 - weeks of gestation) and late (after 32 weeks of gestation) to determine if different patterns of ancillary resource use were present as the frequency of contact with prenatal care providers increases late in gestation. It was hypothesized that increased contact with prenatal care providers late in gestation might decrease use of ancillary services. The second sensitivity analysis limited the sample to women who reported only having a single type of care provider throughout their pregnancy as it was hypothesized that women who received the majority of their prenatal care from a family physician or midwife but were referred to an obstetrician later in pregnancy might have other medical risk factors that would influence ancillary service use.

Table 1 Access to ancillary services

Type of service	Referral type	Cost
Chiropractor	Self-referral or practitioner-referral	Chiropractic care is not covered by provincial health insurance. Patients can pay out of pocket or through a supplemental health insurance plan.
Emergency Department	Self-referral or practitioner-referral	Cost is covered by provincial health insurance.
Family Physician	Self-referral or practitioner-referral	Cost is covered by provincial health insurance.
Hospitalized Overnight	Practitioner-referral	Cost is covered by provincial health insurance.
Nurse Telephone Advice Line	Self-referral	Cost is covered by provincial health insurance.
Nutritionist/Dietician	Self-referral or practitioner-referral	Most dietary counseling is not covered by provincial health insurance. Patients can pay out of pocket or through a supplemental health insurance plan.
Physiotherapist	Self-referral or practitioner-referral	Most physiotherapy is not covered by provincial health insurance. Patients can pay out of pocket or through a supplemental health insurance plan.
Psychologist/Psychiatrist	Practitioner-referral	Costs for a psychiatrist are covered by provincial health insurance. Patients can pay out of pocket or through a supplemental health insurance plan to see a psychologist.
Social Worker	Practitioner-referral	Cost is covered by government.
Specialist Physician (other than an obstetrician)	Practitioner-referral	Cost is covered by provincial health insurance.
Walk-In Clinic	Self-referral	Cost is covered by provincial health insurance.

Results

Type of prenatal care provider

Overall, 536 women (59.1%) received their prenatal care from a family physician or a low-risk maternity clinic; 286 (31.5%) saw an obstetrician; 82 (9.0%) saw a midwife; and 3 (0.3%) received their prenatal care from another source (i.e. walk-in clinic). Due to the low proportion of women who received their prenatal care from another source, these participants have been removed from all further analyses. Two hundred and seventy-one women (22.0%) reported seeing multiple prenatal care providers throughout the course of their pregnancy and were categorized as receiving prenatal care from a family physician, midwife or obstetrician as outlined in the methods section.

Participant characteristics

As seen in Table 2, the majority of women had a partner, were born in Canada, have completed post-secondary education and had an annual household income of at least $60,000. Women did not differ across groups, except women who received their prenatal care from a midwife were significantly more likely to be Caucasian (p = 0.03). Women who participated in the All Our Babies cohort are representative of the pregnant population in Canada in terms of parity, pre-pregnancy BMI, and number of prenatal care visits; however, women in the All Our Babies study tend to be slightly older, better educated and have a higher household income [18].

Contact with prenatal care providers

While the median number of prenatal visits was not significantly different between groups (p = 0.37), participants who received their prenatal care from an obstetrician were significantly more likely to have less than 6 prenatal visits, the minimum number of prenatal visits recommended by the Society of Obstetricians and Gynecologists of Canada [19] and Health Canada's Guidelines for Family-Centred Maternity and Newborn Care [20], throughout the course of their pregnancy (5.6%) compared to participants who received their prenatal care from a family physician (2.4%) or a midwife (2.4%) (p = 0.03). Participants who received their prenatal care from a midwife were significantly more likely to have their first prenatal visit in the first trimester (97.6%), than participants who received their prenatal care from a family physician (85.4%) or an obstetrician (88.1%) (p = 0.007).

Use of ancillary health services during pregnancy

Seven hundred and seventy nine women (85.8%) reported using at least one ancillary service during the course of their pregnancy, and this did not differ based on the type of prenatal care provider (p = 0.88). Women who received their prenatal care from a midwife accessed fewer types of ancillary services (median 2, range 0–7) than women who accessed their prenatal care from a family physician (median 3, range 0–11) or an obstetrician (median 3, range 0–9) (p = 0.04).

Women who received their prenatal care from an obstetrician were significantly more likely to visit a walk-in clinic than women who received their prenatal care from a family physician (OR = 1.51, 95% CI: 1.11-2.05) (Table 3). Women who received their prenatal care from a midwife were significantly less likely to go to the emergency department (OR = 0.47, 95% CI: 0.24-0.89) or call a telephone nurse advice line (OR = 0.30, 95% CI: 0.18-0.50) compared to women who received their prenatal care from a family physician, and were significantly more likely to visit a chiropractor (OR = 4.07, 95% CI: 2.49-6.67) (Table 3).

Sensitivity analysis

Two sensitivity analyses were conducted. The first examined health resource utilization early and late in gestation; the results were in the same direction as those

Table 2 Participant characteristics

Characteristic	Type of prenatal care provider			p-value
	Family physician N = 536 N (%)	Midwife N = 82 N (%)	Obstetrician N = 286 N (%)	
Maternal Age ≥35 years	94 (18.2)	15 (18.5)	61 (21.9)	0.45
Previously been pregnant	322 (60.1)	56 (68.2)	186 (65.0)	0.19
Currently has a partner	532 (99.4)	82 (100.0)	284 (99.3)	0.75
Caucasian Ethnicity	415 (77.7)	74 (90.2)	220 (76.9)	**0.03**
Born in Canada	419 (78.3)	69 (84.1)	216 (75.5)	0.24
Completed Post-Secondary Education	427 (80.0)	63 (76.8)	224 (78.3)	0.74
Currently working or attending school	345 (64.4)	49 (59.8)	169 (59.1)	0.29
Annual Household Income ≥ $60,000	438 (84.9)	68 (85.0)	234 (84.5)	0.99
Own their home	434 (81.0)	69 (84.1)	221 (77.3)	0.32

Table 3 Use of ancillary health services during pregnancy

Type of ancillary health service	Type of prenatal care provider							
	Family physician		Midwife			Obstetrician		
	N = 536		N = 82			N = 286		
	N (%)	OR (95% CI)	N (%)	Unadjusted OR (95% CI) *p value*	Adjusted OR (95% CI) *p value*	N (%)	Unadjusted OR (95% CI) *p value*	Adjusted OR (95% CI) *p value*
Chiropractor	139 (25.9)	1.0 (ref)	48 (58.5)	**4.03 (2.50-6.52) $p < 0.001$**	**4.07 (2.49-6.67) $p < 0.001$**	64 (22.4)	0.82 (0.59-1.16) $p = 0.26$	0.80 (0.56-1.13) $p = 0.21$
Emergency Department	150 (28.0)	1.0 (ref)	12 (14.6)	**0.44 (0.23-0.84)$p = 0.01$**	**0.47 (0.24-0.89) $p = 0.02$**	98 (34.3)	1.34 (0.99-1.83) $p = 0.06$	1.31 (0.96-1.80) $p = 0.09$
Family Physician	387 (72.2)	1.0 (ref)	57 (69.5)	0.88 (0.53-1.46) $p = 0.61$	0.96 (0.57-1.61) $p = 0.88$	204 (71.3)	0.96 (0.70-1.32) $p = 0.79$	0.92 (0.66-1.27) $p = 0.61$
Hospitalized Overnight	28 (5.2)	1.0 (ref)	5 (6.1)	1.18 (0.44-3.14) $p = 0.74$	1.24 (0.46-3.36) $p = 0.67$	20 (7.0)	1.36 (0.75-2.47) $p = 0.30$	1.29 (0.70-2.38) $p = 0.41$
Nurse Telephone Advice Line	322 (60.1)	1.0 (ref)	25 (30.5)	**0.29 (0.18-0.48) $p < 0.001$**	**0.30 (0.18-0.50) $p < 0.001$**	179 (62.6)	1.11 (0.33-1.49) $p = 0.48$	1.15 (0.84-1.55) $p = 0.38$
Nutritionist/Dietician	38 (7.1)	1.0 (ref)	5 (6.1)	0.85 (0.32-2.23) $p = 0.74$	1.00 (0.38-2.68) $p = 0.99$	26 (9.1)	1.31 (0.78-2.21) $p = 0.31$	1.30 (0.76-2.21) $p = 0.34$
Physiotherapist	48 (9.0)	1.0 (ref)	9 (11.0)	1.25 (0.59-2.66) $p = 0.56$	1.32 (0.59-2.95) $p = 0.50$	21 (7.3)	0.81 (0.47-1.37) $p = 0.43$	0.80 (0.46-1.40) $p = 0.43$
Psychologist/Psychiatrist	44 (8.2)	1.0 (ref)	6 (7.3)	0.88 (0.36-2.14) $p = 0.78$	0.99 (0.40-2.43) $p = 0.98$	22 (7.7)	0.93 (0.55-1.59) $p = 0.80$	0.92 (0.53-1.59) $p = 0.77$
Social Worker	15 (2.8)	1.0 (ref)	1 (1.2)	0.43 (0.06-3.29) $p = 0.42$	0.55 (0.07-4.34) $p = 0.57$	14 (4.9)	1.79 (0.35-3.76) $p = 0.13$	1.58 (0.74-3.39) $p = 0.24$
Specialist Physician (other than an obstetrician)	97 (18.1)	1.0 (ref)	10 (12.2)	0.63 (0.31-1.26) $p = 0.19$	0.66 (0.33-1.34) $p = 0.25$	63 (22.0)	1.28 (0.30-1.82) $p = 0.18$	1.27 (0.88-1.82) $p = 0.20$
Walk-In Clinic	178 (33.2)	1.0 (ref)	20 (24.4)	0.65 (0.38-1.11) $p = 0.11$	0.74 (0.43-1.28) $p = 0.28$	119 (41.6)	**1.43 (1.07-1.93) $p = 0.02$**	**1.51 (1.11-2.05) $p = 0.01$**

* Analyses are adjusted for maternal age, education, ethnicity, gravidity and use of prescription medications during pregnancy.

presented in Table 3, hence only the overall findings are presented. The same pattern of service utilization early and late in gestation, irrespective of the type of prenatal care provider, suggests that ancillary service use is not influenced by the frequency of contact with the prenatal care provider. The second sensitivity analysis examined health resource utilization only among women who had a single type of prenatal care provider. The results were also in the same direction as the overall findings, but the relationship between seeing an obstetrician and visiting the emergency department became statistically significant (OR = 1.51, 95% CI 1.03-2.21), suggesting that women who were attended to exclusively by an obstetrician may have other medical risk factors necessitating use of emergency services compared to women who may have received a single consultation from an obstetrician and received the bulk of their prenatal care from a midwife or family physician.

Discussion

This study of low-risk pregnant women, who were largely cared for by physicians (less than 10% of women received their prenatal care from a midwife), shows that regardless of prenatal care provider, the majority of women access at least one ancillary service during the course of their pregnancy. This speaks to the opportunity for coordination of care across multiple services and settings to ensure that women receive consistent information, to avoid duplication of services, and to assist prenatal care providers in attending to the broader needs of pregnant women. Statistically significant differences were seen for some, but not all, ancillary services based on the type of prenatal care provider. Despite restriction to a medically low-risk population and statistical adjustment for baseline differences between groups and for pregnancy-related factors that might predict service utilization such as gravidity and the use of prescription medications, it cannot be ascertained whether these differences are the result of different practice styles of midwives, family physicians and obstetricians or if they are due to unmeasured maternal factors that are associated with the type of prenatal care provider they may choose or, in some cases, require. Alternatively, these findings may suggest that many women who are pregnant will still present with a gestalt of health-related needs which need to be addressed or monitored throughout pregnancy.

Our findings with regards to the association between the type of prenatal care provider and the number of prenatal care visits and the timing of first prenatal visit are comparable to those reported in the Maternity Experiences Survey [13]. O'Brien et al. found that women who received their prenatal care from a midwife were more likely to access care early and had more prenatal visits [13]. A qualitative study examining midwifery care concluded that women who seek midwifery care wanted to pursue a more 'natural approach' to pregnancy and childbirth [21]. This same study found that women who chose midwifery desired to distance themselves from biomedical interventions [21]. The National Maternity Care Attitudes Study found that nulliparous women who received their prenatal care from obstetricians, midwives, and family physician represented different populations of women in terms of both demographic characteristics and attitudes towards the use of medical interventions during labour and delivery [22]. While few demographic differences were observed in this study, attitudinal differences may be reflected in our findings, as women who received their prenatal care from a midwife were not any less likely to access ancillary services but they were less likely to access biomedical services provided through emergency departments and nurse telephone advice lines and more likely to access complementary and alternative medicine (CAM) resources such as chiropractic care. CAM use in Canada is common; 12.4% of the general population reporting that they had accessed at least one CAM service in the past year, with chiropractic care being the fourth most common type of CAM service used (following massage, acupuncture and homeopathy) [23]. While women have been found to be twice as likely to assess CAM services in Canada as men [23], population-based estimates of CAM use in the context of pregnancy are lacking. A study comprising women who contacted the Motherisk program (a teratogen information service based in Toronto Ontario Canada) found that approximately 60% of women used CAM treatments to alleviate nausea and vomiting in pregnancy [24]. A Quebec study examining the use of herbal products in pregnancy estimated that 9% of pregnant women used an herbal supplement alone or in combination with prescription medications [25]. Differences in participant recruitment strategies and baseline characteristics likely explain some, but not all, of the differences in these rates. Unfortunately data on use of CAM services other than chiropractic care was not available in the current study; understanding the prevalence, predictors and outcome of CAM use during pregnancy is an important area for future research.

Women who obtained their prenatal care from an obstetrician would typically have been referred to this level of care due to higher underlying medical or fetal risk than is typically seen in the population of pregnant women cared for by family physicians. Attempts were made to restrict this sample to women at low medical risk; however, these women may have had underlying medical or obstetrical risk factors that influenced their use of ancillary services, particularly walk-in clinics and the emergency department. Additionally, it is possible that some visits classified as emergency department visits were actually obstetrical triage visits, thereby supporting a hypothesis of possible increased risk status in this population. After 20 - weeks of gestation, labour and delivery triage is done on the obstetrical wards and not in the emergency room, even though women might initially present at the emergency room [26]. Alternatively, increased use of walk-in clinics and the emergency department may be related to the availability of after-hours pregnancy-related care. This should be explored in future studies. The consistency of findings between the main analysis that includes women who ever saw an obstetrician for prenatal care and the sensitivity analysis that examined women who only saw an obstetrician for prenatal care also supports the hypothesis of increased medical and/or fetal risk in this group.

As midwifery becomes more established, it is likely that the proportion of women choosing this option for prenatal care will increase. Data from the Canadian Maternity Experiences Survey suggests that women who receive their prenatal care from midwives are more likely to be over the age of 35, have completed post-secondary education and to have used folic acid before pregnancy compared to women who receive their prenatal care from obstetricians or family physicians [13]. Midwives were publicly funded in Alberta as of April 1, 2009 (midway through the recruitment period for this study) [1]. Other studies have found an increase in the use of midwifery services once these services were insured [1]. The increased capacity of midwives to provide prenatal and intra-partum care will be important, as it is estimated that only 11% of family physicians in Canada provide intra-partum care [27], and of those who do not currently offer this service to their patients, 25% have indicated that nothing could convince them to provide intra-partum care [4].

This trend of high resource utilization and accessing multiple unrelated services during pregnancy is likely to continue, regardless of the type of prenatal care provider, as the proportion of pregnancies in older women and women with underlying medical disease continues to increase [2,28]. This study points to the need for increased coordination of care as women see multiple health professionals throughout their pregnancies both for their prenatal care and for ancillary services, who may be providing them with conflicting advice. Yet, despite the increased risk for complications in these pregnancies [29], few, if any, guidelines exist for Canadian prenatal care providers to help guide them in when their patients should be referred to other ancillary services in pregnancy. The Society of Obstetricians and Gynecologists of Canada's 'Guidelines for Care During Pregnancy and Childbirth' contains no references to when women should be referred to other sources of care [19]. While the Health Canada Guidelines for Family-Centred Maternity and Newborn Care speak to the need for appropriate referral to other services and outline that there could potentially be many types of care providers involved in the provision of prenatal care, they stop short of indicating when a referral should be made and what services pregnant women should, or should not, be referred to [20].

Limitations

There are limitations to this study. All service use is self-reported; however, as this sample is limited to women with vaginal delivery and appropriate length of gestation, and this data was collected prospectively, the possibility of recall bias is minimized. Unfortunately, data was not collected on whether ancillary services use was related to pregnancy or not, merely whether it occurred in the prenatal period, so we cannot determine if women were self-referring to ancillary care services or were going at the recommendation of their prenatal care provider. This is important as many of the ancillary services examined in this study would not require referral; thus observed differences may be related to the type of prenatal care provider women chose, and not because of the type of prenatal care received from different providers. This study was limited to women living in a single province during a transition period from regulated midwifery to regulated and provincially reimbursed midwifery. It is unknown if these results can be generalized to other provinces where midwifery is more established. Misclassification bias is also possible if women were unable to accurately report who their prenatal care provider was. We presume that women would be most likely to report that they saw an obstetrician, when they really saw a family physician, which would bias the results towards the null. Misclassification is also possible for the 22% of women who reported seeing multiple types of prenatal care providers; for example, a woman who received the majority of her prenatal care from a family physician and had a single visit to an obstetrician would be classified in this study as receiving her prenatal care from an obstetrician. However, as our findings were robust when limited to women with a single type of care provider, this is unlikely to change our conclusions. Additionally, this study attempted to recruit women from the general population of pregnant women (the majority of whom can be classified as low medical risk) and efforts were made to further restrict this analysis to women with uncomplicated pregnancies; however, residual confounding by pregnancy-related or general medical complications is possible. This may be particularly relevant for women whose primary prenatal care provider was an obstetrician, who typically would have been referred to this level of care provider.

Conclusion

In conclusion, understanding what ancillary care services women access during pregnancy is an important step in measuring women's access to non-obstetric services during pregnancy. Prenatal care is a complex entity and referral pathways between care providers and services are not always clear. This can lead to the provision of fragmented care and create opportunities for errors and loss of information. All types of care providers have a role in addressing the full range of health needs that pregnant women experience. Future studies should examine the referral patterns of prenatal care providers and the content of prenatal care in relation to ancillary service use.

Competing interests

None of the authors have any competing interests to declare.

Authors' contributions

ST designed the overall study and secured funding. AM designed this sub-study, conducted the analysis and drafted the manuscript. All authors participated in the interpretation of findings; critically reviewed the manuscript and approved the final version for submission.

Acknowledgements

The All Our Babies study was supported by an Alberta Innovates Health Solutions Team Grant (Preterm Birth and Healthy Outcomes Team). The funder did not play a role in the design, collection, analysis, and interpretation of data; in the writing of the manuscript; and in the decision to submit the manuscript for publication. During the course of this study Amy Metcalfe held a studentship from the Canadian Institutes of Health Research (CIHR) Strategic Training Program in Genetics, Child Development and Health; she currently holds a CIHR fellowship award. Suzanne Tough holds a Health Scholar award from Alberta Innovates Health Solutions.

Author details

[1]Department of Obstetrics and Gynecology, University of British Columbia, BC Women's and Children's Hospital, 4500 Oak St, Vancouver, BC V6H 3N1, Canada. [2]Division of Maternal Fetal Medicine, Department of Obstetrics and Gynecology, University of British Columbia, 13750 96 Avenue, Surrey, BC V3V 1Z2, Canada. [3]Mental Health Screening and Early Identification, Addiction & Mental Health, Alberta Health Services, 10101 Southport Road SW, Calgary, AB, Canada. [4]Departments of Pediatrics and Community Health Sciences, University of Calgary Child Development Centre, c/o 2888 Shaganappi Trail NW, Calgary, AB T3B 6A8, Canada.

References

1. O'Brien B, Harvey S, Sommerfeldt S, Beischel S, Newburn-Cook C, Schopflocher D: **Comparison of costs and associated outcomes between women choosing newly integrated autonomous midwifery care and matched controls: a pilot study.** *J Obstet Gynaecol Can* 2010, **32**(7):650–656.
2. Zelmer J, Leeb K: **Challenges for providing maternity services: the impact of changing birthing practices.** *Healthcare Quarterly* 2004, **7**(3):21–23.
3. Chan BTB: **The declining comprehensiveness of primary care.** *CMAJ* 2002, **166**(4):429–434.
4. Smith C, Brow JB, Stewart M, Trim K, Freeman T, Beckhoff C, Kasperski MJ: **Ontario care providers' considerations regarding models of maternity care.** *J Obstet Gynaecol Can* 2009, **31**(5):401–408.
5. Coco A: **How often do physicians address other medical problems while providing prenatal care?** *Annals of Family Medicine* 2009, **7**(2):134–138.
6. Sword W, Heaman MI, Brooks S, Tough S, Janssen PA, Young D, Kingston D, Helewa ME, Akhtar-Danesh N, Hutton E: **Women's And care providers' perspectives of quality prenatal care: a qualitative descriptive study.** *BMC Pregnancy Childbirth* 2012, **12**:29.
7. Durand MA, Stiel M, Boivin J, Elwyn G: **Information and decision support needs of parents considering amniocentesis: interviews with pregnant women and health professionals.** *Health expectations: an international journal of public participation in health care and health policy* 2010, **13**(2):125–138.
8. Bai J, Gyaneshwar R, Bauman A: **Models of antenatal care and obstetric outcomes in sydney south west.** *Aust N Z J Obstet Gynaecol* 2008, **48**:454–461.
9. Jackson EA, Francke L, Vsilenko P: **Management of gestational diabetes by family physicians and obstetricians.** *J Fam Pract* 1996, **43**(4):383–388.
10. Monari F, Di Mario S, Facchinetti F, Basevi V: **Obstetricians' And midwives' attitudes toward cesarean section.** *Birth* 2008, **35**(2):129–135.
11. Matthias MS: **The impact of uncertainity on decision making in prenatal consultations: obstetricians' and midwives' perspectives.** *Heal Commun* 2010, **25**:199–211.
12. Tan WM, Klein MC, Saxell L, Shirkoohy SE, Asrat G: **How do physicians and midwives manage the third stage of labour?** *Birth* 2008, **35**(3):220–229.
13. O'Brien B, Chalmers B, Fell D, Heaman M, Darling EK, Herbert P: **The experience of pregnancy and birth with midwives: results from the canadian maternity experiences survey.** *Birth* 2011, **38**(3):207–215.
14. Janssen PA, Saxell L, Page LA, Klein MC, Liston RM, Lee SK: **Outcomes of planned home birth with registered midwifeversus planned hospital birth with midwife or physician.** *CMAJ* 2009, **181**(6–7):377–383.
15. Klein MC, Kaczorowski J, Hall WA, Fraser WD, Liston RM, Eftekhary S, Brant R, Masse LC, Rosinski J, Mehrabadi A, *et al:* **The attitudes of canadian maternity care practitioners towards labour and birth: many differences but important similarities.** *J Obstet Gynaecol Can* 2009, **31**(9):827–840.
16. Khan-Neelofur D, Gulmezoglu M, Villar J, WHO Antenatal Care Trial Research Group: **Who should provide routine antenatal care for low-risk women, and how often? a systematic review of randomized controlled trials.** *Paediatric and Perinatal Epidemiology* 1998, **12**(Suppl 2):7–26.
17. McDonald SD, Pullenayegum E, Bracken K, Chen AM, McDonald H, Malott A, Hutchison R, Haley S, Lutsiv O, Taylor VH, *et al:* **Comparison of midwifery, family medicine, and obstetric patients' understanding of weight gain during pregnancy: a minority of women report correct counselling.** *J Obstet Gynaecol Can* 2012, **34**(2):129–135.
18. McDonald SW, Lyon AW, Benzies KM, McNeil DA, Lye SJ, Dolan SM, Pennell CE, Bocking AD, Tough SC: **The All Our babies pregnancy cohort: design, methods, and participant characteristics.** *BMC Pregnancy and Childbirth* 2013, **13**(Suppl 1):S2.
19. Schuurmans N, Gagne GP, Ezzat A, Colliton I, MacKinnon CJ, Dushinski B, Caddick R, Lalonde AB, Kinch RAH: **Healthy beginnings: guidelines for care during pregnancy and childbirth.** In *Clinical practice guidelines.* Society of Obstetricians and Gynaecologists of Canada; 1998.
20. Health Canada: *Family-centred maternity and newborn care: national guidelines.* Ottawa: Minister of Public Works and Government Services; 2000.
21. Parry DC: **"We wanted a birth experience, not a medical experience": exploring Canadian Women's Use of midwifery.** *Health Care for Women International* 2008, **29**:784–806.
22. Klein MC, Kaczorowski J, Hearps SJC, Tomkinson J, Baradaran N, Hall WA, McNiven P, Brant R, Grant J, Dore S, *et al:* **Birth technology and maternal roles in birth: knowledge and attitudes of Canadian women approaching childbirth for the first time.** *J Obstet Gynaecol Can* 2011, **33**(6):598–608.
23. Metcalfe A, Williams J, McChesney J, Patten SB, Jette N: **Use of complementary and alternative medicine by those with a chronic disease and the general population - results of a national population based survey.** *BMC Complementary Altern Med* 2010, **10**(58).
24. Hollyer T, Boon H, Georgousis A, Smith M, Einarson A: **The use of CAM by women suffering from nausea and vomiting during pregnancy.** *BMC Complementary and Alternative Medicine* 2002, **2**(5).
25. Moussally K, Oraichi D, Berard A: **Herbal products use during pregnancy: prevalence and predictors.** *Pharmacoepidemiology and Drug Safety* 2009, **18**:454–461.

26. De Coster C, Quan H, Elford R, Li B, Mazzei L, Zimmer S: **Follow-through after calling a nurse telephone advice line: a population-based study.** *Fam Pract* 2010, **27:**271–278.
27. Klein MC, Kaczorowski J, Tomkinson J, Hearps S, Baradaran N, Brant R: **Family physicians who provide intrapartum care and those who do not: very different ways of viewing childbirth.** *Can Fam Physician* 2011, **57:**e139–147.
28. Public Health Agency of Canada: *Canadian perinatal health report, 2008 edition.* Ottawa: Government of Canada; 2008.
29. Joseph KS, Allen A, Dodds L, Turner L, Scott H, Liston R: **The perinatal effects of delayed childbearing.** *Obstet Gynecol* 2005, **105**(6):1410–1418.

22

DELAY on first antenatal care visit and its associated factors among pregnant women in public health facilities of Debre Markos town, North West Ethiopia

Atsede Alle Ewunetie[1*], Alemtsehay Mekonnen Munea[2], Belsity Temesgen Meselu[3], Muluye Molla Simeneh[1] and Bekele Tesfaye Meteku[4]

Abstract

Background: Delay on timely initiation of antenatal care has a great impact on adverse pregnancy out comes. However, evidences in Ethiopia revealed that majority of pregnant mothers did not start their first visit as recommrnded by WHO. The aim of this study was to assess delay and associated factors of first antenatal care visit among pregnant mothers at public health facilities of Debremarkos town, North West Ethiopia.

Methods: An institutional based crosss-sectional study was conducted from February to March, 2014 in public health facilities of Debremarkos town North west Ethiopia. A total of 320 pregnant mothers who were sure of their last menstrual periods were interviewed with a structured questionnaire. Data entry was done using Epi data 3.1 and analysis was done using SPSS version 20. Descriptive statistics, binary and multivariable logistic regression analyses were employed to identify the magnitude and factors associated with delay on timely initiation of the first antenatal care visit.

Results: The proportion of respondents who made their first antenatal care visit after 16 weeks of gestation was found to be 33.4%. Mothers residing in rural settings (AOR = 2.8 [95% CI:1.54–5.44]), not attained formal education(AOR = 2.2 [95% CI:1.10–4.68]),with unintended pregnancy (AOR = 3.6 [95% CI:2.00–6.80]) and who perceived that the right initiation time of the first antenatal care visit is beyond 16 weeks of gestation (AOR = 3.9 [95% CI:1.61–9.76]) were more likely delayed on their first antenatal care visit .

Conclusion: Residence, educational status, intention of pregnancy and perception on the right time of first antenatal care visit initiation were found to be predictors of delay on timely initiatin of first antenatal care visit. Therefore, the Zonal health department should strengthen awareness creation about timely initiation of first antenatal care visit and family planning to prevent unintended pregnancy in the community especially in the rural settings.

Keywords: Delay on timely initiation of antenatalcare, Unintended, Pregnancy

* Correspondence: atsialle@gmail.com
[1]Department of Public Health, College of Health Sciences, Debre Markos University, Debre Markos, Ethiopia
Full list of author information is available at the end of the article

Background

Many health problems of pregnant women are preventable, detectable, and treatable if they attained antenatal care (ANC) adequately [1]. The traditional approach of the ANC is a high risk approach which intended to classify pregnant women at low risk or high risk based on predetermined criteria and involved many ANC visits. This approach was hard to implement effectively since many women had at least one risk factor, and not all developed complications; at the same time, some low risk women did develop complications. It is a burden on the healthcare system. As a result, many developing countries, including Ethiopia, are adopting focused antenatal care (FANC) approach. The newly proposed, FANC recommends four ANC visits for most pregnant women. Ideally, the first visit is in the first trimester but not after 16 weeks of gestation [2, 3].

The recommendation sets out from the fact that first trimester pregnancy stage is the fastest developmental period of the fetus, in which all organs become well developed and needs special attention [4, 5]. However, too many women make their first antenatal visit with the pregnancy already compromised or at risk from smoking, inappropriate nutrition, ingestion of a variety of drugs, including pharmaceutical preparations, genitourinary tract infections, anemia and poor dental health [5].

Women present for antenatal care early in their pregnancy period allow enough time for essential and feasible interventions, prevention of complications and early identification of underlying conditions [6]. It also used to prevent, diagnose and treat sexually transmitted infections and work on the elimination of new Human Immune Deficiency Virus infections among new borne through providing integrated quality prevention of mother to child transmission [7–9].

Early attendance of ANC provides a better hemoglobin concentration through nutritional advice, prevention and early treatment of malaria and timely iron foliate supplementation [10, 11]. Beside this, it increases the opportunity of pregnant mothers to have more prenatal care visits, sufficient tests and advice during pregnancy and a skilled birth attendant [12, 13].

Mothers who start ANC after 22 weeks gestation, missed over four routine antenatal visits, who did not seek care or who concealed their pregnancy were manifest 17% of maternal deaths [14]. Suboptimal antenatal care was also found to be the major contributory factor for still birth in India [15]. Mothers who sought antenatal care before the end of the third month had infants who weighed heavier compared to the infants of mothers who sought care later [11, 16, 17].

Even though there is improvement on antenatal care coverage and the World Health Organization recommendation is initiating ANC visit in the first trimester, the time of initiation of first ANC visit is varied throughout the world. In the Ethiopian context, it is recommended that the first ANC visit should be ideally taken place before 16 weeks of pregnancy (2). In order to improve maternal health care service utilization; all governmental health institutions of Ethiopia are providing focused antenatal care service for all pregnant mothers who come to the health institutions free of charge. Early initiation of antenatal care is promoted by health extension workers and health professionals in both urban and rural Keble's. Beside women developmental armies who are delegated in the community have their own role in community mobilization regarding to antenatal care service utilization.

According to the Ethiopia demographic, health survey, over 34% of pregnant women were attending antenatal care at least once. But, only 19% had four or more antenatal care visits during their entire pregnancy, and 11% of women made their first antenatal care visit before the fourth month of pregnancy nationwide [3]. In order to improve maternal and child health, identifying timing of first antenatal care visit among pregnant mothers and factors that affect initiation of first ANC visit is paramount. This study is designed to assess delay on first antenatal care visit among pregnant mothers and factors that affect initiation of first ANC.

Methods

Study design and data sources

An institutional based cross sectional study design was employed from February 1st through March 30, 2014 in public health facilities of Debremarkos town. Debremarkos town is the capital of East Gojjam Zone, which is located 300 km North West of Addis Ababa and 265 km away from regional capital Bahir Dar.

The study populations were pregnant women who visited public health facilities of Debremarkos town for antenatal care and randomly selected during the study period. Those pregnant mothers who were seriously ill or not aware their menstrual period were excluded from the study. The sample size was determined using single population proportion formula with the following assumptions: the proportion of delayed ANC is 74% from previous study conducted in Debre Birhan (18), maximum acceptable marginal error of 5%, an alpha level of 0.05 and a none response rate 10% were used to obtain a sample size of 326.

All public health facilities (one referral Hospital and three health centers) in Debremarkos town were included in the study. The total sample size was proportionally allocated to health facilities based on average monthly flow of pregnant mothers for ANC in each heath facility. The study subjects were recruited by using systematic random sampling technique after identification of the first study subject by simple random sampling method. Multiple enumerations due to referral were avoided using filtering questions.

The outcome variable of the study was delay on initiation of first ANC visit and the explanatory variables included Socio-demographic factors (age, religion, ethnicity, marital status, educational status, average monthly income), Obstetric factors (parity, History of obstetric complication, history of Previous ANC visit and intention of pregnancy),Enabling factors (accessibility of information about ANC and interaction with healthprofessional) and Reinforcing factors (perception of mothers on the advantage of the ANC, timing of ANC visit and frequency of the ANC; reasons that initiate mothers to start ANC after 16 weeks, a decision made to seek ANC, intention of partner to watrds ANC service utilization).

Delay on initiation of first antenatal care visit is initiation of first ANC visit in public health facilities which have skilled health personnel after 16 weeks of gestation.

Data were collected using structured interviewer administered questionnaire adopted from literatures and contextualized to the local situations and study objectives. The data collection tool was translated into the local language (Amharic) and pretested on 5% of the actual sample size out of the study area. Four diploma nurses and one public health professional were involved as data collector and supervisor respectively after taking 1 day training.

Ethical considerations

The study was conducted after obtaining ethical clearance from Bahir Dar University, College of medicine and Health sciences, Research Ethics Committee and letter of support from Amhara regional health bureau ethical review committee. Formal Permission paper was given to woreda health office, Debremarkos Referal Hosipital and responsible persons in each health institution accordingly. Verbal informed consent also obtained from the study participants after explaining the purpose of study. Participants were informed on their full right to skip any question or terminate their participation at any stage. Participants were also assured that there will be no harm or benefit of being participating in this study. All the information from the respondents was kept confidential.

Data processing and analysis

The data were cleaned, coded and entered in Lauritsen JM, Bruus M, Myatt M. Epi Data.A comprehensive tool for validated entry and documentation of data. 2003; 3 and transferred to IBM SPSS Statistics for Windows, Version 20.0. Armonk, NY: IBM Corp for analysis. Both descriptive and inferential statistics were used to summarize the data. Those variables found to be statistically significant ($p < 0.2$) in the binary logistic regression analyses were entered into the multivariable logistic regression model and statistical significance was considered at $p < 0.05$.The strength of association was assessed by odds ratio (OR) with 95% confidence interval.

Results

The response rate was 98.1%.The mean (±SD)age of respondents was 26.3(± 5.1).Among all respondents, 311 (97.2%) were Amhara in ethnic group and majority 299(93.4%) of mothers were orthodox Christian followers (Table 1).

Of all respondents, 107 (33.4%) made their first ANC visit after 16 weeks of gestation. The mean time was 14. 5 (± 6.5) weeks with the range of 4 to 36 weeks. The median and the pick time was 12 weeks of gestation. Above

Table 1 Socio demographic characterstics of pregnant mothers who were attending ANC in the public health facilities of Debremarkos town, Feburary-March 2014($n = 320$)

Varaible		Frequency	Percent
Residence	Rural	69	21.6
	Urban	251	78.4
Age	15–19	16	5.0
	20–24	104	32.5
	25–29	121	37.8
	30–34	55	17.2
	≥35	24	7.5
Ethinicity	Amhara	311	97.2
	Others	9	2.8
Relegion	Orthodox chrstian	299	93.4
	Muslim /Protestant	21	6.6
Marital status	Never married	14	4.4
	Married	293	91.6
	Divorced/widowed	13	4
Educational status	Have no formal education	98	30.6
	Primary education	51	15.9
	Secondary education	87	27.2
	Tertiary education	84	26.3
Occupation	Government employee	81	25.3
	House wife	49	15.3
	Merchant	118	36.9
	Farmer	42	13.1
	Daily labourer	17	5.3
	Students / depende on family	13	4.1
Monthly income	< 1000 ETB(<Q1)	124	38.8
	1000–2987.50ETB	116	36.2
	> 2987.50ETB(>Q3)	80	25.0

Others = Oromo/Tigrie/Agew

half (51.2%) of mothers were start their first ANC visit in the first trimester (Fig. 1) .

Among the total respondents,174 (54.4%) were multiparous. Of these, 126 (74.2%) reported that they had had experience of ANC for the preceding pregnancy. For those who had had ANC visit on preceding pregnancy, 43 (34%) visited the ANC clinic for the first time after 16 weeks of gestation in the current pregnancy. From 68 (21.2%) of mothers who had unintended pregnancy, 25 (36.8%) indicated that they had interest in interrupting their pregnancy (Table 2).

The available health facilities were health centers for 220 (68.8%) of respondents, Hospital for 60(10.8%) of respondents and health posts for 40(12.4%) of respondents. Of all respondents, 182 (56.9%) were advised for ANC on current pregnancy. Of these, only 38 (20.9%) had information on the time of first ANC visit. From those who had information on initiation time of ANC, 2 (5.3%) were informed to start their first visit after 16 weeks of gestation (Table 3).

A majority, 27 (85.3%) of respondents perceived that the ANC is important for both maternal and child health. Among delayed respondents 18 (16.8%) were initiated ANC by considering the time of their visit at the right time (Fig. 2).

Among respondents 264 (82.5%) were decided to seek ANC service jointly with their partners.From all, 287(89.4%) partners supported the need of ANC for every pregnant mothers.

The bivariate analysis showed that pregnant mothers who were residing in rural areas[Crude Odds Ratio (COR) = 3.4, 95% Confidence Interval (CI): 2.01–6.07], not attained formal education[COR = 4.5,95% CI: 2.33–8.67], farmers [COR = 7. 8, 95% CI: 3.37–18.05], having less than 1000 ETB average monthly income[COR = 2.7, 95% CI: 1.45–5.37],experience

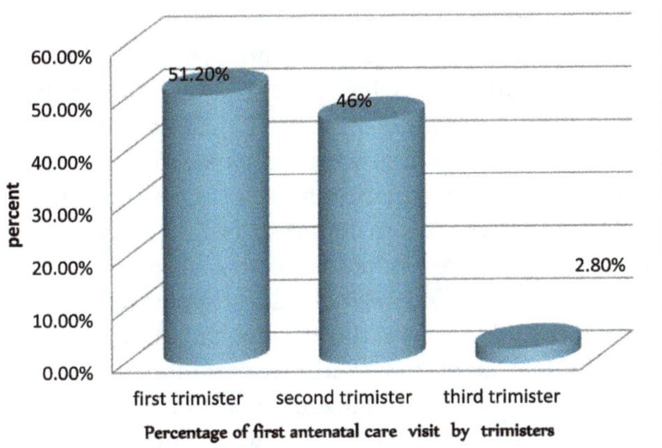

Fig. 1 Distribution of first ANC visits among pregnant mothers in public health facilities in Debremarkos in each trimester between February 2014 and March 2014

Table 2 Obstetric history of pregnant mothers, who were attending ANC in the public health Facilities of Debre Markos town, Feburary – March, 2014 ($n = 320$)

Variable		Frequency	Percent
Gravidity ($n = 320$)	Primigravida	146	45.6
	Multi gravida	174	54.4
Parity (n = 320)	No parity	158	49.4
	≥1 parity	162	50.6
Children born alive ($n = 174$)	0	17	9.8
	1–3	135	77.6
	≥4	22	12.6
Death of children ($n = 157$)	Yes	30	19.1
	No	127	80.9
spontanous abortion (n = 174)	Yes	35	20.1
	No	139	79.9
stillbirth ($n = 174$)	Yes	18	10.3
	No	156	89.7
History of ANC (n = 174)	Yes	126	72.4
	No	48	27.6
ANC initiation time on Previous pregnancy ($n = 126$)	≤16 Weeks	115	91.3
	> 16 Weeks	11	8.7
Type of pregnancy N = 320	Planned	252	78.8
	Unplanned	68	21.2
Intended to intrupt unplannedPregnancy $N = 68$	Yes	25	36.8
	No	43	63.2

Table 3 Availablity and accessability of health information among mothers who were attending ANC in the public health facilities of Debremarkos town, Feburary-March 2014 ($n = 320$)

Variable		Frequency	Percent
Health education about ANCon previous pregnancy (n = 126)	Yes	85	67.5
	No	41	32.5
Advised for ANC ($n = 320$)	Yes	182	56.9
	No	138	43.1
By whom you were advised ($n = 182$)	Husbands	105	57.7
	Healtrhextention Workers	28	15.4
	Relatives	20	11
	Friends/nigbours	29	15.9
Advised on initiation time ($n = 128$)	Yes	38	20.9
	No	144	79.1
Advised time($n = 38$)	≤16 weeks	36	94.7
	> 16 weeks	2	5.3

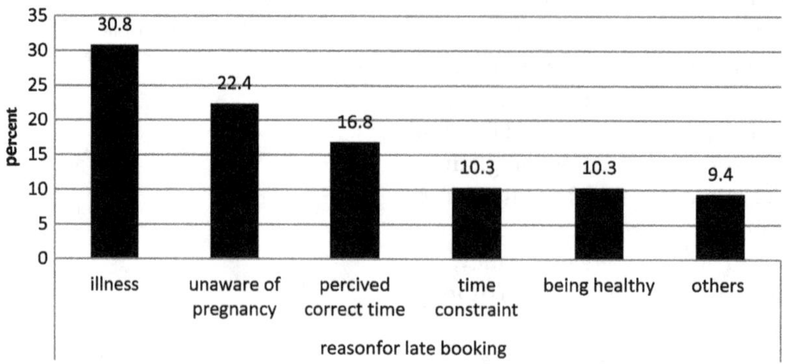

Fig. 2 Reasons for delay on first ANC visit among pregnant mothers who attended ANC in the public health facilities of Debre markos town between February 2014 and March 2014

one or more births [COR = 1.9, 95% CI: 1.22–3.15], not planned their pregnancy [COR = 3.9, 95% CI: 2.25–6.89], having a history of stillbirth [COR = 2.6, 95% CI: 1.01–6.90] and those who perceived that the right time of first ANCvisit is after 16 weeks of gestation [COR = 3.8, 95% CI: 1.69–9.76] were more likely delayed on initiation of the first ANC visit. After adjusting for the potential cofounders; multivariable logistic regressionanalysis indicated that residence, educational status, intention of pregnancy and perception on the right time of first ANC visit were significantly associated with delayed first ANC visit.

Mothers who were residing in rural areas, not attainding formal education, having unplanned pregnancy and perciving the right time of ANC initiation as greater than 16 weeks of gestation were more likely delayed on first ANC visit (Adjusted Odds Ratio (AOR) =2.8 [95% CI:1.54–5. 44]), (AOR = 2.2 [95%CI:1.10–4.68]),(AOR = 3.6 [95% CI: 2.00–6.80]) and (AOR = 3.9[95%CI:1.61–9.76]) respectivelly (Table 4).

Discussion

For many of the essential interventions in ANC, it is crucial to have early identification of underlying conditions. The first ANC visit should be as early as possible in pregnancy [10]. However, evidence in Ethiopia indicated that delayed ANC initiation time among pregnant mothers was high [18–21] .In our study,one third 107 (33.4%) of respondents were delayed to start their first ANC visit with in the first 16 weeks of pregnancy. This finding is higher as compared to a study done in Bengazie (27%, 2007) [22] . This might be due to difference in educational status of mothers between Bengazie and ours. But this finding is comparatively lower than the findings studied in Ndola (68.6%) and Mpongwe (72%) districts of Zambia [23] and South East Tanzania (81.5%) [24], EDHS,2011(89%) [25], Jimma University Specialized Hospital (60.1%) [26], Kembata tembaro Zone (68.6%) [27] and Dembech district of East Gojjam Zone,North west Ethiopia (94.2%) [28] .The possible explanation for this observed difference might be due to study population composition in which proportion of mothers residing in rural areas of current study were lower than other studies.

The finding also showed a significant association of residence and delay on timely initiation of ANC. Those mothers who were residing in rural areas were 2.8 times more likely delayed than urban mothers. Among all respondents, 56% of rural and 27% of urban residents were start ANC after 16 weeks of gestation. Ethiopian demographic and health survey, 2011, revealed that urban mothers made their first visit earlier (4.4 months) than rural mothers (5.5 months) [25]. This finding is also in agreement with the study done in Vietnam in which rural mothers were attained ANC latter and used fewer visits [29].

The possible reason might be better educational status of urban mothers than rular mothers. Because, in our study, 60% of rural mothers were not attaned formal education compared with 23% of urban mothers. The other reason might be availability of alternative health care facilities and having a better chance of health information in urban areas than rular areas. How ever, in contrary to our result,there was no significant difference in the proportionof delayed ANC attendance between urban and rular areas of Zambia [23].The reason for this difference might be the presence of more active mobile maternity service in rular than urbans areas of Zambia.

Educational status was found to have significant association with delayed initation of first ANC visit. Those mothers who had no formal education were delay two times more likely than those who had teritiary education. This is consistent with studies done in Gondar, Kembata tembaro zone,Tanzania and Ghana [11, 24, 27, 30] in which women who had lower education or none booked later than those with higher education.The reason might be high chance of exposure for information in case of educated mothers.

Table 4 Factors associated with delay on first ANCvisit among pregnant mothers who were attending ANC in public health institutions of Debremarkos town,2014(n = 320)

Variable		Delayed		COR(CI)	AOR(C I)	P-Value
		Yes (%)	No (%)			
Residence						
	Rular	39(12.2)	30(9.4)	3.4(2.01–6.07)	2.8(1.54–5.44)[a]	0.001
	Urban	68(21.2)	183(57.2)	1.0	1.0	
Educational status						
	Had no formaleducation	54(16.9)	44(13.8)	4.5(2.33–8.67)	2.2 (1.10–4.68)[a]	0.027
	Primary education	16(5)	35(10.9)	1.6(0.76–3.68)	1.4(0.65–3.42)	
	Secondary education	19(5.9)	68(21.3)	1.0(0.49–2.12)	0.8(0.40–1.87)	
	Tertiary education	18(5.6)	66(20.6)	1.0	1.0	
Occupation						
	Government employee	18(5.6)	63(19.7)	1.0	1.0	
	Merchant	12(3.8)	37(11.6)	1.1(0.49–2.61)	0.9(0.30–2.98)	
	House wife	34(10.6)	84(26.3)	1.4(0.73–2.73)	1.0(0.37–2.94)	
	Farmer	29(9.1)	13(4.1)	7.8(3.37–18.05)	2.2(0.52–9.51)	
	Daily labourer	9(2.8)	8(2.5)	3.9(1.32–11.67)	1.5(0.33–7.21)	
	Student / dependonfamily	5(1.6)	8 (2.5)	2.1(0.63–7.51)	1.1(0.22–5.69)	
Monthly Income						
	< 1000 ETB	51(15.9)	73(22.8)	2.7(1.45–5.37)	1.5(0.66–3.59)	
	1000–2987.50 ETB	40(12.5)	76(23.8)	2.1(1.07–4.10)	1.4(0.66–3.30)	
	> 2987.50 ETB	16(5)	64(20)	1.0	1.0	
Parity						
	No parity	41(12.8))	117(36.6)	1.0	1.0	
	≥1 parity	66(20.6)	96(30)	1.9(1.22–3.15)	1.4(0.86–2.56)	
Types of pregnancy						
	Planned	67(20.9)	185(57.8)	1.0	1.0	
	Unplanned	40(12.5)	28(8.8)	3.9(2.25–6.89)	3.6(2.00–6.80)[a]	0.000
Histrory of still birth						
	No still birth	97(30.3)	205(64.1)	1.0	1.0	
	≥ 1 still birth	10 (3.1)	8(2.5)	2.6(1.01–6.90)	1.6(0.54–5.10)	
Perceived time for 1st ANC visit						
	≤16 weeks	90(28.1)	203(63.4)	1.0	1.0	
	> 16 weeks	17(5.3)	10 (3.1)	3.8(1.69–8.70)	3.9(1.61–9.76)[a]	0.003

[a]Statistical significant at 5% alpha level

Eventhough parity had no association with delayed initiation of ANC in our study, 40.7% of multiparous and 25.9% of nuliparous mothers were start thier first ANCvisit after 16 weeks of gestation.But, it was one of the factors for delayed initiation of ANC in different studies [13, 31, 32].

Intention of pregnancy was significantly associated with delay on initiation of first ANC visit. In this study, women with un planned pregnancy were 3.6 times more likely delayed to initiate first ANC visit than those mothers with planned pregnancy.This finding was inline with a study done in Kembata tembaro Zone [26]. Findings in different studies also in agreement with the association of unplanned pregnancy and delayed initiation of first ANC visit [18, 32–35]. The possible reason might be mothers having intended pregnancy are much cautious and eger to know their pregnancy status and less likely delayed than those who had unintended pregnancy.

Intention of abortion in case of unintended pregnancymight also increased the chance of delayed initiation of ANC.Because, above half 14(56%) of pregnant mothers with unintended pregnancy, who looked for abortion did their first ANC visit after 16 weeks of gestation in our study.

Perception on the right time of ANC initiation was found to be significantly associated with delayed ANC visit. Those mothers who perceived that the right initiation period of first ANC visit is beyond 16 weeks of gestation, were four times delayed than their counter part.

The Possible reason might be decreased exposure for information related to ANC initiation time. Because, in this study only 38(11.8%) of mothers have got information about initiation time of ANC from other persons. Other similar studies also suggested that proper information and advice on pattern of ANC utilization is important to book early [33]; where as, not knowing the right gestational age at which to start the first antenatal care visit was the commonest reason for late ANC attendance [36]. So, appropriate perception of the initial ANC visit was a factor for an early ANC visit. This is inagreement with a study done in Gondar University Hospital [30].

Limitation of the study

The study design is not strong enough to identify determinant factors.

Conclusion

The magnitude of delay on initiation of first ANC visit was still high but it is lower than studies conducted in other areas of Africa and Ethiopia.The time of initiation was ranges from first timester to third trimester and the mean gestational age on initation of first ANC was arround second trimester. According to this study residence, educational status, intention of pregnancy and perception on initiation time of ANC were influencing mothers on timely initiation of first ANC visit. Awarness creation towards timely initiation of first ANC visit and family planning utilization to prevent unplanned pregnancy should be strengthen by Zonal health department in the community specially for the reproductive age group and rural residents. Ministry of education should also improve women education by strengthening adult education in the community. Further study is recommended in the rural community.

Acknowledgements

First and for most thanks to the Almighty GOD who is our power. Our gratitude extends to East Gojjam Zone Plan and Economy department, East Gojjam zone health department, Debremarkos town adminstrative health office and health facilities.

We would like to thank Bahir Dar University and Debre Markos University for their financial and technical support.

We are also grateful to data collectors and study participants for giving us their valuable time.

Authors' contributions

AA drafted the proposal, did the analysis, wrote the results and prepared the manuscript. AM participated on editing, analysis and write up of the result. BT, MM and BT were involved on data analysis and manuscript preparation. All authors read and approved the final manuscript.

Competing interests

The authors declare that they have no competing interests.

Author details

[1]Department of Public Health, College of Health Sciences, Debre Markos University, Debre Markos, Ethiopia. [2]Department of Public Health, College of Medicine and Health Science, Bahir Dar University, Bahir Dar, Ethiopia. [3]Department of Midwifery College of Health Sciences, Debremarkos University, Debre Markos, Ethiopia. [4]Department of Nursing, College of Health Sciences, Debre Markos University, Debre Markos, Ethiopia.

References

1. World Health Organization. Global health observatory (GHO) data. URL. Available form: http://www.who.int/gho/publications/world_health_statistics/2011/en/. 2015 Mar.
2. Ethiopian Federal Ministry of health. Antenatal Care Module: Providing Focused antenatalcare,FMOH.. http://www.open.edu/openlearncreate/mod/oucontent/view.php?id=44&printable=1.
3. Khanna J, Bergsjo P, Lashley K, Peters C, Sherrat D, Villar J. WHO antenatal care randomized trial: manual for the implementation of the new model. 2002. http://apps.who.int/iris/bitstream/10665/42513/1/WHO_RHR_01.30.pdf.
4. WHO. Essential Antenatal,perinatal and post partum care training module :promoting effective preinatal care. Copenhagen: World Health Organization regional office for Europe; 2002.
5. Abou-Zahr CL, Wardlaw TM, World Health Organization. Antenatal care in developing countries: promises, achievements and missed opportunities: an analysis of trends, levels and differentials, 1990–2001. 2003.
6. FMOH. Accelerated Plan for Scaling up PMTCT Services in Ethiopia, Federal Minstry Of Health, Addis Ababa, Ethiopia. 2014.
7. Bollini P, Quack-Lötscher K. Guidelines-based indicators to measure quality of antenatal care. J Eval Clin Pract. 2013;19(6):1060–6.
8. World Health Organization. Global update on HIV treatment 2013: results, impact and opportunities. 2013.
9. East Gojjam zone health department: Annual report of East Gojjam zone health department, Debre markos, Ethiopia. 2013. Unpublished local report.
10. Lawn J, Kerber K. Opportunities for African newborns: practical data policy and programmatic support for newborn care in Africa. 2006.
11. Tayie FA, Lartey A. Antenatal care and pregnancy outcome in Ghana, the importance of women\'s education. African Journal of Food, Agriculture, Nutrition and Development. 2008;8(3):291-303.
12. Hueston WJ, Gilbert GE, Davis L, Sturgill V. Delayed prenatal care and the risk of low birth weight delivery in US. J Community Health. 2003;28(3):199–208.
13. Abeje G, et al. Factors associated with institutional delivery service utilization among mothers in Bahir Dar city adminstration, Amhara region. Reprod Health. 2014;11(22):3–7.
14. Bragg R, Action M. Money and Maternity: charging vulnerable pregnant women for NHS care. Maternity Action and Medact. 2013;26:1-9.
15. Saxena V, Bansal S, Chaturvedi J, Kalra BP, Chandra V, Kansal S. Investigating causes and factors associated with stillbirth by verbal autopsy in Uttarakhand. Indian J Prev Soc Med. 2011;42:14–8.
16. Alibekova R, Huang JP, Chen YH. Adequate prenatal care reduces the risk of adverse pregnancy outcomes in women with history of infertility: a nationwide population-based study. PLoS One. 2013;8(12):e84237.
17. Gebremariam A. Factors predisposing to low birth weight in JimmaHospital southwestern Ethiopia. East Afr Med J. 2005;8(1):554.
18. Zegeye AM, Bitew BD, Koye DN. Prevalence and determinants of early antenatal care visit among pregnant women attending antenatal care in Debre Berhan health institutions, Central Ethiopia. Afr J Reprod Health. 2013;17(4):130–6.

19. Pell C, Meñaca A, Were F, Afrah NA, Chatio S, Manda-Taylor L, Hamel MJ, Hodgson A, Tagbor H, Kalilani L, Ouma P. Factors affecting antenatal care attendance: results from qualitative studies in Ghana, Kenya and Malawi. PLoS One. 2013;8(1):e53747.
20. Kebede B, Gebeyehu A, Andargie G. Use of previous maternal health services has a limited role in reattendance for skilled institutional delivery: cross-sectional survey in Northwest Ethiopia. Int J Womens Health. 2013;5:79.
21. Fenta M. Assessment of factors affecting utilization of maternal health care services in Ayssaita and Dubti towns, afar regional state, north East Ethiopia. Master thesis, 2005.
22. Ziyo FY, Matly FA, Mehemd GM, Dofany EM. Relation between prenatal care and pregnancy outcome at Benghazi. Sudanese J Public Health. 2009;4(4): 403–10.
23. Banda I, Michelo C, Hazemba A. Factors associated with late antenatal care attendance in selected rural and urban communities of the Copperbelt province of Zambia. Med J Zambia. 2012;39(3):29–36.
24. Gross K, Alba S, Glass TR, Schellenberg JA, Obrist B. Timing of antenatal care for adolescent and adult pregnant women in South-Eastern Tanzania. BMC Pregnancy Childbirth. 2012;12(1):16.
25. Demographic E. Health survey (2011) Addis Ababa. Ethiopia and Calverton: Central Statistical Agency and ICF International; 2012.
26. Ewnetu W, Assegid S, Wondafrash W, Ewnetu H. Factors associated with late antenatal care initiation in an Ethiopian clinic. Research. 2015.
27. Tekelab T, Berhanu B. Factors associated with late initiation of antenatal care among pregnant women attending antenatal Clinic at Public Health Centers in Kembata Tembaro zone, southern Ethiopia. Sci Technol Arts Res J. 2014;3(1):108–15.
28. Gedefaw M, Muche B, Aychiluhem M. Current status of antenatal care utilization in the context of data conflict: the case of Dembecha District, Northwest Ethiopia. Open J Epidemiol. 2014;4(04):208.
29. Toan TK. Antenatal and delivery care utilization in urban and rural contexts in Vietnam. A study in two health and demographic surveyllance sites. Gothenburg, Sweden. 2012.
30. Belayneh T, Adefris M, Andargie G. Previous early antenatal service utilization improves timely booking: cross-sectional study at university of Gondar hospital, northwest Ethiopia. J Pregnancy. 2014;2014:1-7.
31. UmberJalil B, Yasmeen K, Razia N. Relation ship between maternal hemoglobin and prenatal out come, Pakistan railway hospital ,Rawalpindi. Rawal Med J. 2007;32:102–4.
32. Exavery A, Kanté AM, Hingora A, Mbaruku G, Pemba S, Phillips JF. How mistimed and unwanted pregnancies affect timing of antenatal care initiation in three districts in Tanzania. BMC Pregnancy Childbirth. 2013;13(1):35.
33. Tariku A, Melkamu Y, Kebede Z. Previous utilization of service does not improve timely booking in antenatal care: cross sectional study on timing of antenatal care booking at public health facilities in Addis Ababa. Ethiop Journal Health Dev. 2010;24(3).227-233.
34. Birmeta K, Dibaba Y, Woldeyohannes D. Determinants of maternal health care utilization in Holeta town, Central Ethiopia. BMC Health Serv Res. 2013;13(1):256.
35. Dibaba Y, Fantahun M, Hindin MJ. The effects of pregnancy intention on the use of antenatal care services: systematic review and meta-analysis. Reprod Health. 2013;10(1):50.
36. Kisuule I, Kaye DK, Najjuka F, Ssematimba SK, Arinda A, Nakitende G, Otim L. Timing and reasons for coming late for the first antenatal care visit by pregnant women at Mulago hospital, Kampala Uganda. BMC Pregnancy Childbirth. 2013;13(1):121.

Permissions

All chapters in this book were first published in P&C, by BioMed Central; hereby published with permission under the Creative Commons Attribution License or equivalent. Every chapter published in this book has been scrutinized by our experts. Their significance has been extensively debated. The topics covered herein carry significant findings which will fuel the growth of the discipline. They may even be implemented as practical applications or may be referred to as a beginning point for another development.

The contributors of this book come from diverse backgrounds, making this book a truly international effort. This book will bring forth new frontiers with its revolutionizing research information and detailed analysis of the nascent developments around the world.

We would like to thank all the contributing authors for lending their expertise to make the book truly unique. They have played a crucial role in the development of this book. Without their invaluable contributions this book wouldn't have been possible. They have made vital efforts to compile up to date information on the varied aspects of this subject to make this book a valuable addition to the collection of many professionals and students.

This book was conceptualized with the vision of imparting up-to-date information and advanced data in this field. To ensure the same, a matchless editorial board was set up. Every individual on the board went through rigorous rounds of assessment to prove their worth. After which they invested a large part of their time researching and compiling the most relevant data for our readers.

The editorial board has been involved in producing this book since its inception. They have spent rigorous hours researching and exploring the diverse topics which have resulted in the successful publishing of this book. They have passed on their knowledge of decades through this book. To expedite this challenging task, the publisher supported the team at every step. A small team of assistant editors was also appointed to further simplify the editing procedure and attain best results for the readers.

Apart from the editorial board, the designing team has also invested a significant amount of their time in understanding the subject and creating the most relevant covers. They scrutinized every image to scout for the most suitable representation of the subject and create an appropriate cover for the book.

The publishing team has been an ardent support to the editorial, designing and production team. Their endless efforts to recruit the best for this project, has resulted in the accomplishment of this book. They are a veteran in the field of academics and their pool of knowledge is as vast as their experience in printing. Their expertise and guidance has proved useful at every step. Their uncompromising quality standards have made this book an exceptional effort. Their encouragement from time to time has been an inspiration for everyone.

The publisher and the editorial board hope that this book will prove to be a valuable piece of knowledge for researchers, students, practitioners and scholars across the globe.

List of Contributors

Tommy Carlsson
Department of Women's and Children's Health, Uppsala University, SE-75237 Uppsala, Sweden
BMC, Husargatan 3, D11:1, SE-75237 Uppsala, Sweden

Elisabet Mattsson
Department of Women's and Children's Health, Uppsala University, SE-75237 Uppsala, Sweden
Department of Health Care Sciences, Ersta Sköndal University College, SE-10061 Stockholm, Sweden

Megan Kash-Macdonald
Population, Policy and Practice, UCL Great Ormond Street Institute of Child Health, 30 Guilford Street, WC1N 1EH, London, UK

Abigail Easter
Centre for Implementation Science, Health Service and Population Research, Institute of Psychiatry, Psychology & Neuroscience, King's College London, London, UK

Amanda Bye
Population, Policy and Practice, UCL Great Ormond Street Institute of Child Health, 30 Guilford Street, WC1N 1EH, London, UK
Centre for Implementation Science, Health Service and Population Research, Institute of Psychiatry, Psychology & Neuroscience, King's College London, London, UK
Department of Midwifery, Florence Nightingale Faculty of Nursing, Midwifery & Palliative Care, King's College London, London, UK

Jill Shawe
Institute of Health and Community, University of Plymouth, Devon, UK

Nadia Micali
Population, Policy and Practice, UCL Great Ormond Street Institute of Child Health, 30 Guilford Street, WC1N 1EH, London, UK
Child and Adolescent Psychiatry Division, Department of Child and Adolescent Health, Geneva University Hospital, Geneva, Switzerland
Department of Psychiatry, Faculty of Medicine, University of Geneva, Geneva, Switzerland

Debra Bick
Department of Women and Children's Health, School of Life Course Sciences, Faculty of Life Sciences and Medicine, King's College London, London, UK

Michael Boah and Emmanuel A. Ayamga
Ghana Health Service, Kassena Nankana West District Health Directorate, Paga, Upper East Region, Ghana

Abraham B. Mahama
UNICEF- Ghana Country Office, Accra, Ghana

An Chen, Henni Tenhunen and Paul Lillrank
Institute of Healthcare Engineering, Management and Architecture (HEMA), Department of Industrial Engineering and Management, Aalto University, Maarintie 8, 00076 Espoo, Finland

Antti Peltokorpi
Department of Civil Engineering, Aalto University, Rakentajanaukio 4, 02150 Espoo, Finland

Seppo Heinonen and Vedran Stefanovic
Department of Obstetrics and Gynaecology, Helsinki University Hospital and University of Helsinki, Haartmaninkatu 2, 00290 Helsinki, Finland

Paulus Torkki
Institute of Healthcare Engineering, Management and Architecture (HEMA), Department of Industrial Engineering and Management, Aalto University, Maarintie 8, 00076 Espoo, Finland
Department of Public Health, Faculty of Medicine, Helsinki University, Biomedicum 1, 00290 Helsinki, Finland

S. Darius Tandon, Erin A. Ward, Mya Carter and Jaime Hamil
Northwestern University Feinberg School of Medicine, 750 N. Lake Shore Drive, 6th Floor, Chicago, IL 60614, USA

Julie A. Leis
James Bell Associates, 3033 Wilson Blvd, Suite 650, Arlington, VA 22201, USA

Hannah Snyder and Huynh-Nhu Le
Department of Psychology, George Washington University, 2125 G. St. NW, Washington, DC 20052, USA

Tamar Mendelson
Department of Mental Health, Johns Hopkins University Bloomberg School of Public Health, 624 N. Broadway, Room 853, Baltimore, MD 21205, USA

Deborah F. Perry
Center for Child and Human Development, Georgetown University, 3300 Whitehaven St., Suite 3300, Washington, DC 20057, USA

Daniel Gyamfi, Kwabena Owusu Danquah, Ernest Adankwah and Gertrude Akua Amissah
Department of Medical Laboratory Technology, Faculty of Allied Health Sciences, Kwame Nkrumah University of Science and Technology, Kumasi, Ghana

Yaw Amo Wiafe and Angela Odame
Department of Sonography, Faculty of Allied Health Sciences, Kwame Nkrumah University of Science and Technology, Kumasi, Ghana

Marjolein Zweekhorst
Athena Institute, Faculty of Science, Vrije Universiteit, Amsterdam, The Netherlands

Vincent De Brouwere
Department of Public Health, Institute of Tropical Medicine, Maternal and Reproductive Health Unit, Antwerp, Belgium

Azucena Bardají
ISGlobal, Hospital Clínic- Universitat de Barcelona, Barcelona, Spain

Ibukun-Oluwa Omolade Abejirinde
Athena Institute, Faculty of Science, Vrije Universiteit, Amsterdam, The Netherlands
Department of Public Health, Institute of Tropical Medicine, Maternal and Reproductive Health Unit, Antwerp, Belgium
ISGlobal, Hospital Clínic- Universitat de Barcelona, Barcelona, Spain

Renate Douwes
Simavi, Amsterdam, The Netherlands

Rudolf Abugnaba-Abanga
Presbyterian Health Services-North, Bolgatanga Upper East Region Ghana

Jos van Roosmalen
Athena Institute, Faculty of Science, Vrije Universiteit, Amsterdam, The Netherlands
Department of Obstetrics, Leiden University Medical Centre, Leiden, The Netherlands

Abraham Yeneneh and Atinkut Alamirrew
College of Medicine and Health Sciences Institute of Public Health, Department of Health Informatics, University of Gondar, Gondar, Ethiopia

Kassahun Alemu and Abel Fekadu Dadi
College of Medicine and Health Sciences, Institute of Public Health, Department of Health Informatics, Department of Epidemiology and Biostatistics, University of Gondar, Gondar, Ethiopia

Muhabaw Shumye Mihret, Miteku Andualem Limenih and Temesgen Worku Gudayu
Department of Midwifery, College of Medicine and Health Sciences, University of Gondar, Gondar, Ethiopia

Ann Yang, Selena An, Diwakar Mohan, Jennifer Callaghan-Koru, Marissa Silverman and Peter J. Winch
Department of International Health, Johns Hopkins Bloomberg School of Public Health, Baltimore, MD, USA

Amnesty LeFevre
Department of International Health, Johns Hopkins Bloomberg School of Public Health, Baltimore, MD, USA
School of Public Health and Family Medicine, Division of Epidemiology and Biostatistics, University of Cape Town, Cape Town, South Africa

Rose Mpembeni and Idda Mosha
School of Public Health and Social Sciences, Muhimbili University of Health and Allied Sciences, Dar es Salaam, Tanzania

Charles Kilewo
School of Public Health and Social Sciences, Muhimbili University of Health and Allied Sciences, Dar es Salaam, Tanzania
Department of Obstetrics and Gynaecology, Muhimbili University of Health and Allied Sciences, Dar es Salaam, Tanzania

Giulia Besana and Chrisostom Lipingu
Jhpiego Tanzania, Dar es Salaam, PO, Tanzania

Asha S. George
Department of International Health, Johns Hopkins Bloomberg School of Public Health, Baltimore, MD, USA
School of Public Health, University of the Western Cape, Bellville, South Africa

A. Kater-Kuipers, E. M. Bunnik and I. D. de Beaufort
Department of Medical Ethics and Philosophy of Medicine, Erasmus MC, University Medical Centre Rotterdam, Room 24.17, Wytemaweg 80, 3015 CN Rotterdam, The Netherlands

R. J. H. Galjaard
Department of Clinical Genetics, Erasmus MC, University Medical Centre Rotterdam, Wytemaweg 80, 3015 CN Rotterdam, The Netherlands

Tigistu Toru
Mizan Aman college of health science, Mizan Aman, Ethiopia

Fantaye Chemir and Susan Anand
School of nursing and midwifery, Jimma University, Jimma, Ethiopia

Sanjit Roy and Md. Aminul Haque
Department of Population Sciences, University of Dhaka, Dhaka 1000, Bangladesh

Kihinetu Gelaye Wudineh, Azezu Asres Nigusie, Shumiye Shiferaw Gesese, Azimeraw Arega Tesu and Fentahun Yenealem Beyene
Department of Midwifery, College of Medicine and Health Sciences, Bahir Dar University, Bahir Dar, Ethiopia

Amanda Daley
Sport, Exercise and Health Sciences, Loughborough University, Epinal Way, Loughborough, Leicestershire LE11 3TU, UK

Muhammad Riaz
Population Health Research Institute, University of Leicester, University Road, Leicester LE1 7RH, UK

Sarah Lewis
Division of Epidemiology and Public Health and UK Centre for Tobacco and Alcohol Studies, University of Nottingham, Nottingham NG5 1PB, UK

Paul Aveyard
Nuffield Department of Primary Care Health Sciences, Radcliffe Observatory Quarter, University of Oxford, Woodstock Road, Oxford OX2 6GG, UK

Tim Coleman
Division of Primary Care and UK Centre for Tobacco and Alcohol Studies, University of Nottingham, Nottingham NG5 1PB, UK

Isaac Manyonda
Department of Obstetrics and Gynecology, St George's University of London and St George's NHS Trust, Blackshaw Road, London SW17 0QT, UK

Robert West
Health Behaviour Research Centre, Department of Epidemiology and Public Health, UCL, Gower Street, London WC1E 6BT, UK

Beth Lewis
School of Kinesiology, University of Minnesota, Minneapolis, MN 55455, USA

Bess Marcus
Department of Family and Preventive Medicine, University of California, San Diego, CA 92093-0628, USA

Adrian Taylor
Plymouth University Peninsula Schools of Medicine and Dentistry, Plymouth Science Park, Plymouth, Devon PL6 8BX, UK

Judith Ibison and Andrew Kent
Institute of Medical and Biomedical Education, St George's University of London, Cranmer Terrace, London SW17 ORE, UK

Michael Ussher
Population Health Research Institute, St George's University of London, Cranmer Terrace, London SW17 ORE, UK
Institute for Social Marketing, University of Stirling, Stirling, Stirling FK9 4LA, UK

Binu Gurung, Louise J. Jackson, Mark Monahan and Tracy E. Roberts
Health Economics Unit, Institute of Applied Health Research, College of Medical and Dental Sciences, University of Birmingham, Edgbaston, Birmingham B15 2TT, UK

Ruth Butterworth
Cheshire and Mersey Specialist Perinatal Mental Health Service, Thorn Road Clinic, Thorn Road, Runcorn WA7 5HQ, UK

Karol J. Marwa
Department of Pharmacology, Catholic University of Health and Allied Sciences, Mwanza, Tanzania

Deodatus Ruganuza
Department of Parasitology, Catholic University of Health and Allied Sciences, Mwanza, Tanzania

Agnes Njalika and Deogratias Katabalo
School of Pharmacy, Catholic University of Health and Allied Sciences, Mwanza, Tanzania

Erasmus Kamugisha
Department of Biochemistry, Catholic University of Health and Allied Sciences, Mwanza, Tanzania

Jui-Ming Liu
Division of Urology, Department of Surgery, Taoyuan General Hospital, Ministry of Health and Welfare, Taoyuan, Taiwan
Department of Medicine, National Yang-Ming University, Taipei, Taiwan
Graduate Institute of Life Sciences, National Defense Medical Center, Taipei, Taiwan

Feng-Hsiang Chiu
American-Sino Women's & Children's, Hospital (SongYuan), Shanghai City, China
Lihuili Eastern Hospital, Ningbo Medical Center, Ningbo City, Zhejiang province, China

Yueh-Ping Liu
Department of emergency Medicine, National Taiwan University Hospital, Taipei, Taiwan

Shu-Pin Chen
Division of Genetics and endocrinology, Chang Gung Children's Hospital, Taoyuan, Taiwan

Hsun-Hao Chan
Division of Urology, Department of Surgery, Yumin medical corporation Yumin hospital, Nantou, Taiwan

Jing-Jung Yang
Department of Psychiatry, Cardinal Tien Hospital, New Taipei City, Taiwan
Institute of Biomedical Engineering, College of Medicine and College of Engineering, National Taiwan University, Taipei, Taiwan

Fung-Wei Chang
Superintendent, Tri-Service General Hospital Penghu Branch, National Defence Medical Center, Penghu Branch, Taiwan

Ren-Jun Hsu
Graduate Institute of Life Sciences, National Defense Medical Center, Taipei, Taiwan
Biobank Management Center of the Tri-Service General Hospital, National Defense Medical Center, Taipei, Taiwan
Department of Pathology and Graduate Institute of Pathology and Parasitology, the Tri-Service General Hospital, National Defense Medical Center, No. 161, Sec. 6, Minquan E. Road, Neihu District, Taipei 114, Taiwan

Li Jiao-ling, Geng Xiu-ping, Li Xiao-fen, Yang Bo-yang and Fang Qian
Department of Ultrasound, GZ Women & Children Medical Centre, Jinsui Road 9, Guangzhou 510623, China

Chen Kun-shan
Department of Invasive Technology, GZ Women & Children Medical Centre, Guangzhou 510623, China

He Qiu-ming
Neonatal Intensive Care Unit, GZ Women & Children Medical Centre, Guangzhou 510623, China

Brenda MY Leung
Department of Community Health Sciences, University of Calgary, Calgary, AB, Canada

Bonnie J Kaplan and Suzanne Tough
Department of Community Health Sciences, University of Calgary, Calgary, AB, Canada
Department of Paediatrics, University of Calgary, 2888 Shaganappi Trail SW, Calgary, AB, Canada

Catherine J Field, Mariel Fajer Gomez and Linda J McCargar
Department of Agricultural, Food and Nutritional Science, University of Alberta, Edmonton, AB, Canada

Misha Eliasziw
Department of Community Health Sciences, University of Calgary, Calgary, AB, Canada
Department of Public Health and Community Medicine, Tufts University, Boston, MA, USA

Lisa Gagnon
Department of Psychiatry, University of Calgary, Calgary, AB, Canada

Amy Metcalfe
Department of Obstetrics and Gynecology, University of British Columbia,
BC Women's and Children's Hospital, 4500 Oak St, Vancouver, BC V6H 3N1, Canada

Kristen Grabowska
Division of Maternal Fetal Medicine, Department of Obstetrics and Gynecology, University of British Columbia, 13750 96 Avenue, Surrey, BC V3V 1Z2, Canada

Carol Weller
Mental Health Screening and Early Identification, Addiction & Mental Health, Alberta Health Services, 10101 Southport Road SW, Calgary, AB, Canada

Suzanne C Tough
Departments of Pediatrics and Community Health Sciences, University of Calgary Child Development Centre, c/o 2888 Shaganappi Trail NW, Calgary, AB T3B 6A8, Canada

Atsede Alle Ewunetie and Muluye Molla Simeneh
Department of Public Health, College of Health Sciences, Debre Markos University, Debre Markos, Ethiopia

Alemtsehay Mekonnen Munea
Department of Public Health, College of Medicine and Health Science, Bahir Dar University, Bahir Dar, Ethiopia

Belsity Temesgen Meselu
Department of Midwifery College of Health Sciences, Debremarkos University, Debre Markos, Ethiopia

Bekele Tesfaye Meteku
Department of Nursing, College of Health Sciences, Debre Markos University, Debre Markos, Ethiopia

Index

www.ingramcontent.com/pod-product-compliance
Lightning Source LLC
LaVergne TN
LVHW080704210926
848485LV00003B/416